Sex Hormones, Exercise and Women

Anthony C. Hackney
Editor

Sex Hormones, Exercise and Women

Scientific and Clinical Aspects

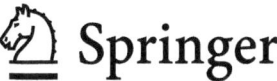
Springer

Editor
Anthony C. Hackney, PhD, DSc
Department of Nutrition
University of North Carolina
Chapel Hill, NC, USA

Department of Exercise & Sport Science
University of North Carolina
Chapel Hill, NC, USA

ISBN 978-3-319-83079-7   ISBN 978-3-319-44558-8   (eBook)
DOI 10.1007/978-3-319-44558-8

© Springer International Publishing Switzerland 2017
Softcover reprint of the hardcover 1st edition 2016
This work is subject to copyright. All rights are reserved by the Publisher, whether the whole or part of the material is concerned, specifically the rights of translation, reprinting, reuse of illustrations, recitation, broadcasting, reproduction on microfilms or in any other physical way, and transmission or information storage and retrieval, electronic adaptation, computer software, or by similar or dissimilar methodology now known or hereafter developed.
The use of general descriptive names, registered names, trademarks, service marks, etc. in this publication does not imply, even in the absence of a specific statement, that such names are exempt from the relevant protective laws and regulations and therefore free for general use.
The publisher, the authors and the editors are safe to assume that the advice and information in this book are believed to be true and accurate at the date of publication. Neither the publisher nor the authors or the editors give a warranty, express or implied, with respect to the material contained herein or for any errors or omissions that may have been made.

Printed on acid-free paper

This Springer imprint is published by Springer Nature
The registered company is Springer International Publishing AG
The registered company address is: Gewerbestrasse 11, 6330 Cham, Switzerland

This work is dedicated to my good friend and mentor, the late Dr. Atko Viru, of Tartu University, Estonia.

Preface

In the late 1970s medical science was beginning to understand that exercise training, while normally an extremely positive physiological stimulus, could also have some drawbacks. Landmark research studies by scientists such as Dr. Barbara Drinkwater, Dr. Anne Loucks, and Dr. Michelle Warren, as well as others, demonstrated that exercise training could be a causative factor in disrupting the endocrine control of a woman's reproductive system leading to the development of "athletic amenorrhea" (secondary amenorrhea). This medical condition is now recognized as part of the conditions associated with the Female Athletic Triad.

The basic premise of the research work on the development of athletic amenorrhea in women can be conceptualized as follows:

Exercise → Female Reproductive Hormones → Physiologic Consequences (negative)

That is, aspects of exercise and exercise training modulate the functioning of the female reproductive hormones. This modulating influence can be highly negative, leading to low estrogen and progesterone states and disruption of normal ovary function and menstruation. Contemporary research has demonstrated that the critical aspects initiating the sequence of such events are energy availability (i.e., development of a low energy availability state; recently designated as part of the Reduced Energy Deficient in Sports conditions [REDS] by an International Olympic Committee medical commission).

As a young professional I found the research on athletic amenorrhea an exciting and fascinating aspect of exercise endocrinology. But my curiosity also caused me to think about the relationship in a different fashion and ask the question—If exercise affects reproductive hormones, could the reproductive hormones have physiological effects unrelated to reproduction that influences the capacity of women to exercise? This seemed a logical question to me as many hormones have more than one physiological effect/impact, and structurally many reproductive hormones have chemical structures similar to many metabolic and water balance hormones. In other words I wondered:

Female Reproductive Hormones → Exercise → Physiologic Consequences
(negative/positive?)

After studying the research literature, it was apparent that animal researchers had been asking this question and seeing that the female reproductive hormones did affect physiological systems and processes that affected exercise capacity. At that time, nearly 30 years ago, the human-based literature was extremely sparse. With that, I and a number of other researchers began to pursue the question of whether the female reproductive hormones have physiological impacts on the bodily systems that are essential to the exercise capacity of women exercisers.

In asking this question, to myself, the underlying premise was not to examine women to see why in some activities men are better. But, more to understanding the unique physiology of women and whether female sex hormones might account for some of the variance in physiological performance between amenorrheic and eumenorrheic women, and within women across the age span as they experience menarche to menopause. That has been my interest in pursuing this absorbing topic and why I wanted to develop this book.

This book was developed with hope that the select group of professionals writing the various chapters could address this last question. Like nearly all written works, this one could be improved and be made better, but I am extremely proud and thankful to the authors who contributed and put forth so much hard work. Each discussed topic provides current insight into the state-of-the-art research in the respective topic area. It is hoped the reader will be as excited and fascinated after reading the individual topics as the authors were in writing them. I also hope the insights provided here will inspire new researchers to ask questions about the roles of female sex hormones in exercise and pursue investigations to seek answers to those questions.

Chapel Hill, NC, USA   Anthony C. Hackney, PhD, DSc

Acknowledgments

I wish to acknowledge the support of my graduate students who certainly helped me bring this to completion. You are a great group of young professionals.

Thanks

My sincere thanks to all the authors involved with this project. They were wonderful to work with and I appreciate their professionalism. I also wish to sincerely thank my family for their support while I worked on this project.

Contents

1 **The Hypothalamic–Pituitary–Ovarian Axis and Oral Contraceptives: Regulation and Function** 1
Hope C. Davis and Anthony C. Hackney

2 **Sex Hormones and Their Impact on the Ventilatory Responses to Exercise and the Environment** 19
Joseph W. Duke

3 **Sex Hormones and Substrate Metabolism During Endurance Exercise** 35
Laurie Isacco and Nathalie Boisseau

4 **Sex Hormone Effects on the Nervous System and their Impact on Muscle Strength and Motor Performance in Women** 59
Matthew S. Tenan

5 **Estrogen and Menopause: Muscle Damage, Repair and Function in Females** 71
Peter M. Tiidus

6 **Nutritional Strategies and Sex Hormone Interactions in Women** 87
Nancy J. Rehrer, Rebecca T. McLay-Cooke and Stacy T. Sims

7 **The Effect of Sex Hormones on Ligament Structure, Joint Stability and ACL Injury Risk** 113
Sandra J. Shultz

8 **Sex Hormones and Physical Activity in Women: An Evolutionary Framework** 139
Ann E. Caldwell and Paul L. Hooper

9 **Sex Hormones and Environmental Factors Affecting Exercise** 151
Megan M. Wenner and Nina S. Stachenfeld

10	Exercise, Depression-Anxiety Disorders and Sex Hormones	171
	Shannon K. Crowley	
11	Stress Reactivity and Exercise in Women	193
	Tinna Traustadóttir	
12	Sex Hormones, Cancer and Exercise Training in Women	209
	Kristin L. Campbell	
13	The Effects of Acute Exercise on Physiological Sexual Arousal in Women	227
	Cindy M. Meston and Amelia M. Stanton	
14	Sex Hormones, Menstrual Cycle and Resistance Exercise	243
	Yuki Nakamura and Katsuji Aizawa	
15	Effects of Sex Hormones and Exercise on Adipose Tissue	257
	Victoria J. Vieira-Potter	
16	Exercise in Menopausal Women	285
	Monica D. Prakash, Lily Stojanovska, Kulmira Nurgali and Vasso Apostolopoulos	
Index		309

Contributors

Katsuji Aizawa, Ph.D. Senshu University, Kanagawa, Japan

Vasso Apostolopoulos, Ph.D. Centre for Chronic Disease, College of Health and Biomedicine, Victoria University, Melbourne, VIC, Australia

Nathalie Boisseau, Ph.D. Laboratory of the Metabolic Adaptations to Exercise under Physiological and Pathological Condition, Clermont Auvergne University, Clermont-Ferrand, France

Ann E. Caldwell, Ph.D. Anschutz Health and Wellness Center, University of Colorado Denver, School of Medicine, Aurora, CO, USA

Kristin L. Campbell, P.T., M.Sc., Ph.D. Department of Physical Therapy, Faculty of Medicine, University of British Columbia, Vancouver, BC, Canada

Centre of Excellence in Cancer Prevention, School of Population and Public Health, Faculty of Medicine, University of British Columbia, Vancouver, BC, Canada

Shannon K. Crowley, Ph.D. Department of Exercise Science, North Carolina Wesleyan College, Rocky Mount, NC, USA

Hope C. Davis, M.A. Human Movement Science Curriculum, University of North Carolina, Chapel Hill, NC, USA

Joseph W. Duke, Ph.D. Department of Biological Sciences, Northern Arizona University, Flagstaff, AZ, USA

Anthony C. Hackney, Ph.D., D.Sc. Department of Nutrition, University of North Carolina, Chapel Hill, NC, USA

Department of Exercise & Sport Science, University of North Carolina, Chapel Hill, NC, USA

Paul L. Hooper, Ph.D. Department of Anthropology, Emory University, Atlanta, GA, USA

Laurie Isacco, Ph.D. Laboratory of Prognostic Markers and Regulatory Factors of Cardiovascular Diseases and Exercise Performance Health Innovation Platform, University of Bourgogne Franche-Comte, Besançon, France

Rebecca T. McLay-Cooke, B.Ph.Ed., B.Sc., M.Sc. Department of Human Nutrition, University of Otago, Dunedin, Otago, New Zealand

Cindy M. Meston, Ph.D. Department of Psychology, The University of Texas at Austin, Austin, TX, USA

Yuki Nakamura, Ph.D. St. Margaret's Junior College, Tokyo, Japan

Kulmira Nurgali, M.B.B.S., Ph.D. College of Health & Biomedicine, Victoria University, Melbourne, VIC, Australia

Monica D. Prakash, Ph.D. Centre for Chronic Disease, College of Health and Biomedicine, Victoria University, Melbourne, VIC, Australia

Nancy J. Rehrer, B.A., M.Sc., Ph.D. School of Physical Education Sport & Exercise Sciences, University of Otago, Dunedin, Otago, New Zealand

Sandra J. Shultz, Ph.D., A.T.C. Department of Kinesiology, University of North Carolina at Greensboro, Greensboro, NC, USA

Stacy T. Sims, B.A., M.Sc., Ph.D. Health, Sport and Human Performance, University of Waikato, Adams Centre for High Performance, Mount Maunganui, New Zealand

Nina S. Stachenfeld, Ph.D. Department of Obstetrics, Gynecology and Reproductive Sciences, The John B. Pierce Laboratory and Yale School of Medicine, New Haven, CT, USA

Amelia M. Stanton, B.A. Department of Psychology, The University of Texas at Austin, Austin, TX, USA

Lily Stojanovska, M.Sc., Ph.D. Centre for Chronic Disease, College of Health and Biomedicine, Victoria University, Melbourne, VIC, Australia

Matthew S. Tenan, Ph.D. United States Army Research Laboratory, Aberdeen Proving Ground, Adelphi, MD, USA

Peter M. Tiidus, B.Sc., M.Sc., Ph.D. Faculty of Applied Health Sciences, Brock University, St. Catharines, ON, Canada

Tinna Traustadóttir, Ph.D. Department of Biological Sciences, Northern Arizona University, Flagstaff, AZ, USA

Victoria J. Vieira-Potter, Ph.D. Department of Nutrition and Exercise Physiology, University of Missouri, Columbia, MO, USA

Megan M. Wenner, Ph.D. Department of Kinesiology and Applied Physiology, University of Delaware, Newark, DE, USA

Chapter 1
The Hypothalamic–Pituitary–Ovarian Axis and Oral Contraceptives: Regulation and Function

Hope C. Davis and Anthony C. Hackney

Introduction

Over the past few generations female participation in sports has continued to increase, which has resulted in a greater need for research in the area of sports medicine, physiological effects, and consequences of exercise by women. Specific further work is still needed particularly in the area of reproductive endocrinology. The female reproductive system is a complex physiological system consisting of many hormonal and regulatory components. Thus, it is imperative for exercise scientists who wish to study the female reproductive system to have a strong knowledge base of the controlling regulatory axis of the system, referred to as the Hypothalamic–Pituitary–Ovarian (HPO) axis.

The intent of this chapter is to provide such background information about the neuroendocrine basics of the female reproductive system relative to: the hypothalamus, the pituitary, the ovary, and the uterus. The chapter focuses on providing a brief review of the essential endocrinology of the menstrual cycle in health females as well as providing information about oral contraceptive (OC) function and use. This context provides an essential framework for discussions provided in subsequent chapters in this book.

H.C. Davis, M.A.
Human Movement Science Curriculum, University of North Carolina, Chapel Hill, NC, USA

A.C. Hackney, Ph.D., D.Sc. (✉)
Department of Nutrition, University of North Carolina, Chapel Hill, NC, USA

Department of Exercise & Sport Science, University of North Carolina,
Chapel Hill, NC, USA
e-mail: ach@email.unc.edu

Hypothalamic–Pituitary System

Proper functioning of the reproductive system is critical not only to reproductive health, but overall health in women. Abnormal reproductive health can sometimes be characterized by amenorrhea and, or other medical maladies (see later discussion, this chapter).

Regulation of the female reproductive system consists of complex interactions between endocrine feedback loops of the hypothalamus, pituitary, and ovary. Although there is debate whether the hypothalamus or pituitary is the most important regulator in the process, there is no denying that all three neuroendocrine glands must work together to ensure proper functioning (Sam and Frohman 2008).

The signaling process begins in the hypothalamus, where gonadotropin-releasing hormone (GnRH) is released into the blood stream and travels to the pituitary gland. The pituitary responds by releasing gonadotropin hormones, specifically luteinizing hormone (LH) and follicle stimulating hormone (FSH) in females. The anterior pituitary also releases growth hormone (GH), thyroid-stimulating hormone (TSH), prolactin, and adrenal corticotrophin hormone in response to a variety of other hypothalamic stimuli; these other hormones control primarily growth-development, metabolism, and responses to stress. The posterior pituitary produces hormones as well, namely oxytocin and antidiuretic hormone (ADH; also called vasopressin). Oxytocin controls lactation as opposed to growth and development, and ADH functions with aldosterone (released by adrenal cortex) to maintain fluid and electrolyte balance (Brooks et al. 2005). In healthy women GnRH is released in a pulsatile manner, and consequently FSH and LH are released in a similar pulsatile pattern from the anterior pituitary (Speroff and Fritz 2005).

Current research suggests that a set of brain peptides encoded by the *Kiss1* gene, known more commonly as kisspeptin, may be an important upstream regulator in GnRH release in humans as well as many other mammalian species (Lapatto et al. 2007). Kisspeptin neurons in the hypothalamus modulate the prepubescent LH surge that occurs in females as well as the actions of sex steroids on GnRH neurons (Gu and Simerly 1997). This regulation of the reproductive axis is illustrated by the reproductive defects that exist in mice and other mammals when the kisspeptin receptor gene is disrupted (Dungan et al. 2007). Additional physiological parameters, such as metabolic disruptions (e.g., under nutrition), can decrease kisspeptin expression, which in turn can suppress reproductive functioning (Castellano et al. 2005; Luque et al. 2007).

Sex Steroid Hormones

Estrogen

Estrogen is one of the two major reproductive hormones released as a result of the HPO axis activity. Estrogen refers to a group of similarly structured steroid hormones that are produced primarily in the ovaries of females. The estrogen group is made up of estrone, estriol, and estradiol-β-17, the latter of which contributes primarily to reproductive function (Wierman 2007). These estrogens have physiological roles in both males and females, including soft tissue, skeletal muscle, and the epidermis (Wierman 2007). The estrogens (estrone and estriol) are essentially produced locally in target tissue (peripheral conversion) such as adipose cells. Estradiol-β-17, the estrogen primarily produced at the ovaries, is responsible for primary and secondary female sex characteristics and therefore is the main estrogen discussed in this chapter.

As previously stated, the HPO axis is the main regulator of estrogen production in women. The pituitary release of FSH and LH results in binding to the ovarian receptors for these hormones, which induces the production and secretion of both estrogen and progesterone (see later section; Ferin 1996).

Specifically within the ovary, LH binds to LH receptor cites on the thecal cells. When stimulated, they convert available cholesterol into androgens (McNatty et al. 1979). These androgens are then transported to the granulosa cells where FSH binds to FSH receptors, thus stimulating conversion of androgens into estradiol-β-17 via aromatase enzymes (Hillier 1987).

Estrogen gradually increases during the follicular phase of the menstrual cycle in order to support the developing oocyte (McNatty et al. 1979). Once the egg is released from the ovary, the follicle shifts from estrogen to progesterone production and estrogen levels slowly decrease throughout the luteal phase of the cycle. Although the ovary will still produce estradiol-β-17 during the cycle, it will be in conjunction with progesterone, thus decreasing the overall concentration and effectiveness of estrogen (see discussion later section).

Recent studies have found that natural mutation of estrogen receptors (ERs) or deficiency of aromatase (the enzyme that converts androgens to estradiol-β-17 in the ovary and some peripheral tissues) results in tissue specific deficits, including the vascular system, central nervous system, gastrointestinal tract, immune system, skin, kidney, and lungs (Couse and Korach 1999; Curtis and Korach 2000; Eddy et al. 1996; Hewitt and Korach 2003; Matsumoto et al. 2005; Robertson et al. 1999). Lastly, physiological estradiol-β-17 can increase lipolysis and inhibit glycogen utilization during rest and acute exercise (Hackney 1999). It is thought that estradiol-β-17 may directly alter enzymatic activity or indirectly affect insulin sensitivity thereby affecting glycogen usage (Bunt 1990). Estrogens not only control primary and secondary sex characteristics in females, but also regulate a number of functions throughout female and male target tissues in the body through its direct and indirect impacts on other neuroendocrine agents (Bunt 1990; see Fig. 1.1 and 1.2).

Progesterone

Progesterone is the second major reproductive hormone produced and regulated via the HPO axis. Progesterone is the major progestogen (steroid hormone classification) and is produced predominately by the ovaries, but it is also produced locally in some tissues. Similarly to estradiol-β-17, LH regulates progesterone production within the ovary. During the luteal phase of the menstrual cycle, LH

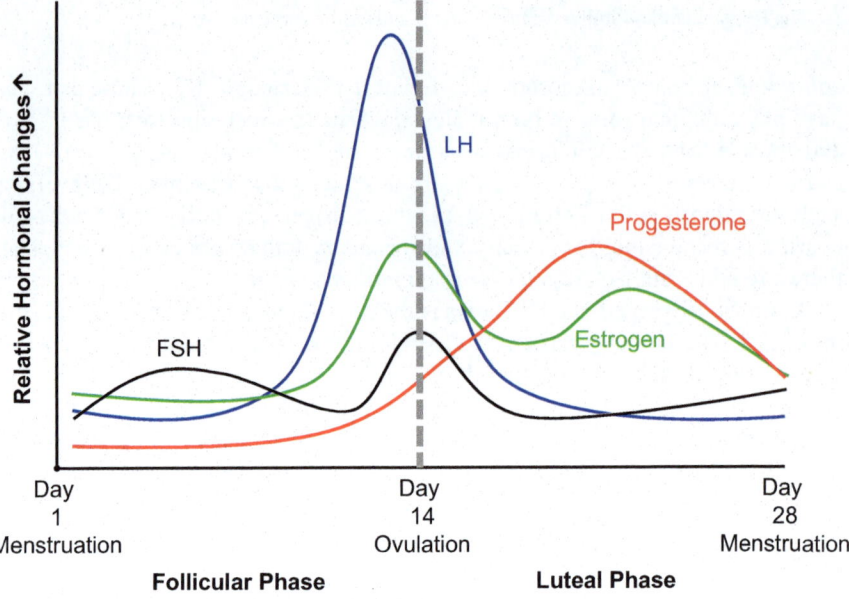

Fig. 1.1 Figure displays the typical key regulatory hormone changes associated with the menstrual cycle in a healthy eumenorrheic woman

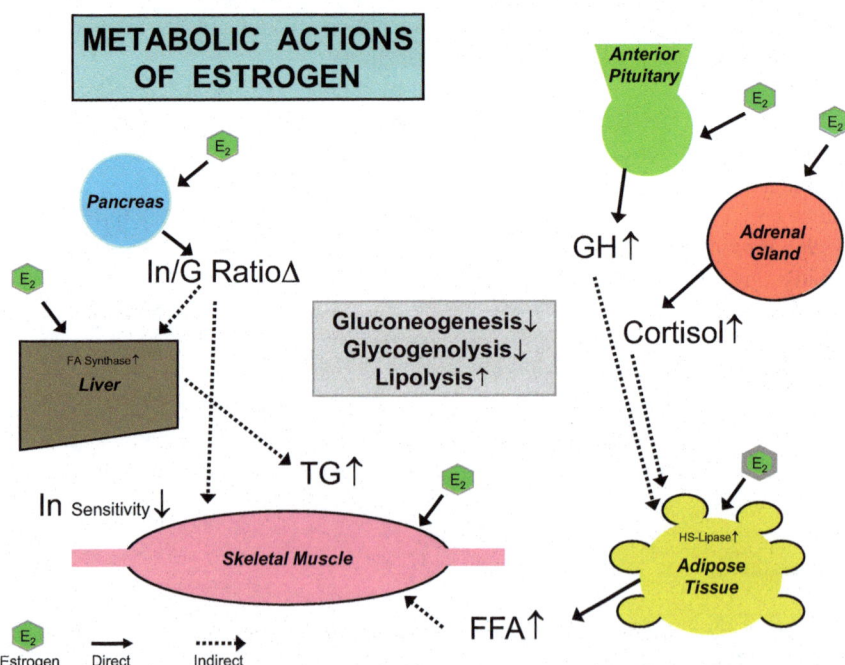

Fig. 1.2 Figure illustrates of the direct (*solid line arrows*) and indirect (*dashed line arrows*) effects of estrogen (E_2) on a variety of hormones and physiologic processes associated with many critical aspects of regulating energy metabolism and energy substrate availability. Abbreviations: *FFA* free fatty acids, *G* glucagon, *GH* growth hormone, *In* insulin, *TG* triglycerides. Symbols: ↑ = increase; ↓ = decrease; Δ = delta (change)

stimulates LH receptors on luteinized granulosa cells of the ovary, leading to the conversion of cholesterol to both progesterone and estrogen (Filicori 1999). Progesterone stabilizes the endometrial lining in preparation for fertilization and pregnancy (Filicori 1999). When progesterone concentrations are high, progesterone can inhibit binding of estrogen to an ER by blocking the binding site . This causes the conversion of estradiol-β-17 to estrone, a less active form of estrogen (Erickson et al. 1985). Progesterone also has important effects on the central nervous system, vascular tissue, and other target tissues (Mani et al. 1997; please see other chapters in book for details).

The Ovary

As previously stated, the ovary is responsible for the production of estrogen and progesterone, but it is also responsible for the maturation and release of the oocytes, or eggs, during the luteal phase of the menstrual cycle. The ovary is made of the outer cortex, the inner medulla, and the hilum, but it is the outer cortex that is considered the functional component of the ovary. This outer portion contains the follicles that produce and release mature eggs as well as estrogen and progesterone (Speroff and Fritz 2005).

Oocytes

The oocytes in the outer cortex begin to develop around the seventh week of fetal life. Oogonias, or germ cells, form along the gonadal ridge of the fetus surrounded by a developing follicle. This follicle is made of a fluid-filled cavity surrounded by granulosa and thecal cells. These oogonias undergo rapid mitosis and can reach up to six to seven million in the ovary. The oogonias will become oocytes and diminish in number via follicular atresia throughout a female's lifetime (Himelstein-Braw et al. 1976; Motta et al. 1997). When the oocytes in the ovary have been depleted, a woman will undergo menopause (typically the fourth to fifth decade of life) and stop releasing eggs from the ovaries. Interestingly, the majority of these oocytes will be depleted before females reach puberty. Just 300,000–500,000 oocytes exist at the start of puberty, and only 400–500 will actually go through ovulation, with the rest starting the process but undergoing programmed apoptosis prior to release from the follicle (Himelstein-Braw et al. 1976; Motta et al. 1997).

Ovulation and Ovarian Hormone Production

At the onset of puberty, the hypothalamus begins to release GnRH in a pulsatile fashion, thus releasing the gonadotropins, FSH and LH (see earlier overview in this chapter). As noted, these hormones result in the release of the sex steroid hormones progesterone and estrogen at the ovary as well as the designation of which follicle will complete ovulation.

Within each follicle, thecal cells have LH receptors which when stimulated convert cholesterol to androgen. The androgen then moves to the layer of granulosa cells where it serves as a substrate and produces estrogen via intracellular aromatase enzymes stimulated by FSH (Hillier 1987).

Each month, between 3 and 11 follicles begin to grow independently of hormone influence (Gougeon 1986). Increasing levels of FSH induces granulosa cells to increase the number of FSH receptors on their cell membranes (Mais et al. 1986). This feed forward regulatory system exponentially increases sensitivity of FSH in the granulosa cells, and the cell with the most receptors and therefore the highest sensitivity to FSH will become the dominant follicle during the menstrual cycle. The dominant follicle then secretes an increased amount of estrogen in response to the increased androgen substrate supply in order to support the oocyte (McNatty et al. 1979).

Luteinization, the process of progesterone production to prepare the endometrial lining for development of an embryo, is dependent on LH. In turn, LH stimulates LH receptors on the granulosa cells, which leads to the conversion of cholesterol to progesterone and estrogen (Filicori 1999). Circulating progesterone levels can also block FSH and LH receptors in order to prevent new follicle growth during this time (Nippoldt et al. 1989).

Additionally, there are several less widely known reproductive sex hormones that should be mentioned. Granulosa cells produce inhibin, which inhibits FSH secretion in remaining follicles that have not been selected as the dominant follicle, and activin, which stimulates FSH and increases the sensitivity of FSH at the ovary (Kitaoka et al. 1988). Follistatin is an additional hormone that inhibits activin and is released by the anterior pituitary (Besecke et al. 1997).

The Menstrual Cycle

The fluctuating production and release of these reproductive hormones over approximately 28 days is known as the menstrual cycle. It consists primarily of low-estrogen (follicular) and high-estrogen (luteal) phases, which are divided by the ovulatory period (~mid-cycle). Day One begins on the first day of menses (bloody discharge), or the first day of withdrawal bleeding, and is the start of the follicular phase. During this time the dominant follicle is selected (see earlier discussion). This stage is characterized by increasing FSH and low-estrogen due to regression of the corpus luteum from the previous cycle. With increased sensitivity of FSH due to FSH receptors on the granulosa cells, a dominant follicle is selected and begins to secrete estrogen. Mid-cycle, a positive feedback loop emerges as increasing estrogen levels from the follicle stimulate the LH surge characteristic of the luteal phase (Pauerstein et al. 1978). Following ovulation, progesterone is released in a pulsatile manner from the follicle in response to the LH surge. The follicle then becomes the corpus luteum within the uterus (Vande Wiele et al. 1970). If fertilization occurs, the embryo remains in the endometrium and develops into a fetus. If no fertilization occurs the corpus luteum is degraded via proteolytic enzymes (Brannian and Stouffer 1991). This is accompanied by a fall in estrogen and progesterone and the onset of menstruation. The entire cycle takes approximately 28 days, although the cycle ranges from 21 to 35 days (Nelson 2014) in a healthy adult female. Then the cycle begins again with the start of menstruation and the follicular phase. Figure 1.1 gives an illustrative display of the major circulating hormonal changes over the menstrual cycle.

The Uterus

During the menstrual cycle, an oocyte travels from the ovary to the uterus, where it is either fertilized or shed along with the menstrual tissue. This section provides a basic overview of the anatomy and function of the uterus and its key role within the menstrual cycle.

Anatomy

The anatomy of the uterus consists of the fundus, the corpus, the cornu, and the cervix. The uppermost region of the uterus consists of the fundus, and it is the usual site of embryo development if fertilization occurs. The corpus is the body, and the cornu is the site of the insertion of the fallopian tubes. The cervix is the bottom most portion and connects the uterus to the vagina (Smout et al. 1969). The uterus has three layers: the mesometrium, which is the innermost layer, the myometrium, and the endometrium, which is the outermost layer. Each layer consists of multiple smooth muscles (Smout et al. 1969).

Uterine Phases

The uterus goes through two phases during a menstrual cycle as well: the proliferative phase corresponds with the follicular phase while the secretory phase aligns with the luteal phase of the ovary. In the proliferative phase, circulating estrogen contributes to endometrial gland growth as well as stroma and endothelial cell number growth (Ludwig and Spornitz 1991). Post ovulation, progesterone levels increase corresponding to the secretory phase of the uterus. Circulating progesterone blocks the binding site on estrogen receptors, thus suppressing endometrial growth. Progesterone also causes the conversion of estradiol-β-17 to estrone (Falany and Falany 1996). Nearing the end of the cycle, the corpus luteum disappears. The stroma and glands undergo apoptosis, and the endometrium shrinks causing the spiral arteries to oscillate between vasospasm and vasodilation. This change can cause tissue ischemia and inflammation and leads to an increase in local prostaglandin production, which cause menstrual cramps and ultimately help to extrude menstrual tissue (Markee 1978). Additionally, decreasing progesterone leads to matrix metalloproteinase release, further breaking down the endometrial layer during menstruation (Irwin et al. 1996).

Oral Contraceptives

Effectiveness

Despite their somewhat controversial side effects, oral contraceptives (OCs) are used by an estimated 100 million females around the world to prevent unwanted pregnancy (Christin-Maitre 2013; Hanson and Burke 2012). Oral contraceptives work basically by producing high estrogen levels during a female's follicular phase. The mid-cycle gonadotropin (LH, FSH) surge is then inhibited and ovulation does not occur (Speroff et al. 1983).

Motivation, or the extent to which a female wishes to prevent pregnancy, is a large predictor in OC success. Age, socioeconomic status, and education are all inversely related to failure rates in OC usage (Mishell 1989). For example, first year failure rate is around 3 % (Mishell 1989), but this rate jumps to 4.7 % for users under the age of 22 years (Ory 1982). Failures can also occur occasionally even if the user takes all of the prescribed OCs on their schedule. About half of females discontinue use of an OC within 1 year and fail to begin using another contraceptive method, which can increase rate of unwanted pregnancy (Hatcher et al. 1988).

Composition

Most OCs are composed of at least one estrogen and one progestin (synthetic progestogens), although the types and concentrations vary from pill to pill.

Estrogens

The two most common estrogens found in OCs in the USA are ethinyl estradiol (EE) and mestranol. While EE is activated upon oral administration, mestranol requires demethylation in the liver to become pharmacologically active (Goldzieher et al. 1980). In order to account for this delay, OCs contain at least 50 μg of mestranol; however, both forms of estrogen use in OCs are equally potent for clinical purposes (Goldzieher et al. 1975).

Progestins

There are five types of progestins commonly found in OCs in the USA: norethindrone, norethindrone acetate, ethynodiol diacetate, norgestrel, and norethynodrel. Norgestrel is the most potent of these hormonally, while the other four are essentially equipotent.

Clinically it is known that norethynodrel has a strong estrogenic effect with no antiestrogenic or androgenic effect (Harris 1969), while norgestrel has little or no estrogenic effects. Norethindrone acetate and norgestrel have large antiestrogenic effects, and ethynodiol diacetate has a low antiestrogenic effect with a low androgenic effect (Hatcher et al. 1988). OCs with high androgenic effect are usually reserved for specific-cases in patients.

Combinations

Since the 1960s, when OCs first became available in the USA, the total dose of hormones used has gradually been reduced. Estrogen has lowered from 50 to 150 µg down to less than 50 µg, while progestin has been reduced from 1 to 10 mg to less than 1 mg. Additionally, triphasic and biphasic OCs have been created to better mimic the female menstrual cycle and maintain reproductive health.

Biphasic OCs were created after the initial reduction in steroid dosage in an effort to decrease to a greater extent the side effects caused by OCs, as it is known that side-effects discourage compliance (Hillard 1992). Biphasic and triphasic OCs mimic the rise and fall of estrogen of a normal menstrual cycle, and lower the overall monthly steroid dosage (Upton 1983). However, some observational studies have reported less cycle control and higher incidence of pregnancy in biphasic and triphasic OCs (Ketting 1988; Kovacs et al. 1989). Since biphasic and triphasic pills are not widely available outside of the USA, there is currently not enough evidence to support that biphasic or triphasic OCs are better or more effective than monophasic OCs in preventing unwanted pregnancies (Van Vliet et al. 2006a, b, 2011). There is evidence to suggest that triphasic OCs containing levonorgestrel result in less breakthrough bleeding than in biphasic OCs that contain norethindrone (Van Vliet et al. 2006a, b). Additionally, triphasic OCs typically have lower progestins and therefore fewer metabolic effects; however, this does not appear to change incidence of spotting or bleeding compared to monophasic OCs (Foster 1989).

Progestin-Only

Progestin only pills are less effective than combination OCs as ovulation is not consistently inhibited under this drug regimen. However, this may be the best option for females who are currently breastfeeding, as progestin alone does not diminish the duration of lactation as combination OCs do (Committee on Drugs 1981; Lonnerdal et al. 1980). This is important as decreased breast milk production may lead to decreased infant weight gain and altered milk composition (Lonnerdal et al. 1980).

Instructions for Use

Traditionally, females took the first OC pill on Day Five of the menstrual cycle or on the first Sunday after menstruation began. Now it is common to take the first pill on Day One of the cycle. This may reduce the risk of becoming pregnant during the first month on the OC. If there is absolutely no chance of pregnancy, then the pill can be started immediately at any time. A backup contraception method is recommended for the first month on the OC. This is especially true if the first OC dose is taken later than Day five of the menstrual cycle.

Combined OCs are taken for 21 days, followed by 7 days of placebo pill when menstruation occurs. Furthermore, patients are guided to take the placebo pills during the 7 days off as a reminder to promote compliance. If a patient forgets a pill, she should take it as soon as she remembers without postponing the next pill. More than two missed days may result in spotting, in which case a back-up contraception method is also recommended. Additionally in this situation, it may be necessary for OCs use to be stopped for 1 week and restarted at a new cycle.

Progestin-only pills are taken every day, with no days off for withdrawal bleeding. Spotting and amenorrhea are common in patients using this method (Committee on Drugs 1981).

Adverse Effects

Although there are many reported severe side effects of OC use, much of the data is from high-estrogen OC pills, and this data may not reflect newer OC pills formulations with different compositions. Some of the major adverse effects are discussed briefly below.

Cardiovascular Risk

Venous thromboembolism (deep vein thrombosis) and pulmonary embolism are two to eight times more likely in OC users; this risk is directly related to the dosage of estrogen taken. Thrombotic and hemorrhagic strokes are five times more likely in women taking OCs than in control groups; however, varicose veins are no longer a contraindication. Many of these risks can still continue after OC use ends, so patients should continue to receive screenings for risk factors after discontinuing OC use (Layde and Beral 1981).

Mortality risks are associated with OC users who are older in age (over 35 years) and smoke (Layde and Beral 1981; Tietze and Lewit 1979). Mortality risks are related not only to age, but also to other cardiovascular risk factors such as cholesterol, blood pressure, and diabetes mellitus (Layde and Beral 1981; Tietze and Lewit 1979). For example, myocardial infarction risks increase 350–800 times for a female smoker between 41 and 45 years of age compared to a nonsmoker between the ages of 27 and

37 (Jick et al. 1978). Hypertension is two to three times more likely in women taking OCs. Normally the increase in blood pressure is about 1–5 % (Fisch et al. 1972), but in some cases major increases can occur (Harris 1969; Tobon 1972).

In the past, OCs were not recommended for women over 40, but the American College of Obstetricians and Gynecologists now states that healthy women through the age of 44 years can continue use of OCs if screened for cardiovascular risk factors (Mishell 1989). In healthy women, there is no detected increase in stroke or myocardial infarction (Porter et al. 1985; Porter et al. 1987).

Neoplastic Effects

One common concern with OC use is increased risk of cancer due to findings from current research involving hormone replacement therapy. However, contrastingly OCs may have a protective effect for ovarian and endometrial cancer (Lee 1987; Lee et al. 1987). Studies on breast cancer risk factors are still being conducted, though at this time the UK Committee on Safety of Medicines and the US Food and Drug Administration do not strongly recommend changing OC prescription based on breast cancer risk factors (Cancer risks of oral contraception 1989; Cases/controls, breast cancer, and the pill 1989).

Cervical cancer risk may increase on OC use, although this is hard to determine since research is confounded by numerous factors including: age at first sexual intercourse, number of sexual partners, exposure to human papillomavirus, frequency of cytological screening, use of barrier contraceptives or spermicides, and cigarette smoking (Celentano et al. 1987). Whether or not OCs are the cause of cervical cancer, OC users are generally at higher risk for cervical neoplasia and should get regular screening of cervical cytology, especially if they have used OCs for over 5 years (Mishell 1989).

Malignant melanoma has been also studied in OC users, since melanocytes respond to female sex hormones. If OCs are a risk factor for this form of cancer, it appears to be at a relative low level (Mattson et al. 1986).

Metabolic Effects

Estrogens tend to increase high-density lipoprotein (HDL) cholesterol and lower low-density lipoprotein (LDL) cholesterol, while progestins have the opposite effect. Most multiphasic OCs, as well as low-dose OCs, have low progestin doses to decrease any adverse effects on serum lipids for this reason (Foster 1989; Patsch et al. 1989).

OCs may increase the risk of diabetes mellitus cases in already susceptible women. High doses tend to result in abnormal glucose-tolerance tests in 4–16 % of females, while low-dose OCs do not alter glucose, insulin or glucagon levels in healthy women or women with a history of gestational diabetes (Kung et al. 1987; van der Vange et al. 1987).

Miscellaneous Effects: Adverse

OCs may precipitate gallstone disease symptoms in susceptible women (Layde et al. 1982), but do not increase risk of bladder disease. Research shows that inadvertently using OCs shortly after conception as well as conceiving shortly after ending OC use does not increase chance of congenital abnormalities (Wilson and Brent 1981; Wiseman and Dodds-Smith 1984).

It is normal for there be a delay in fertility after ending OC use; however, a lack of menstruation for more than 6 months could be indicative of an underlying problem (Vessey et al. 1983). *Chlamydia trachomatis* is more prevalent in women using OCs, but this may be because females on OCs are more likely to have intercourse. Meanwhile, pelvic infection is typically reduced in OC users. Biochemical research suggests that OCs may induce tryptophan oxygenase activity, which can cause a pyridoxine (vitamin B_6) deficiency (Slap 1981). A vitamin deficiency can alter moods in many patients and increase risk of depression, though it appears that low-dose OCs usually do not result in a vitamin B_6 deficiency (van der Vange et al. 1989).

It is known that the anterior cruciate ligament (ACL) also contains ERs. Several research studies suggest that estrogen binding on the ACL may alter muscle and ligament stiffness throughout the menstrual cycle. It was thought OC use could inhibit fluctuations because of a constant estrogen dose; however, one recent study suggests muscle properties including stiffness are not affected by hormonal fluctuation or OC use (Bell et al. 2011). This topic is discussed in detail in a later chapter by Schultz in this book.

Minor Side Effects

Nausea, breakthrough bleeding, and amenorrhea are common side effects of OC use. Generally, these symptoms should mitigate within 3 months of use. Breakthrough bleeding in the first half of the cycle is a result of too low of a dose of estrogen, and this is normally modified with a supplemental estrogen dose rather than switching to a higher dose estrogen pill. Bleeding in the second half is a result of either progestin or estrogen deficiency. Generally changing to a more potent progestin (norgestrel) can solve this problem. Increasing the progestin component of an OC dose may solve amenorrhea as well. The progestin increase will thicken the endometrial build-up and induce bleeding.

Nausea is generally caused by the estrogen in the OC dose and can be solved by taking the OC dose at night and with food or by switching to a lower dose of estrogen. A low-dose OC may also alleviate water retention which is a widely experienced side effect.

Drug Interactions

Antibiotics and anticonvulsants may interact with OC dosages and result in accidental pregnancy. This is caused by select hepatic enzyme induction, which lowers estrogen to a degree that ovulation is not prevented (Mattson et al. 1986). With the exception of rifampin, these accidental pregnancies are very low in long-term antibiotic users. Topical antibiotics, however, do not appear to increase these risks and should not be a major concern for OC users (Mattson et al. 1986).

Non-contraceptive Benefits

Ovarian and endometrial cancers are reduced by 50 % in OC users, as well as ectopic pregnancy and primary dysmenorrhea. Risks decrease for pelvic inflammatory disease as well as ovarian cysts. Iron deficiency anemia is less common since OC users tend to bleed less, and menstrual irregularities and premenstrual symptoms are also decreased. Rheumatoid arthritis and toxic shock syndrome may also occur with lower frequency as well (Mishell 1989).

Choosing a Pill: Summary

An OC selection should provide the lowest effective dose of both estrogen and progestin and should minimize side effects. A good recommended initial dose is 35 µg of estrogen and 0.5–1 mg of norethindrone as is found in a majority of triphasic OCs. Higher doses should be reserved for patients with specific issues (e.g., patients should be screened initially within 3 months of starting an OC, and yearly or biennially for check-up screening to ensure a safe and efficacious dosage is being used) (Committee on Gynecologic Practices, ACOG 2013).

The HPO axis is a complex regulatory axis that controls the female menstrual cycle as well as other aspects of female health mentioned above. OCs introduce additional estrogen and progestin hormones into the female body during the follicular phase in order to inhibit the mid-cycle gonadotropin surge and subsequent ovulation. Although there are some known minor side effects that may occur with OC use, overall it is an easy, noninvasive, and relatively low risk way to prevent unwanted pregnancy.

Summary and Conclusions

The HPO axis is the major regulator of the female reproductive system. This regulation begins when GnRH is released from the hypothalamus at the onset of puberty, which stimulates LH and FSH production at the anterior pituitary. These hormones then bind to ovarian receptors, stimulating the release of the female reproductive hormones estrogen and progesterone. This regulation process is quite precise and complicated, and several upstream regulators (e.g., brain peptide) such as kisspeptin control it. In sum, a fully functional HPO axis is critical to fertility and overall female reproductive health.

Regulation of the reproductive axis can also be influenced by OCs, which are used by females worldwide to prevent unwanted pregnancy. OCs work by increasing estrogen concentrations during the follicular phase of a female's cycle. High estrogen levels then prevent the mid-cycle gonadotropin surge necessary for ovulation. OCs are still considered somewhat controversial due to potentially adverse side effects (as well as due to some societal and cultural issues), and more research should be conducted on OC use in the future to learn more about these side effects. There is also a tremendous need for more research on the interaction of exercise metabolism and performance with OC usage, as scant rigorous scientific evidence exists, some of which is presented in later chapters in this book.

References

Bell DR, Blackburn JT, Ondrak KS, et al. The effects of oral contraceptive use on muscle stiffness across the menstrual cycle. Clin J Sport Med. 2011;21:467–73.
Besecke LM, Guendner MJ, Sluss PA, et al. Pituitary follistatin regulates activin- mediated production of follicle stimulating hormone during the rat estrous cycle. Endocrinology. 1997;138:2841–8.
Brannian JD, Stouffer RL. Cellular approaches to understand the function and regulation of the primate corpus luteum. Semin Reprod Endocinol. 1991;9:341–51.
Brooks GA, Fahey TD, Baldwin KM. Exercise physiology: human bioenergetics and its applications. New York: McGraw-Hill; 2005.
Bunt JC. Metabolic actions of estradiol: significance for acute and chronic exercise responses. Med Sci Sports Exerc. 1990;22:286–90.
Cancer risks of oral contraception. Lancet. 1989;1:84.
Cases/controls, breast cancer, and the pill. Lancet. 1989;1:1000.
Castellano JM, Navarro VM, Fernandez-Fernandez R, et al. Changes in hypothalamic KiSS-1 system and restoration of pubertal activation of the reproductive axis by kisspeptin in undernutrition. Endocrinology. 2005;146:3917–25.
Celentano DD, Klassen AC, Weisman CS, et al. The role of contraceptive use in cervical cancer: the Maryland cervical cancer case-control study. Am J Epidemiol. 1987;126:592–604.
Christin-Maitre S. History of oral contraceptive drugs and their use worldwide. Best Pract Res Clin Endocrinol Metab. 2013;27(1):3–12.
Committee on Drugs. American academy of pediatrics: breastfeeding and contraception. Pediatrics. 1981;68:138–40.
Committee on Gynecologic Practices: Understanding and using the U.S. selected practice recommendations for contraception use, 2013. American College of Obstetricians and Gynecologists. Number 577, November 2013.
Couse JF, Korach KS. Estrogen receptor null mice: what have we learned and where will they lead us? Endocr Rev. 1999;20:358–417.
Curtis SH, Korach KS. Steroid receptor knockout models: phenotypes and responses illustrate interactions between receptor signaling pathways in vivo. Adv Pharmacol. 2000;47:357–80.
Dungan HM, Gottsch ML, Zeng H, et al. The role of kisspeptin-GPR54 signaling in the tonic regulation and surge release of gonadotropin-releasing hormone/luteinizing hormone. J Neurosci. 2007;27:12088–95.
Eddy EM, Washburn TF, Bunch DO, et al. Targeted disruption of the estrogen receptor gene in male mice causes alteration of spermatogenesis and infertility. Endocrinology. 1996;137:4796–805.
Erickson GF, Magoffin DA, Dyer CA, et al. The ovarian androgen producing cells: a review of structure/function relationships. Endocr Rev. 1985;6:371–99.

Falany JL, Falany CN. Regulation of estrogen sulfotransferase in human endometrial adenocarcinoma cells by progesterone. Endocrinology. 1996;137:1395–401.
Ferin M. The menstrual cycle: an integrative view. In: Adashi EY, Rock JA, Rosenwaks Z, editors. Reproductive endocrinology, surgery, and technology, vol. 1. Philadelphia: Lippincott-Raven; 1996. p. 103–21.
Filicori M. The role of luteinizing hormone in folliculogenesis and ovulation induction. Fertil Steril. 1999;71:405–14.
Fisch IR, Freedman SH, Myatt AV. Oral contraceptives, pregnancy, and blood pressure. JAMA. 1972;222:1510.
Foster DC. Low-dose monophasic and multi-phasic oral contraceptives: a review of potency, efficacy, and side effects. Semin Reprod Endocrinol. 1989;7:205–12.
Goldzieher JW, de la Pena A, Chenault CB, et al. Comparative studies of the ethynyl estrogens used in oral contraceptives III: effect of plasma gonadotropins. Am J Obstet Gynecol. 1975;122:626–36.
Goldzieher JW, Dozier TS, de la Pena A. Plasma levels and pharmacokinetics of ethynyl estrogens in various populations II: mestranol. Contraception. 1980;21:17–27.
Gougeon A. Dynamics of follicular growth in the human: a model from preliminary results. Hum Reprod. 1986;1:81–7.
Gu GB, Simerly RB. Projections of the sexually dimorphic anteroventral periventricular nucleus in the female rat. J Comp Neurol. 1997;384:142–64.
Hackney AC. Influence of oestrogen on muscle glycogen utilization during exercise. Acta Physiol Scand. 1999;67(3):273–4.
Hanson SJ, Burke AE. Fertility control: contraception, sterilization, and abortion. In: Hurt KJ, editor. The Johns Hopkins manual of gynecology and obstetrics. 4th ed. Philadelphia: Lippincott Williams & Wilkins; 2012.
Harris PWR. Malignant hypertension associated with oral contraceptives. Lancet. 1969;2:466.
Hatcher RA, Guest F, Stewart F, et al. Contraceptive technology 1988–1989. 14th ed. New York: Irvinton Publishers Inc; 1988.
Hewitt SC, Korach KS. Oestrogen receptor knockout mice: roles for oestrogen receptors alpha and beta in reproductive tissues. Reproduction. 2003;125:143–9.
Hillard PJA. Oral contraception noncompliance: the extent of the problem. Adv Contracept. 1992;8 Suppl 1:13–20.
Hillier SG. Intrafollicular paracrine function of ovarian androgen. J Steroid Biochem. 1987;27:351–7.
Himelstein-Braw R, Byskov AG, Peters H, et al. Follicular atresia in the infant human ovary. J Reprod Fertil. 1976;46:55–9.
Irwin JC, Kirk D, Gwatkin RB, et al. Human endometrial matrix metalloproteinase-2, a putative menstrual proteinase. Hormonal regulation in cultured stromal cells and messenger RNA expression during the menstrual cycle. J Clin Invest. 1996;97:438–47.
Jick H, Dinan B, Rithman KJ. Oral contraceptives and nonfatal myocardial infarction. JAMA. 1978;239:1403–6.
Ketting E. The relative reliability of oral contraceptives: findings of an epidemiological study. Contraception. 1988;37:343–8.
Kitaoka M, Kojima I, Ogata E. Activin-A: a modulator of multiple types of anterior pituitary cells. Biochem Biophys Res Commun. 1988;157:48–54.
Kovacs GT, Riddoch G, Duncombe P, et al. Inadvertent pregnancies in oral contraceptive users. Med J Aust. 1989;150:549–51.
Kung AW, Ma JTC, Wong VCW, et al. Glucose and lipid metabolism with triphasic oral contraceptives in women with history of gestational diabetes. Contraception. 1987;35:257–69.
Lapatto R, Pallais JC, Zhang D, et al. Kiss1/mice exhibit more variable hypogonadism than gpr54/mice. Endocrinology. 2007;148:4927–36.
Layde PM, Beral V. Further analyses of mortality in oral contraceptive users: royal college of general practitioners oral contraception study. Lancet. 1981;1:541–6.

Layde PM, Vessey MP, Yeates D. Risk factors for gallbladder disease: a cohort study of young women attending family planning clinics. J Epidemiol Community Health. 1982;36:274–8.

Lee NC. Combination oral contraceptive use and risk of endometrial cancer: the cancer and steroid hormone study of the centers for disease control and the national institute of child health and human development. JAMA. 1987;257:796–800.

Lee NC, Wingo PA, Gwinn ML, et al. The reduction in risk of ovarian cancer associated with oral contraceptive use: the cancer and steroid hormone study of the centers for disease control and the national institute of child health and human development. N Engl J Med. 1987;316:650–5.

Lonnerdal B, Forsum E, Hambraues L. Effect of oral contraceptives on composition and volume of breast milk. Am J Clin Nutr. 1980;33:816–24.

Ludwig H, Spornitz UM. Microarchitecture of the human endometrium by scanning electron microscopy: menstrual desquamation and remodeling. Ann N Y Acad Sci. 1991;622:28–46.

Luque RM, Kineman RD, Tena-Sempere M. Regulation of hypothalamic expression of KiSS-1 and GPR54 genes by metabolic factors: analyses using mouse models and a cell line. Endocrinology. 2007;148:4601–11.

Mais V, Kazer RR, Cetel NS, et al. The dependency of folliculogenesis and corpus luteum function on pulsatile gonadotropin secretion in cycling women using a gonadotropin-releasing hormone antagonist as a probe. J Clin Endocrinol Metab. 1986;62:1250–5.

Mani SK, Blaustein JD, O'Malley BW. Progesterone receptor function from a behavioral perspective. Horm Behav. 1997;31:244–55.

Markee JE. Menstruation in intraocular endometrial transplants in the Rhesus monkey. Am J Obstet Gynecol. 1978;131:558–9.

Matsumoto T, Takeyama K, Sato T, et al. Study of androgen receptor functions by genetic models. J Biochem (Tokyo). 2005;138:105–10.

Mattson RH, Cramer JA, Darney PD, et al. Use of oral contraceptives by women with epilepsy. JAMA. 1986;256:238–40.

McNatty KP, Makris A, DeGrazia C, et al. The production of progesterone, androgens, and estrogens by granulosa cells, thecal tissue, and stromal tissue from human ovaries in vitro. J Clin Endocrinol Metab. 1979;49:687–99.

Mishell DR. Contraception. N Engl J Med. 1989;320:777–87.

Motta PM, Makabe S, Nottola SA. The ultrastructure of human reproduction. I. The natural history of the female germ cell: origin, migration and differentiation inside the developing ovary. Hum Reprod Update. 1997;3:281–95.

Nelson LM. Menstruation and the menstrual cycle fact sheet. The National Women's Health Information Center. 2014. http://www.womenshealth.gov/publications/our-publications/fact-sheet/menstruation.cfm. Accessed 13 Dec 2015.

Nippoldt TB, Reame NE, Kelch RP, et al. The roles of estradiol and progesterone in decreasing luteinizing hormone pulse frequency in the luteal phase of the menstrual cycle. J Clin Endocrinol Metab. 1989;69:67–76.

Ory HW. The noncontraceptive health benefits from oral contraceptive use. Fam Plann Perspect. 1982;14:182–4.

Patsch W, Brown SA, Gotto AM, et al. The effect of triphasic oral contraceptives on plasma lipids and lipoproteins. Am J Obstet Gynecol. 1989;161:1396–401.

Pauerstein CJ, Eddy CA, Croxatto HD, et al. Temporal relationships of estrogen, progesterone, and luteinizing hormone levels to ovulation in women and infrahuman primates. Am J Obstet Gynecol. 1978;130:876–86.

Porter JB, Hunter JR, Jick H, et al. Oral contraceptives and nonfatal vascular disease. Obstet Gynecol. 1985;66:1–4.

Porter JB, Jick H, Walker AM. Mortality among oral contraceptive users. Obstet Gynecol. 1987;70:29–32.

Robertson KM, O'Donnell L, Jones ME, et al. Impairment of spermatogenesis in mice lacking a functional aromatase (cyp 19) gene. Proc Natl Acad Sci U S A. 1999;96:7986–91.

Sam S, Frohman LA. Normal physiology of hypothalamic pituitary regulation. Endocrinol Metab Clin North Am. 2008;37(1–22):vii.

Slap GB. Oral contraceptives and depression (Impact, prevalence and cause). J Adolesc Health Care. 1981;2:53–64.

Smout CFV, Jacoby F, Lillie EW. Gynecological and obstetrical anatomy, descriptive & applied. Baltimore: Williams & Wilkins; 1969.

Speroff L, Fritz MA. Clinical gynecologic endocrinology and infertility. 7th ed. Philadelphia: Lippincott Williams & Wilkins; 2005.

Speroff L, Glass RH, Kase NG. Clinical gynecologic endocrinology and infertility. 3rd ed. Baltimore: Williams & Wilkins; 1983.

Tietze C, Lewit C. Life risks associated with reversible methods of fertility regulation. Int J Gynaecol Obstet. 1979;16:456–9.

Tobon H. Malignant hypertension, uremia, and hemolytic anemia in a patient on oral contraceptives. Obstet Gynecol. 1972;40:681–5.

Upton GV. The phasic approach to oral contraception: the triphasic concept and its clinical application. Int J Fertil. 1983;28:121–40.

van der Vange N, Kloosterboer HJ, Haspels AA. Effect of seven low-dose combined oral contraceptive preparations on carbohydrate metabolism. Am J Obstet Gynecol. 1987;156:918–22.

van der Vange N, van den Berg H, Kloosterboer HJ, et al. Effects of seven low-dose combined contraceptives on vitamin B_6 status. Contraception. 1989;40:377–84.

Van Vliet HA, Grimes DA, Helmerhorst FM et al. Biphasic versus monophasic oral contraceptives for contraception. Cochrane Database Syst Rev. 2006;(3):Cd002032.

Van Vliet HA, Grimes DA, Helmerhorst FM et al. Biphasic versus triphasic oral contraceptives for contraception. Cochrane Database Syst Rev. 2006;(3):Cd003283.

Van Vliet HA, Grimes DA, Lopez LM et al. Triphasic versus monophasic oral contraceptives for contraception. Cochrane Database Syst Rev. 2011;(11):Cd003553

Vande Wiele RL, Bogumil J, Dyrenfurth I, et al. Mechanisms regulating the menstrual cycle in women. Recent Prog Horm Res. 1970;26:63–103.

Vessey MP, Lawless M, McPherson K, et al. Fertility after stopping use of intrauterine contraceptive device. Br Med J. 1983;286:106.

Wierman ME. Sex steroid effects at target tissues: mechanisms of action. Adv Physiol Educ. 2007;31(1):26–33.

Wilson JG, Brent RL. Are female sex hormones teratogenic? Am J Obstet Gynecol. 1981;141:567–80.

Wiseman RA, Dodds-Smith IC. Cardiovascular birth defects and antenatal exposure to female sex hormones: a reevaluation of some base data. Teratology. 1984;30:359–70.

Chapter 2
Sex Hormones and Their Impact on the Ventilatory Responses to Exercise and the Environment

Joseph W. Duke

Abbreviations

O_2	Oxygen
CO_2	Carbon dioxide
PaO_2	Partial pressure of O_2 in arterial blood
$PaCO_2$	Partial pressure of CO_2 in arterial blood
pH	Blood acidity
OC	Oral contraceptives
BSA	Body surface area
LP	Luteal phase
FP	Follicular phase
VO_2 peak	Peak aerobic capacity
RR	Respiratory rate
V_T	Tidal volume
EILV	End-inspiratory lung volume
EELV	End-expiratory lung volume
WOB	Work of breathing
PAO_2	Partial pressure of O_2 in the alveolus
A-aDO_2	Alveolar-to-arterial difference in PO_2
HVR	Hypoxic ventilatory response
HCVR	Hypercapnic ventilatory response
MPA	Medroxyprogesterone
N_2	Nitrogen
FIO_2	Fraction of inspired oxygen
SaO_2	Arterial O_2 saturation
$P_{ET}CO_2$	End-tidal partial pressure of CO_2

J.W. Duke, Ph.D. (✉)
Department of Biological Sciences, Northern Arizona University, Flagstaff, AZ, USA
e-mail: jwduke615@gmail.com

Introduction

The respiratory system plays an integral role in the first two steps of the oxygen (O_2) transport system. Specifically, it is responsible for the bulk flow of atmospheric air into the lungs and the diffusion of O_2 from alveoli into the pulmonary capillary blood thereby maintaining a sufficiently high arterial partial pressure of O_2 (PaO_2). Additionally, the respiratory system plays a prominent role in regulating the partial pressure of carbon dioxide ($PaCO_2$) in the arterial blood, as well as maintaining blood acidity, i.e., pH. These tasks must be accomplished as energetically efficiently as possible by regulating breathing volumes, rates, and patterns to be as economical as possible. The respiratory system is also intimately linked with the cardiovascular system and pulmonary vascular pressure and resistance must remain low to keep right heart work to a minimum and prevent damage to the alveolar-capillary blood gas interface. Damage of this interface would inevitably have a negative impact on the respiratory system's diffusive ability.

This system is highly integrated and tightly regulated in a narrow range under a variety of physiologic conditions. Aerobic exercise using a significant proportion of total body mass (e.g., running or cycling) significantly increases O_2 demand, which results in compensatory changes to increases O_2 transport. Simulated or natural terrestrial environments like high altitude or hypothermia or hyperthermia also place challenges on O_2 transport and delivery that are met by altering respiratory system activity. There are an infinite number of physiologic and pathophysiologic factors that alter transiently or permanently the responses of the respiratory system. These factors may also positively or negatively impact the system's ability to function in its primary roles described above. To this end, there are also a number of neurochemical factors—hormones and neurotransmitters—altered naturally or pharmacologically, which are known to interact with and affect the respiratory system. Specific to this chapter are the role sex hormones, i.e., progesterone and estrogen, may play as these hormones vary throughout the menstrual cycle with and without oral contraceptive (OC) use in women. Meaning their impact to influence ventilation at rest, during exercise, and/or in response to changes in PaO_2 and/or $PaCO_2$ may be variable throughout the menstrual cycle or with OC use. Such influence and information would be of great interest to scientists and clinicians working in the respiratory physiology area.

Accordingly, this chapter will review the pertinent scientific and clinical literature investigating the effects of sex hormones in women, specifically estrogens and progestogens, on various parameters of the respiratory system. Unfortunately a lot of this work is yet to be done, and therefore, differences between men and women will also be briefly discussed herein. Because it is the sex hormone progesterone that likely mediates critical changes in ventilatory drive, nearly all studies described here compare ventilatory parameters only between the luteal and follicular phases because this is when progesterone is at its highest and lowest, respectively, i.e., when the effect would be its greatest. In this chapter I discuss the following major areas: ventilation at rest and in response to exercise, breathing patterns and respiratory mechanics at rest and during exercise, pulmonary gas exchange efficiency, and ventilatory chemoreception. Within each section I discuss sex differences, the impact of changes in sex hormones, i.e., across the menstrual cycle, and the effect of OC use if data are available.

Chapter 1 of this book outlines, in detail, the changes in sex hormones during a normal menstrual cycle with and without OC use. Therefore, the reader is referred to that chapter for specific information on those topics.

Effect of Sex and Sex Hormones on Resting and Exercise Ventilatory Parameters

Rest and Exercise Ventilation

Effect of Sex

The impact of sex on respiratory structure and function is well known with absolute lung volumes and maximal expiratory airflow rates being lower in women compared to men (ATS 1991; Miller et al. 2005). Generally, it has been well accepted that the basis of these differences is due primarily to stature, but even when corrected for standing height females still have smaller lung volumes and lesser airway function parameters compared to their male counterparts (McClaran et al. 1998; Mead 1980; Thurlbeck 1982). With respect to expiratory airflow rates, the disparity between sexes is likely due to females having smaller airways than their male counterparts even when matched for height (i.e., lung size) (Dominelli et al. 2011, 2015a; Smith et al. 2014; Sheel et al. 2016). The mechanisms regulating in utero and/or postnatal lung develop are beyond the scope of this chapter, but the interested reader should refer to select references (Burri 1974; Burri et al. 1974; Thebaud and Abman 2007; Burri 1999) for more information on the topic. Additionally, why and when lung development begins to differ between males and females, ultimately resulting in males having larger airways (Dominelli et al. 2011, 2015a), is of interest, but also beyond the scope of this chapter. The interested reader is also directed to select references (Thurlbeck 1982; Hibbert et al. 1995; Martin et al. 1987; Pagtakhan et al. 1984) for more information on that topical area.

Ultimately, the smaller respiratory attributes (e.g., lungs and airways) and body size in females compared to males have an effect on resting ventilation and the ventilatory responses to exercise. Studies that have compared resting ventilation between men and women have been equivocal with some reporting no difference (Duke et al. 2014; Guenette et al. 2004; Matsuo et al. 2003; Olfert et al. 2004; Sebert 1983; White et al. 1983) and others reporting that women have a lower resting ventilation (MacNutt et al. 2012). Regardless of whether resting ventilation was statistically different between men and women, most studies have reported only a 1–3.3 L/min difference for minute ventilation, i.e., dead space plus alveolar ventilation (Duke et al. 2014; Guenette et al. 2004; Matsuo et al. 2003; Olfert et al. 2004; White et al. 1983; MacNutt et al. 2012). Body surface area (BSA) has an effect on metabolic rate, i.e., carbon dioxide (CO_2) output, which in turn would have an effect on ventilation at rest so it may be more appropriate to express ventilation, at rest or during exercise, corrected for BSA. When done, the differences in resting ventilation between men and women are either reduced (Sebert 1983; White et al. 1983) or completely abolished (Guenette et al. 2004; MacNutt et al. 2012).

On the contrary, there is a clear consensus on the difference in ventilation during severe and/or maximal exercise between men and women with men having a greater ventilation than women (Dominelli et al. 2015a, b; Guenette et al. 2004, 2009; Matsuo et al. 2003; Olfert et al. 2004; MacNutt et al. 2012; Cory et al. 2015; Wilkie et al. 2015). Again, correcting ventilation during exercise for BSA narrows the difference between men and women, but to a much lesser extent than during rest (Dominelli et al. 2015a, b; Guenette et al. 2004, 2009; Olfert et al. 2004; MacNutt et al. 2012; Cory et al. 2015; Wilkie et al. 2015). The underlying cause for the lower ventilation during maximum exercise in women is due to a several contributing factors. The primary cause for this difference is lung size, which is a function of height/body size (McClaran et al. 1998). However, there is a clear effect of sex on airway diameter such that when men and women of similar lung sizes are compared, the women have a smaller airway luminal area (Mead 1980; Dominelli et al. 2015a; Sheel et al. 2009). Ultimately, this has an effect on the rate of airflow into and out of the lungs because of the profound impact of airway (i.e., tube) diameter on resistance to airflow as governed by Poiseuille's equation. Put another way, because women have smaller airways they have a greater magnitude of airflow resistance, which means that in order to match the ventilatory rate of their male counterparts of a similar lung/body size they would need to generate extraordinarily high intrathoracic pressures that would make ventilation extremely energetically costly (see below).

Effect of Sex Hormones

As described above, experimentally, progesterone has been shown to be a ventilatory stimulant so it stands to reason that normal fluctuations in progesterone that occur throughout the normal menstrual cycle would affect resting and exercise ventilation such that ventilation under any condition would be highest during the luteal phase (LP) and lowest in the follicular phase (FP). The effect of menstrual cycle phase, i.e., sex hormones, on resting ventilation has been extensively studied, but the findings at present are equivocal. A number of studies have observed ventilation at rest to be significantly greater during the LP compared to the FP (MacNutt et al. 2012; Schoene et al. 1981; Das 1998; Takano 1984; Takano et al. 1981; Williams and Krahenbuhl 1997) while others observed no difference between these phases (Matsuo et al. 2003; White et al. 1983; Beidleman et al. 1999; Regensteiner et al. 1990; da Silva 2006; Hackney et al. 1991; Lebrun et al. 1995; Smekal et al. 2007). Precisely why these findings are equivocal is due to a multitude of factors including, but not limited to, training status, research/exercise protocol used, and how menstrual cycle was monitored, which would impact the researchers' ability to accurately determine what menstrual cycle phase a woman was in such that some could have failed to study individuals when progesterone was at its absolute highest or lowest.

The consensus on the effect of menstrual cycle phase on ventilation during exercise is that there is no effect (Matsuo et al. 2003; Beidleman et al. 1999; Regensteiner et al. 1990; Hackney et al. 1991; Lebrun et al. 1995; Smekal et al. 2007; Casazza et al. 2002; Dombovy et al. 1987; Bryner et al. 1996; De Souza et al. 1990; Lebrun et al. 2003; MacNutt et al. 2012). The lack of an effect persisted while subjects exercised while breathing hypoxic gas (15 % O_2) at sea level (MacNutt et al. 2012) or while in a simulated hypobaric environment (4300 m; (Beidleman et al. 1999)). However, Schoene et al. (1981) and Williams and Karenbuhl (1997) showed that ventilation is greater during the LP compared to the FP. This slight disagreement in the literature is probably due to the reasons mentioned above. Nevertheless, the majority agreement in the literature on the lack of an effect of menstrual cycle phase is convincing though it is peculiar given the known effect of progesterone on ventilation shown experimentally (Behan and Wenninger 2008; Behan et al. 2003; Dempsey et al. 1986). The lack of an effect ultimately demonstrates how complex and tightly regulated ventilation is because the increased ventilation needed to maintain PaO_2, $PaCO_2$, and pH homeostasis during exercise must be done as economically as possible and clearly changes in sex hormones in normally menstruated women appear to be insufficient to disrupt this balance. It is also likely that the feedforward and feedback mechanisms regulating exercise-induced ventilatory drive are too dominant and robust to be altered by sex hormones in physiologic concentrations.

Effects of OC Use

The impact of OC use on athletic performance, metabolic rate at rest and during exercise, and the ventilatory responses to exercise and the environment are only recently being studied extensively. Currently, only a few published studies have examined these parameters. Much needs to be done in this area particularly because of the various types of OC currently used by women. OC's are either synthetic progesterone only or combination synthetic estrogen-progesterone and are either monophasic with the same level(s) of synthetic hormone in each pill or are multiphasic with varying level(s) of synthetic hormones in each pill (see Chapter 1 discussion). Nettlefold et al. (2007) studied women who were regularly taking monophasic OC and found no difference in resting ventilation between the active and inactive pill phases, which represent the LP and FP, respectively. Casazza et al. (2002) studied eumenorrheic women before and after 4 months of triphasic OC use and found no difference in ventilation during peak exercise between the active and inactive pill phases. Similarly, Lebrun et al. (2003) studied highly active women (peak aerobic capacity (VO_2 peak) > 50 mL/kg/min) while they were on a triphasic OC and found no difference in ventilation during peak (i.e., near maximal) exercise.

Ventilatory Pattern and Respiratory Mechanics

Effect of Sex

In general, the ventilatory pattern, that is respiratory rate (RR) and tidal volume (V_T), is variable between individuals regardless of sex as it is common for individuals to utilize different strategies to attain the same ventilatory rate. Nevertheless, the majority of the research has shown that RR does not differ between men and women (Dominelli et al. 2015a, b; Cory et al. 2015; Wilkie et al. 2015; Bryner et al. 1996), but V_T is generally smaller in women (Dominelli et al. 2015a, b; Cory et al. 2015; Guenette et al. 2009; Wilkie et al. 2015), which is unsurprising given that maximum V_T is a function of lung volume and women, on average, have smaller lungs. Thus, similar to resting ventilation, if V_T is corrected for BSA then the magnitude of the sex effect decreases by at least 60% (Dominelli et al. 2015a, b; Guenette et al. 2004, 2009; Cory et al. 2015; Wilkie et al. 2015).

Similar to RR and V_T, operating lung volumes are also variable between individuals regardless of sex. Operating lung volumes refers to where on the continuum of lung volumes between total lung capacity (i.e., lungs completely full) and residual volume (i.e., lungs "empty") an individual is breathing. This is a complex and complicated area of respiratory physiology, but only a brief introduction is provided and the reader is directed to several in depth reviews on the topic (Johnson et al. 1999; Sheel and Romer 2012). Operating lung volumes are quantified by obtaining the volume of air in the lungs at end-inspiration (end-inspiratory lung volume; EILV) and the volume of air left in the lungs at end-expiration (end-expiratory lung volume; EELV) at rest or during exercise and are expressed as a proportion of lung volume, most commonly total lung capacity or vital capacity. Because of the characteristics of the lung tissue and chest wall, at rest individuals breathe at approximately halfway between total lung capacity and residual volume and ventilation is minimally costly because expiration is almost entirely passive. When one begins to exercise and ventilation increases this is achieved by inspiring to closer to total lung capacity, i.e., increasing EILV, and expiring more completely, i.e., decreasing EELV. As mentioned at the beginning of this chapter, the respiratory center chooses a ventilatory pattern that is both effective in maintaining homeostasis, but also energetically efficient and thus the operating lung volumes are important to consider. Operating lung volumes are a proxy of respiratory mechanics and have implications for the energetic cost of breathing; i.e., the work of breathing (WOB) (Agostoni and Hyatt 1986; Otis et al. 1950; Otis 1964). Generally, the larger the EILV (i.e., breathing too close to total lung capacity) and/or the smaller the EELV (i.e., breathing too close to residual volume) the greater the energetic cost of a given ventilatory rate. Similar to RR and V_T, EILV and EELV have considerable variation between individuals, but they have been compared in men and women at rest and during exercise.

There have been a few studies to explicitly study the effect of sex on respiratory mechanics, but results on EELV and EILV have been equivocal. Guenette et al. (2007) studied respiratory mechanics in men and women at rest and during maximum exercise. The authors observed women to have a greater EELV ($42 \pm 8\%$ vs. $35 \pm 5\%$

of vital capacity) and EILV (88 ± 5 % vs. 82 ± 7 % of vital capacity) compared to men. Dominelli et al. (2015a) also found EELV to be significantly greater in women compared to men during maximum exercise, but found no difference in EILV. Dominelli et al. (2015b) and Cory et al. (2015) found no difference in operating lung volumes between men and women at rest or during exercise. In addition to studying the effect of sex on operating lung volumes several studies have investigated the effect of sex on the WOB. It has been repeatedly shown that women have a greater WOB during exercise than men particularly when they are ventilating at a high proportion of their ventilatory capacity (Dominelli et al. 2015b; Guenette et al. 2007, 2009). The underlying reason for the greater WOB in women compared to men appears to be due to the greater work needed to overcome airflow resistance (Dominelli et al. 2013, 2015a, b; Guenette et al. 2007, 2009), which is a consequence of women having smaller airways than men (Dominelli et al. 2015a; Sheel et al. 2009).

Effect of Sex Hormones

The effect of menstrual cycle phase on the ventilatory patterns during exercise has been infrequently reported. In those few studies that have reported RR and V_T at rest or during exercise have reported no difference between these parameters during the LP and FP (MacNutt et al. 2012; Das 1998; Bryner et al. 1996). Thus, not only does the total ventilation not change across the menstrual cycle, neither does the strategy utilized to attain that ventilatory rate. Only Nettlefold et al. (2007) have reported RR and V_T at rest in women using OC and reported no effect of pill phase (active vs. inactive) on these parameters. Similarly, Bryner et al. (1996) found no difference in RR during maximal exercise between pill phases. At present, no studies have examined the effect of OC use on EILV, EELV, or the WOB. More work is needed in this area, but the likely outcome is that there will be no effect of sex hormones (endogenous or exogenous) on these parameters due to the inherent variability in RR, V_T, EILV, and EELV combined with the minimal effect on ventilation during exercise.

Pulmonary Gas Exchange

Effect of Sex

The exchange of gas between the blood in the pulmonary circulation and the environment is the primary role of the respiratory system. How effective the respiratory system is in this role is defined by pulmonary gas exchange efficiency, which is quantified as the difference in the partial pressure of O_2 in the alveolar air (PAO_2) and PaO_2 and referred to as the A-aDO_2. If pulmonary gas exchange was completely efficient then the A-aDO_2 would equal 0 Torr meaning that the blood leaving the left ventricle has the same O_2 tension as that in the alveolar air, but this is not the case physiologically. In general, the A-aDO_2 is ~5 Torr at rest and can increase three to fivefold during maximal exercise. The cause(s) of the inefficiency in pulmonary gas exchange is beyond the scope of this chapter, but the interested reader is referred to the seminal review on this topic (Dempsey and Wagner 1999), as well as a comprehensive review (Stickland et al. 2013) and a key book chapter on the topic (Romer et al. 2012).

The vast majority of the studies examining pulmonary gas exchange efficiency have been performed in males so data on females is, at present, lacking. The first study to examine pulmonary gas exchange efficiency in women was done by Harms et al. (1998) in the late 1990's. The authors reported that women appear to have a greater fall in PaO_2 and a greater $A-aDO_2$ during near-maximal exercise compared to men. More recently, Dominelli et al. (2013) reported identical findings in a sample with a wide range of aerobic capacities (VO_2 peak=28–62 mL/kg/min). However, Hopkins et al. (2000) found PaO_2 during maximal exercise in women to not be different from men. Similarly, Olfert et al. (2004) and Duke et al. (2014) found no difference in the $A-aDO_2$ between men and women at rest and during near-maximal exercise breathing air and hypoxic gas (12–12.5 % O_2).

Despite the somewhat equivocal findings in this area, it is generally accepted that the prevalence and extent of pulmonary gas exchange inefficiency is greater in women than in men and that gas exchange impairments occur at a lower relative exercise intensity (Dominelli et al. 2013; Harms et al. 1998). The likely underlying cause of the greater degree of gas exchange inefficiency in women compared to men is the greater extent of mechanical constraints to ventilation in women because of their smaller lungs and airways. In essence, mechanical constraints to ventilation would result in an inadequate hyperventilatory response to exercise, which would likely contribute to the fall in PaO_2. To test this hypothesis, some have used low-density gas (i.e., 80 % helium and 20 % O_2) during exercise to alleviate or abolish the ventilatory constraints that are present. When done, it has been shown that the impairment in pulmonary gas exchange either goes away or is significantly reduced (McClaran et al. 1998; Dominelli et al. 2013; Dempsey et al. 1984). An important thing to keep in mind here is that this would occur in all individuals with small lungs/airways and/or ventilatory constraints and thus is not unique to women.

No studies have examined the effect of sex hormones either via changes during the menstrual cycle or from OC use. Women do tend to have a lower $PaCO_2$, on the basis of having a smaller ventilation, than men, which could affect pulmonary gas exchange efficiency, but there is no evidence to suggest that menstrual cycle phase has an effect on exercise performance, respiratory exchange ratio, and/or blood lactate accumulation during exercise (Smekal et al. 2007). Therefore, any potential effect of sex hormones on pulmonary gas exchange efficiency would either be minimal or of no functional consequence. Nevertheless, many studies still need to be performed in order to better understand the basic sex differences, as well as the effect of menstrual cycle phase, in the area of pulmonary gas exchange. Fortunately, there has been a significant push in the scientific community to either include women in studies and/or study women specifically so hopefully the data addressing this important area of respiratory physiology are forthcoming.

Effect of Sex and Sex Hormones on Ventilatory Chemoresponsiveness

Ventilatory output in response to changes in PaO_2 and $PaCO_2$ is coordinated in the respiratory control center in the brain stem and is done with input from central and various peripheral chemoreceptors. Sex hormones exert their effect on ventilation at the level of the central nervous system by specifically altering the set point, i.e., the point at which ventilation begins to increase, or ventilatory gain, i.e., the output from a given change (Behan and Wenninger 2008; Behan et al. 2003; Dempsey et al. 1986; Tatsumi et al. 1995). Accordingly, it is generally accepted that alterations in ventilatory chemoresponsiveness, as a result of varying levels of progesterone and estrogen through the menstrual cycle or as a consequence of OC use, represent the most robust sex hormone-induced respiratory system changes. Exogenous progesterone in healthy men has been shown to be a ventilatory stimulant (Skatrud et al. 1978) and an effective treatment for patients with breathing disorders like chronic obstructive pulmonary disease and/or obstructive sleep apnea (Dempsey et al. 1986; Tatsumi et al. 1986, 1995; Skatrud et al. 1980; Kimura et al. 1988). In contrast, estrogen alone does not appear to alter the hypoxic ventilatory response (HVR) or hypercapnic ventilatory response (HCVR), but when combined with progesterone appears to potentiate the progesterone-induced changes in ventilation (Tatsumi et al. 1995, 1997; Regensteiner et al. 1989; Brodeur et al. 1986) likely by inducing progesterone receptor expression (Brodeur et al. 1986). The studies referenced above are important contributions to this area of study as they have described how ventilation is affected by sex hormones. However, these studies have largely used pharmacological doses of sex hormones to evoke and quantify a compensatory effect on ventilation and/or ventilatory responsiveness.

Effect of Sex

Differences in the ventilatory responses between men and women to hypoxia and/or hypercapnia have been largely equivocal. Specifically, the hypoxic ventilatory response (HVR) has been shown to be either lesser (Aitken et al. 1986; Mortola and Saiki 1996; Tatsumi et al. 1991) or greater (White et al. 1983; Hirshman et al. 1975) in men compared to women or not different (Guenette et al. 2004; Dahan et al. 1998; Jensen et al. 2005; Jordan et al. 2000; Loeppky et al. 2001; Sajkov et al. 1997; Sarton et al. 1999). Similarly, the HCVR has been shown to be greater (White et al. 1983; MacNutt et al. 2012) in men compared to women or not different (Aitken et al. 1986; Rebuck et al. 1973). There are several potential explanations for variable results between men and women on HVR, but the most prominent and relevant to the current text is that not all have characterized the menstrual cycle phase in which the women were studied.

Hypoxic Ventilatory Response

Effect of Sex Hormones

The data on how and if HVR varies across the menstrual cycle is equivocal. Recently MacNutt et al. (2012) compared the isocapnic HVR between the LP and FP in moderate to well-trained women (VO_2 peak = 43.4 ± 9.5 mL/kg/min) and found no effect of menstrual cycle phase. Likewise, Beidleman et al. (1999), Regensteiner et al. (1990) and Dombovy et al. (1987) observed no difference in HVR in women between the LP and FP. Regensteiner et al. (1990) also examined the effect of medroxyprogesterone (MPA) supplementation on HVR and still did not observe a significant difference between the LP and FP. Some have reported a significantly greater HVR in the LP compared to FP. Specifically Schoene et al. (1981) studied the HVR in athletic (VO_2 peak = 49.6 ± 5.2 mL/kg/min) and nonathletic (35.2 ± 4.2 mL/kg/min) eumenorrheic women between the LP and FP. The researchers found the HVR to be greater in the LP compared to the FP in all women. Interestingly, Schoene et al. (1981) also found the HVR to be lower in the LP in athletes compared to nonathletes, demonstrating a clear effect of training status on ventilatory chemoresponsiveness that is also observed in men (Harms and Stager 1995). White et al. (1983) studied the HVR in women during the LP and FP, as well as in men. They reported a significantly greater HVR in the LP compared to the FP in women and a significantly greater HVR in men compared to women in the FP only, i.e., FP was the lowest, LP was in the middle, and men were the highest. Similarly, Takano (1984) observed a significantly greater HVR in the LP compared to the FP.

There are a few potential reasons as to why these data are equivocal on the effect of menstrual cycle phase, i.e., high or low levels of progesterone, on the HVR. First, there is significant heterogeneity in fitness levels of women being studied. Because endurance training attenuates the HVR (Harms and Stager 1995), comparing fit women with unfit men may bias the results in favor of a difference in HVR. Second, the method by which HVR is determined varies between studies. Nearly all studies utilize an isocapnic test that requires a substantial resting period (up to 30 min) to establish a true resting ventilation before gradually flowing 100% nitrogen (N_2) into a gas reservoir to decrease the fraction of inspired O_2 (FIO_2) from 0.21 (21%) to ~0.05 (5%) over 5–10 min. However, the means by which a numerical value is obtained and stated as the HVR is assessed differently between studies. One method (i.e., "A" method) quantifies HVR based upon the shape of the hyperbolic relationship between ventilation and PAO_2 (Weil et al. 1970). The greater the "A" value, the greater the ventilatory response to decreased FIO_2 (i.e., PAO_2). The second method (i.e., "slope" method) quantifies HVR as the slope of the least squares regression line between arterial O_2 saturation (SaO_2) and ventilation such that the HVR units are liters per minute per % fall in SaO_2 and reported as positive numbers by convention. Generally, researchers tend to rely on the slope method more frequently than the A method because of ease of computation, but strong agreement has been reported between methods ($r=0.70$–0.97; (Moore et al. 1984; Townsend et al. 2002). Nevertheless, it is conceivable that an individual may have a high A parameter, but a low slope value (Townsend et al. 2002).

Effect of OC Use

The impact of various OC's on the HVR has not been rigorously studied. Regensteiner et al. (1989) is the only study to date to investigate the effect of OC use, per se, on the HVR. They studied postmenopausal women while they took estrogen, progesterone, or both (i.e., in actuality a hormone replacement therapy intervention) and found only the combination of hormones to have a significant effect on HVR. Clearly, more work needs to be done in this area to better elucidate the effect, if any, OC use has on the HVR.

Hypercapnic Ventilatory Response

Effect of Sex Hormones

Similar to HVR, findings on changes in HCVR across the menstrual cycle remain equivocal. MacNutt et al. (2012) used a standard rebreathing method without prior hyperventilation to assess CO_2 sensitivity, i.e., HCVR quantified as the slope of the least squares regression line between ventilation and the end-tidal partial pressure of CO_2 ($P_{ET}CO_2$). Using this method they found no difference in HCVR across menstrual cycle phases. Similarly findings of no difference on HCVR between the LP and FP have been reported by Beidleman et al. (1999), White et al. (1983), as well as Regensteiner et al. (1990) even during MPA supplementation. Slatkovska et al. (2006) and Takano et al. (1981) also found no difference in HCVR between the LP and FP when they used both hypoxic and hyperoxic HCVR protocols. However, Dombovy et al. (1987), Schoene et al. (1981), Dutton et al. (1989), and Williams and Krahenbuhl (1997) all found HCVR to be greater in the LP compared to the FP. Similar to HVR there appears to be a fitness effect on HCVR because only the nonathletic women demonstrated a menstrual cycle phase effect (Schoene et al. 1981; Harms and Stager 1995; Byrne-Quinn et al. 1971; Martin et al. 1979).

There are multiple methodological ways to assess the HCVR and a main point of difference is whether or not the subjects perform a prior hyperventilation before the rebreathing aspect of the procedure. This is done to lower $P_{ET}CO_2$ from ~40 to 20–25 Torr and would allow one to observe and measure basal ventilation, as well as observe and quantify the CO_2 threshold, that is the $P_{ET}CO_2$ at which ventilation increases linearly (Duffin 2011; Mateika et al. 2004). Why a researcher would or would not choose to use a select HCVR protocol with a prior hyperventilation in their research design is beyond the scope of this chapter, but the interested reader is directed to reviews on the topic (Duffin 2011; Duffin et al. 2000). Nevertheless the appropriate interpretation of alterations in the CO_2 threshold is that a lower threshold implies an enhanced chemoresponsiveness to hypercapnia and a higher threshold implies a delayed or depressed chemoresponsiveness to hypercapnia. Similar to HCVR and HVR, findings on the CO_2 threshold have been equivocal. The CO_2 threshold has been shown to be lower in women compared to men (MacNutt et al. 2012; Beidleman et al. 1999). Additionally, MacNutt et al. (2012) and Beidleman et al. (1999) found the CO_2 threshold to be significantly lower in the LP compared to the FP, while others have observed there to be no difference in CO_2 threshold between the LP and FP (Takano et al. 1981; Regensteiner et al. 1990; Dombovy et al. 1987; Slatkovska et al. 2006; Dutton et al. 1989) even with MPA supplementation (Regensteiner et al. 1990).

Effect of OC Use

The impact of various OC's on the HCVR has not been rigorously studied. Nettlefold et al. (2007) studied the hyperoxic and hypoxic HCVR in 12 women who were taking various monophasic OC's during the active and inactive pill phase, i.e., the LP and FP, respectively. They found no difference between pill phases in CO_2 threshold or slope for either HCVR test. The only other study that investigated the effect of OC, per se, did so in postmenopausal women taking estrogen, progesterone, or both (Regensteiner et al. 1989). They found no effect on CO_2 threshold or HCVR slope for estrogen or progesterone alone. However, when taking both estrogen and progesterone they observed a decreased CO_2 threshold and a significantly steeper HCVR slope. Clearly, more work needs to be done in this area with particular focus on the different types of OC's.

Summary

In summary, the data discussed above outlines the current knowledge and understanding of the scientific community on the sex differences in the responses of the respiratory system to exercise and the environment, as well as describes the available (but limited) literature examining the effects of changes in sex hormones on these respiratory system responses. At present, the existing data is largely equivocal in a number of important areas such as ventilation at rest and the ventilatory response to hypoxia and hypercapnia. This is probably due to the variability of hormonal levels in subjects within and between studies, fitness level of subjects, differences in testing procedure and protocols being used. Additionally, the variability, i.e., individuality, of responses to hormones also provides another degree of complexity. On the contrary, the data are in agreement that there is a sex effect on the ventilatory response to exercise. As described at length above, this is due to women having smaller lungs and airways compared to men. Similarly, changes in sex hormones via the menstrual cycle or with OC use do not appear to have an effect on the ventilatory responses to exercise. Nevertheless, the understanding of basic sex differences and the effect of variations in sex hormones on these ventilatory parameters is incomplete, but these data may be forthcoming with the increased focus on including women as subjects in research studies. Future work should focus on developing consistency in research protocols and rigorously monitoring the menstrual cycle to ensure that measurements are taken during the time of the greatest and lowest concentration of progesterone.

Additionally, it would be helpful to gain an understanding of how the responses described above do or do not vary during the ovulatory phase of the menstrual cycle, which has not been examined in exercise studies.

References

Agostoni E, Hyatt RE. Static behavior of the respiratory system. In: Macklem PT, Mead J, editors. Handbook of physiology. Bethesda: American Physiological Society; 1986.

Aitken ML, Franklin JL, Pierson DJ, Schoene RB. Influence of body size and gender on control of ventilation. J Appl Physiol. 1986;60(6):1894–9.

ATS. Lung function testing: selection of reference values and interpretative strategies. American Thoracic Society. Am Rev Respir Dis. 1991;144:1202–18.

Behan M, Wenninger JM. Sex steroidal hormones and respiratory control. Respir Physiol Neurobiol. 2008;164(1-2):213–21.

Behan M, Zabka AG, Thomas CF, Mitchell GS. Sex steroid hormones and the neural control of breathing. Respir Physiol Neurobiol. 2003;136(2-3):249–63.

Beidleman BA, Rock PB, Muza SR, Fulco CS, Forte Jr VA, Cymerman A. Exercise VE and physical performance at altitude are not affected by menstrual cycle phase. J Appl Physiol. 1999;86(5):1519–26.

Brodeur P, Mockus M, McCullough R, Moore LG. Progesterone receptors and ventilatory stimulation by progestin. J Appl Physiol. 1986;60(2):590–5.

Bryner RW, Toffle RC, Ullrich IH, Yeater RA. Effect of low dose oral contraceptives on exercise performance. Br J Sports Med. 1996;30(1):36–40.

Burri PH. The postnatal growth of the rat lung. 3. Morphology. Anat Rec. 1974;180(1):77–98.

Burri PH. Lung development and pulmonary angiogenesis. In: Gaultier C, Bourbon JR, Post M, editors. Lung development. New York: Oxford University Press; 1999. p. 122–55.

Burri PH, Dbaly J, Weibel ER. The postnatal growth of the rat lung. I. Morphometry. Anat Rec. 1974;178(4):711–30.

Byrne-Quinn E, Weil JV, Sodal IE, Filley GF, Grover RF. Ventilatory control in the athlete. J Appl Physiol. 1971;30(1):91–8.

Casazza GA, Suh SH, Miller BF, Navazio FM, Brooks GA. Effects of oral contraceptives on peak exercise capacity. J Appl Physiol. 2002;93(5):1698–702.

Cory JM, Schaeffer MR, Wilkie SS, Ramsook AH, Puyat JH, Arbour B, et al. Sex differences in the intensity and qualitative dimensions of exertional dyspnea in physically active young adults. J Appl Physiol. 2015;119(9):998–1006.

da Silva SB, de Sousa Ramalho Viana E, de Sousa MB. Changes in peak expiratory flow and respiratory strength during the menstrual cycle. Respir Physiol Neurobiol. 2006;150(2-3):211–9.

Dahan A, Sarton E, Teppema L, Olievier C. Sex-related differences in the influence of morphine on ventilatory control in humans. Anesthesiology. 1998;88(4):903–13.

Das TK. Effects of the menstrual cycle on timing and depth of breathing at rest. Indian J Physiol Pharmacol. 1998;42(4):498–502.

De Souza MJ, Maguire MS, Rubin KR, Maresh CM. Effects of menstrual phase and amenorrhea on exercise performance in runners. Med Sci Sports Exerc. 1990;22(5):575–80.

Dempsey JA, Wagner PD. Exercise-induced arterial hypoxemia. J Appl Physiol. 1999;87(6):1997–2006.

Dempsey JA, Hanson P, Henderson KS. Exercise-induced arterial hypoxemia in healthy human subjects at sea level. J Physiol. 1984;355:161–75.

Dempsey JA, Olson EB, Skatrud JB. Hormones and neurochemicals in the regulation of breathing. In: Cherniak NS, Widdicombe JG, editors. Handbook of physiology: the respiratory system: control of breathing. Washington, DC: American Physiological Society; 1986.

Dombovy ML, Bonekat HW, Williams TJ, Staats BA. Exercise performance and ventilatory response in the menstrual cycle. Med Sci Sports Exerc. 1987;19(2):111–7.

Dominelli PB, Guenette JA, Wilkie SS, Foster GE, Sheel AW. Determinants of expiratory flow limitation in healthy women during exercise. Med Sci Sports Exerc. 2011;43:1666–74.

Dominelli PB, Foster GE, Dominelli GS, Henderson WR, Koehle MS, McKenzie DC, et al. Exercise-induced arterial hypoxaemia and the mechanics of breathing in healthy young women. J Physiol. 2013;591(Pt 12):3017–34.

Dominelli PB, Molgat-Seon Y, Bingham D, Swartz PM, Road JD, Foster GE, et al. Dysanapsis and the resistive work of breathing during exercise in healthy men and women. J Appl Physiol. 2015a;119(10):1105–13.

Dominelli PB, Render JN, Molgat-Seon Y, Foster GE, Romer LM, Sheel AW. Oxygen cost of exercise hyperpnoea is greater in women compared with men. J Physiol. 2015b;593(8):1965–79.

Duffin J. Measuring the respiratory chemoreflexes in humans. Respir Physiol Neurobiol. 2011;177(2):71–9.

Duffin J, Mohan RM, Vasiliou P, Stephenson R, Mahamed S. A model of the chemoreflex control of breathing in humans: model parameters measurement. Respir Physiol. 2000;120(1):13–26.

Duke JW, Elliott JE, Laurie SS, Beasley KM, Mangum TS, Hawn JA, et al. Pulmonary gas exchange efficiency during exercise breathing normoxic and hypoxic gas in adults born very preterm with low diffusion capacity. J Appl Physiol. 2014;117(5):473–81.

Dutton K, Blanksby BA, Morton AR. CO_2 sensitivity changes during the menstrual cycle. J Appl Physiol. 1989;67(2):517–22.

Guenette JA, Diep TT, Koehle MS, Foster GE, Richards JC, Sheel AW. Acute hypoxic ventilatory response and exercise-induced arterial hypoxemia in men and women. Respir Physiol Neurobiol. 2004;143(1):37–48.

Guenette JA, Witt JD, McKenzie DC, Road JD, Sheel AW. Repiratory mechanics during exercise in endurance-trained men and women. J Physiol. 2007;581:1309–22.

Guenette JA, Querido JS, Eves ND, Chua R, Sheel AW. Sex differences in the resistive and elastic work of breathing during exercise in endurance-trained athletes. Am J Physiol Regul Integr Comp Physiol. 2009;297(1):R166–75.

Hackney AC, Curley CS, Nicklas BJ. Physiological responses to submaximal exercise at the mid-follicular, ovulatory, and mid-luteal phases of the menstrual cycle. Scand J Med Sci Sports. 1991;1:94–8.

Harms C, Stager JM. Low chemoresponsiveness and inadequate hyperventilation contribute to exercise-induced hypoxemia. J Appl Physiol. 1995;79(2):575–80.

Harms CA, McClaran SR, Nickele GA, Pegelow DF, Nelson WB, Dempsey JA. Exercise-induced arterial hypoxemia in healthy young women. J Physiol. 1998;507:619–28.

Hibbert M, Lannigan A, Raven J, Landau L, Phelan P. Gender differences in lung growth. Pediatr Pulmonol. 1995;19(2):129–34.

Hirshman CA, McCullough RE, Weil JV. Normal values for hypoxic and hypercapnic ventilaroty drives in man. J Appl Physiol. 1975;38(6):1095–8.

Hopkins SR, Barker RC, Brutsaert TD, Gavin TP, Entin P, Olfert IM, Veisel S, Wagner PD. Pulmonary gas exchange during exercise in women: effects of exercise type and work increment. J Appl Physiol. 2000;89:721–30.

Jensen D, Wolfe LA, O'Donnell DE, Davies GA. Chemoreflex control of breathing during wakefulness in healthy men and women. J Appl Physiol. 2005;98(3):822–8.

Johnson BD, Weisman I, Zeballos R, Beck K. Emerging concepts in the evaluation of ventilatory limitations during exercise. Chest. 1999;116:488–503.

Jordan AS, Catcheside PG, Orr RS, O'Donoghue FJ, Saunders NA, McEvoy RD. Ventilatory decline after hypoxia and hypercapnia is not different between healthy young men and women. J Appl Physiol. 2000;88(1):3–9.

Kimura H, Tatsumi K, Kunitomo F, Okita S, Tojima H, Kouchiyama S, Masuyama S, Shinozaki T, Mikami M, Watanabe S. Obese patients with sleep apnea syndrome treated by progesterone. Tohoku J Exp Med. 1988;156:151–7.

Lebrun CM, McKenzie DC, Prior JC, Taunton JE. Effects of menstrual cycle phase on athletic performance. Med Sci Sports Exerc. 1995;27(3):437–44.

Lebrun CM, Petit MA, McKenzie DC, Taunton JE, Prior JC. Decreased maximal aerobic capacity with use of a triphasic oral contraceptive in highly active women: a randomised controlled trial. Br J Sports Med. 2003;37(4):315–20.

Loeppky JA, Scotto P, Charlton GC, Gates L, Icenogle M, Roach RC. Ventilation is greater in women than men, but the increase during acute altitude hypoxia is the same. Respir Physiol. 2001;125(3):225–37.

MacNutt MJ, De Souza MJ, Tomczak SE, Homer JL, Sheel AW. Resting and exercise ventilatory chemosensitivity across the menstrual cycle. J Appl Physiol. 2012;112(5):737–47.

Martin BJ, Sparks KE, Zwillich CW, Weil JV. Low exercise ventilation in endurance athletes. Med Sci Sports. 1979;11(2):181–5.

Martin TR, Castile RG, Fredberg JJ, Wohl ME, Mead J. Airway size is related to sex but not lung size in normal adults. J Appl Physiol. 1987;63(5):2042–7.

Mateika JH, Mendello C, Obeid D, Badr MS. Peripheral chemoreflex responsiveness is increased at elevated levels of carbon dioxide after episodic hypoxia in awake humans. J Appl Physiol. 2004;96(3):1197–205. discussion 6.

Matsuo H, Katayama K, Ishida K, Muramatsu T, Miyamura M. Effect of menstrual cycle and gender on ventilatory and heart rate responses at the onset of exercise. Eur J Appl Physiol. 2003;90(1-2):100–8.

McClaran S, Harms CA, Pegelow DF, Dempsey JA. Smaller lungs in women affect exercise hyperpnea. J Appl Physiol. 1998;84(6):1872–81.

Mead J. Dysanapsis in normal lungs assessed by the relationship between maximal flow, static recoil, and vital capacity. Am Rev Respir Dis. 1980;121(2):339–42.

Miller MR, Hankinson J, Brusasco V, Burgos F, Casaburi R, Coates A, Crapo R, Enright P, van der Grinten CPM, Gustafsson P, Jensen R, Johnson DC, MacIntyre N, McKay R, Navajas D, Pedersen OF, Pellegrino R, Viegi G, Wanger J, Force AE. Standardisation of spirometry. Eur Respir J. 2005;26:319–38.

Moore LG, Huang SY, McCullough RE, Sampson JB, Maher JT, Weil JV, et al. Variable inhibition by falling CO_2 of hypoxic ventilatory response in humans. J Appl Physiol. 1984;56(1):207–10.

Mortola JP, Saiki C. Ventilatory response to hypoxia in rats: gender differences. Respir Physiol. 1996;106(1):21–34.

Nettlefold L, Jensen D, Janssen I, Wolfe LA. Ventilatory control and acid-base regulation across the menstrual cycle in oral contraceptive users. Respir Physiol Neurobiol. 2007;158(1):51–8.

Olfert IM, Balouch J, Kleinsasser A, Knapp A, Wagner H, Wagner PD, et al. Does gender affect human pulmonary gas exchange during exercise? J Physiol. 2004;557(Pt 2):529–41.

Otis AB. The work of breathing. In: Fenn WO, Rahn H, editors. Handbook of physiology. Washington, DC: American Physiological Society; 1964.

Otis AB, Fenn WO, Rahn H. Mechanics of breathing in man. J Appl Physiol. 1950;2(11):592–607.

Pagtakhan RD, Bjelland JC, Landau LI, Loughlin G, Kaltenborn W, Seeley G, et al. Sex differences in growth patterns of the airways and lung parenchyma in children. J Appl Physiol. 1984;56(5):1204–10.

Rebuck AS, Kangalee M, Pengelly LD, Campbell EJ. Correlation of ventilatory responses to hypoxia and hypercapnia. J Appl Physiol. 1973;35(2):173–7.

Regensteiner JG, Woodard WD, Hagerman DD, Weil JV, Pickett CK, Bender PR, et al. Combined effects of female hormones and metabolic rate on ventilatory drives in women. J Appl Physiol. 1989;66(2):808–13.

Regensteiner JG, McCullough RG, McCullough RE, Pickett CK, Moore LG. Combined effects of female hormones and exercise on hypoxic ventilatory response. Respir Physiol. 1990;82(1):107–14.

Romer LM, Sheel AW, Harms CA. The respiratory system. In: Farrell PA, Joyner MJ, Caiozzo VJ, editors. ACSM's advanced exercise physiology. Baltimore: Lippincott Williams and Wilkins; 2012. p. 242–96.

Sajkov D, Neill A, Saunders NA, McEvoy RD. Comparison of effects of sustained isocapnic hypoxia on ventilation in men and women. J Appl Physiol. 1997;83(2):599–607.

Sarton E, Teppema L, Dahan A. Sex differences in morphine-induced ventilatory depression reside within the peripheral chemoreflex loop. Anesthesiology. 1999;90(5):1329–38.

Schoene RB, Robertson HT, Pierson DJ, Peterson AP. Respiratory drives and exercise in menstrual cycles of athletic and nonathletic women. J Appl Physiol. 1981;50(6):1300–5.

Sebert P. Heart rate and breathing pattern: interactions and sex differences. Eur J Appl Physiol Occup Physiol. 1983;50(3):421–8.

Sheel AW, Romer LM. Ventilation and respiratory mechanics. Compr Physiol. 2012;2(2):1093–142.

Sheel AW, Guenette JA, Yuan R, Holy L, Mayo JR, McWilliams AM, et al. Evidence for dysanapsis using computed tomographic imaging of the airways in older ex-smokers. J Appl Physiol. 2009;107(5):1622–8.

Sheel AW, Dominelli PB, Molgat-Seon Y. Revisiting dysanapsis: sex-based differences in airways and the mechanics of breathing during exercise. Exp Physiol. 2016;101(2):213–8.

Skatrud JB, Dempsey JA, Kaiser DG. Ventilatory response to medroxyprogesterone acetate in normal subjects: time course and mechanism. J Appl Physiol. 1978;44(6):939–44.

Skatrud JB, Dempsey JA, Bhansali P, Irvin C. Determinants of chronic carbon dioxide retention and its correction in humans. J Clin Invest. 1980;65(4):813–21.

Slatkovska L, Jensen D, Davies GA, Wolfe LA. Phasic menstrual cycle effects on the control of breathing in healthy women. Respir Physiol Neurobiol. 2006;154(3):379–88.

Smekal G, von Duvillard SP, Frigo P, Tegelhofer T, Pokan R, Hofmann P, et al. Menstrual cycle: no effect on exercise cardiorespiratory variables or blood lactate concentration. Med Sci Sports Exerc. 2007;39(7):1098–106.

Smith JR, Rosenkranz SK, Harms CA. Dysanapsis ratio as a predictor for expiratory flow limitation. Respir Physiol Neurobiol. 2014;198:25–31.

Stickland MK, Lindinger MI, Olfert IM, Heigenhauser GJ, Hopkins SR. Pulmonary gas exchange and acid-base balance during exercise. Compr Physiol. 2013;3(2):693–739.

Takano N. Reflex hypoxic drive to respiration during the menstrual cycle. Respir Physiol. 1984;56(2):229–35.

Takano N, Sakai A, Iida Y. Analysis of alveolar PCO2 control during the menstrual cycle. Pflugers Arch. 1981;390(1):56–62.

Tatsumi K, Kimura H, Kunitomo F, Kuriyama T, Watanabe S, Honda Y. Sleep arterial oxygen desaturation and chemical control of breathing during wakefulness in COPD. Chest. 1986;90(1):68–73.

Tatsumi K, Hannhart B, Pickett CK, Weil JV, Moore LG. Influences of gender and sex hormones on hypoxic ventilatory response in cats. J Appl Physiol. 1991;71(5):1746–51.

Tatsumi K, Moore LG, Hannhart B. Influences of sex steroids on ventilation and ventilatory control. In: Dempsey JA, Pack AI, editors. Regulation of breathing. New York: Marcel Dekker; 1995. p. 829–64.

Tatsumi K, Pickett CK, Jacoby CR, Weil JV, Moore LG. Role of endogenous female hormones in hypoxic chemosensitivity. J Appl Physiol. 1997;83(5):1706–10.

Thebaud B, Abman SH. Bronchopulmonary dysplasia: where have all the vessels gone? Roles of angiogenic growth factors in chronic lung disease. Am J Respir Crit Care Med. 2007;175(10):978–85.

Thurlbeck WM. Postnatal human lung growth. Thorax. 1982;37(8):564–71.

Townsend NE, Gore CJ, Hahn AG, McKenna MJ, Aughey RJ, Clark SA, et al. Living high-training low increases hypoxic ventilatory response of well-trained endurance athletes. J Appl Physiol. 2002;93(4):1498–505.

Weil JV, Byrne-Quinn E, Sodal IE, Friesen WO, Underhill B, Filley GF, et al. Hypoxic ventilatory drive in normal man. J Clin Invest. 1970;49(6):1061–72.

White DP, Douglas NJ, Pickett CK, Weil JV, Zwillich CW. Sexual influence on the control of breathing. J Appl Physiol. 1983;54(4):874–9.

Wilkie SS, Dominelli PB, Sporer BC, Koehle MS, Sheel AW. Heliox breathing equally influences respiratory mechanics and cycling performance in trained males and females. J Appl Physiol. 2015;118(3):255–64.

Williams TJ, Krahenbuhl GS. Menstrual cycle phase and running economy. Med Sci Sports Exerc. 1997;29(12):1609–18.

Chapter 3
Sex Hormones and Substrate Metabolism During Endurance Exercise

Laurie Isacco and Nathalie Boisseau

Abbreviations

AMPC	Cyclic adenosine monophosphate
AMPK	Adenosine monophosphate-activated protein kinase
ANP	Atrial natriuretic peptide
CHO	Carbohydrates
CPT-I	Carnitine palmitoyltransferase I
CS	Citrate synthase
E2	17β-estradiol
EE	Ethinyl estradiol
ER	Estrogen receptors
FFA	Free fatty acids
FP	Follicular phase
GH	Growth hormone
GLUT4	Glucose transporter type 4
GMPC	Cyclic guanosine monophosphate
HRT	Hormone replacement therapy
HSL	Hormone-sensitive lipase
IGF-1	Insulin-like growth factor 1
IMCL	Intramyocellular lipid

L. Isacco, Ph.D. (✉)
Laboratory of Prognostic Markers and Regulatory Factors of Cardiovascular Diseases and Exercise Performance Health Innovation Platform, University of Bourgogne Franche-Comte, Besançon, France
e-mail: laurie.isacco@univ-fcomte.fr

N. Boisseau, Ph.D.
Laboratory of the Metabolic Adaptations to Exercise under Physiological and Pathological condition, Clermont Auvergne University, Clermont-Ferrand, France

LP	Luteal phase
LPL	Lipoprotein lipase
MCAD	Medium-chain acylCoA dehydrogenase
MLOR	Maximal lipid oxidation rates
mRNA	Messenger ribonucleic acid
OC	Oral contraceptives
OC−	Oral contraceptive nonusers
OC+	Oral contraceptive users
PDK4	Pyruvate dehydrogenase kinase isozyme 4
PGC-1α	Peroxisome proliferator-activated receptor- γ coactivator 1α
PPAR	Peroxisome proliferator-activated receptor
Ra	Rate of appearance
Rd	Rate of disappearance
RER	Respiratory exchange ratio
SREBP-1c	Sterol regulatory element-binding protein-1c
VO_{2max}	Maximal oxygen consumption
β-HAD	β-hydroxy acyl-CoA dehydrogenase

Introduction

Carbohydrates (CHO) and fat are the main energy sources mobilized to meet the energy demands during muscle contraction. Their relative contribution is modulated by different parameters. Exercise intensity and duration are the main determinants of fuel selection; however, age, diet, physical activity level, weight status, and sex also can influence this choice (Jeukendrup and Wallis 2005; Brooks and Mercier 1994). All, these variables have been extensively studied in athletes for performance enhancement, and also in people with chronic diseases with the aim of improving health and quality of life (Bordenave et al. 2008; Lambert et al. 1997).

Today, sex-related differences, due to the presence of sex-specific steroids, in substrate utilization during exercise are widely acknowledged. Indeed, estrogen and progesterone interact directly and/or indirectly with tissues and organs involved in energy metabolism, such as muscle, liver, and adipose tissue. In women, the natural ovarian hormone fluctuations during the menstrual cycle, the drastic decrease in steroid concentrations at menopause, the use of oral contraceptives (OC), or hormone replacement therapy (HRT) can all influence substrate metabolism during endurance exercise (Isacco et al. 2012a).

The aim of this chapter is to present an overview of the sex differences in substrate metabolism during endurance exercise and to specifically discuss the effects of the menstrual cycle, OC, menopause, and HRT on these metabolic responses.

Sex Differences in Substrate Metabolism During Endurance Exercise

To avoid any flaws, before any comparison of exercise-induced metabolic responses between men and women, the populations' age and training status should be matched and the diet and time since the last training bout must be controlled. The maximal oxygen consumption (VO_{2max}) can be used to match the groups' physical activity level; however, VO_{2max} should be expressed relative to the fat-free mass and not per kilogram of body mass because women have approximately 5–8 % more body fat than men (Tarnopolsky 2008; Carter et al. 2001a). If all these variables are not taken into account, conflicting results may be obtained, as already shown in the literature (Blatchford et al. 1985; Costill et al. 1976; Froberg and Pedersen 1984). Another inherent difficulty is the potential heterogeneity of the hormonal status in the women's group. Different variables, such as the phase of the menstrual cycle, OC use, oligomenorrhea, amenorrhea, menopause, HRT type (to mention just a few), have to be finely controlled to avoid any intra-group discrepancies. Therefore, it is easy to understand why research on exercise-induced health improvement or performance enhancement is predominantly conducted in men and why results obtained in men are frequently applied also to women.

Carbohydrate Metabolism

Many studies investigated sex differences in substrate oxidation rates during moderate-intensity endurance exercise, most of the time in young subjects (~18–30 years old). Overall, through respiratory exchange ratio (RER) measurement, they revealed that, at a given relative work intensity, women show a lower reliance on whole-body CHO oxidation to support energy demands (Tarnopolsky et al. 1990; Tarnopolsky et al. 1995; Romijn et al. 2000; Carter et al. 2001b; Devries et al. 2006; Tremblay et al. 2010). Similarly, stable isotope-based measurement of hepatic glucose turnover showed that women rely less on CHO stores than men, as indicated by the lower glucose rate of appearance (Ra), disappearance (Rd) and metabolic clearance (Carter et al. 2001a; Devries et al. 2006). The origin of this adaptation is still unknown and could be attributed to lower liver glycogenolysis and/or gluconeogenesis in women than men. Conversely, it is not clear whether skeletal muscle glycogen stores are spared in women during moderate-intensity endurance exercise. Some studies did not find any sex difference in muscle CHO utilization after a single bout of cycling exercise (Tarnopolsky et al. 1995; Roepstorff et al. 2002; Zehnder et al. 2005), whereas others found higher net (from muscle biopsies) or estimated glycogen use in men during a running exercise (Carter et al. 2001a; Tarnopolsky et al. 1990). At a higher exercise intensity level

(Wingate protocol: 30s cycle sprint), a muscle glycogen sparing effect (glycogen use reduced by 50%) was detected in women compared with men, but only in Type 1 and not Type 2 skeletal fibers (Esbjornsson-Liljedahl et al. 1999).

Fat Metabolism

For the same relative exercise intensity, women show greater reliance on fat than men, as indicated by their lower RER (Tarnopolsky 2008). As women generally have a higher percentage of body fat, this could theoretically lead to greater free fatty acid (FFA) availability and fat oxidation than in men. However, a decrease in body fat mass favors lipolytic sensitivity. Lipolytic responsiveness is thus enhanced in subjects with low body fat mass (Klein et al. 1994) and decreased in people with obesity (Wolfe et al. 1987).

While stable isotope-based methods show higher lipolysis (i.e., higher glycerol Ra) in women than in men during moderate-intensity prolonged exercise (Carter et al. 2001b), it is not possible to accurately estimate the role of FFA or intramyocellular lipids (IMCL) in the total fat oxidation rates. IMCL concentrations at rest are higher in women than in men (Roepstorff et al. 2002; Roepstorff et al. 2006; Devries et al. 2007; Tarnopolsky et al. 2007) due to the higher lipid droplet content, and not to their larger size (Tarnopolsky et al. 2007). However, it is still unclear whether IMCL utilization is higher (Roepstorff et al. 2002; Roepstorff et al. 2006; Steffensen et al. 2002), lower (Zehnder et al. 2005), or similar (White et al. 2003; Devries et al. 2007) in women and men during moderate-intensity prolonged exercise. FFA utilization is not different in endurance-trained women and men at 25%, 65%, and 85% of VO_{2max} (Romijn et al. 2000) and also in untrained subjects during a single bout of exercise (90 min) performed at 45% VO_{2max} (Burguera et al. 2000). Only Roepstorff et al. (2002) found a greater amount of oxidized FFA in women than in men after 1 h of a 90 min cycling exercise performed at 60% VO_{2max}.

Estrogen-Induced Sex Differences in Substrate Metabolism (Table 3.1)

Studies in rodents and humans suggest that estrogen have a significant role in regulating substrate metabolism at rest and during endurance exercise (Tarnopolsky 2008; Vieira-Potter et al. 2015; Maher et al. 2010; Sladek 1974; Kendrick et al. 1987).

Animals supplemented with 17β-estradiol (E2) show higher activity of lipoprotein lipase (LPL) (Ellis et al. 1994), carnitine palmitoyltransferase I (CPT-I), and short-chain β-hydroxy acyl-CoA dehydrogenase (β-HAD) (Campbell and Febbraio 2001) in skeletal muscle and reduced hepatic glycogen utilization compared with untreated controls (Campbell and Febbraio 2001; Kendrick et al. 1987; Hatta et al. 1988). However, no difference is observed in β-HAD (McKenzie et al. 2000), CPT-I (Berthon et al. 1998), or LPL (Kiens et al. 2004) activities between men supplemented with E2 and women.

Table 3.1 Effect of 17β-estradiol (E2) on substrate metabolism in human and rodent models

E2 supplementation and substrate metabolism		
Population/model	Effects	References
Amenorrheic women	↓ RER during exercise	Ruby et al. (1997)
Men	↓ RER during exercise	Carter et al. (2001a, Devries et al. (2005), Hamadeh et al. (2005)
Men	↓ CHO oxidation during exercise	Hamadeh et al. (2005)
	↑ Fat oxidation during exercise	Hamadeh et al. (2005)
	↑ FFA during exercise	Ruby et al. (1997)
	↓ Ra of glucose during exercise (also in women)	Carter et al. (2001a), Devries et al. (2005), Ruby et al. (1997)
	↓ Rd of glucose during exercise	Carter et al. (2001a), Devries et al. (2005)
	↓ Resting adipose tissue activity	Ellis et al. (1994)
Rats	↑ LPL activity in muscle during exercise	Ellis et al. (1994)
	↑ CPT-I, β-HAD	Campbell and Febbraio (2001)
Sex differences		
Tissue	Effects	References
Muscle	CPT-I ♂ = ♀	Berthon et al. (1998)
	β-HAD ♂ = ♀	Carter et al. (2001b)
	Muscle LPL activity ♂ = ♀	Kiens et al. (2004)
E2 supplementation in men		
Muscle RNA levels	↑ PPAR-α, PPAR-β	Tarnopolsky (2008)
	↑ CPT-I, SREBP-1c	Tarnopolsky (2008)
	↑ GLUT4	Tarnopolsky (2008)
Muscle protein and RNA levels	↑ MCAD (↑ PGC-1α mRNA, ↓ microRNA miR-29b)	Maher et al. (2010)

E2 administration to men (Carter et al. 2001a; Devries et al. 2005; Hamadeh et al. 2005) or to women with amenorrhea (Ruby et al. 1997) decreases RER, CHO kinetics and oxidation rates and increases plasma FFA concentrations and fat oxidation rates during moderate-intensity prolonged exercise (Devries et al. 2005; Hamadeh et al. 2005; Ruby et al. 1997; Carter et al. 2001a). No effect is observed on whole-body lipolysis (Ruby et al. 1997; Carter et al. 2001a) or on muscle glycogen utilization (Tarnopolsky et al. 2001; Devries et al. 2005). Pharmacological suppression and replacement of ovarian hormones in women showed that E2 decreases CHO oxidation rates by reducing muscle glycogen utilization and Rd (muscle uptake) (D'Eon et al. 2002).

E2 increases the messenger ribonucleic acid (mRNA) expression of peroxisome proliferator-activated receptor α and β (PPAR-α, PPAR-β), sterol regulatory element-binding protein-1c (SREBP-1c), CPT-I, glucose transporter type 4

(GLUT4), and glycogen synthase (Tarnopolsky 2008). E2 supplementation in men upregulates peroxisome proliferator-activated receptor-γ coactivator 1 α (PGC-1α) and the microRNA miR-29b (predicted to regulate PGC-1α), leading to increased mitochondrial gene expression of medium-chain acylCoA dehydrogenase (MCAD), which is involved in lipid utilization (Maher et al. 2010).

Menstrual Cycle and Substrate Metabolism During Endurance Exercise

Fluctuations of Ovarian Hormones During the Menstrual Cycle

Female sexual maturity is characterized by an increase in ovarian hormone concentrations leading to the appearance of the menstrual cycle and the secondary sexual characteristics. The menstrual cycle is one of the most important biological rhythms in women. Estrogen (17β-estradiol, estrone, and estriol) and progesterone are the two main ovarian hormones of the menstrual cycle and they fluctuate predictably during 23–28 days (Reilly 2000). They are mainly secreted by the ovaries and to a lesser extent by the adrenal glands (Lebrun 1994).

The menstrual cycle is divided in two distinct phases: follicular phase (FP) (early, mid, and late) and luteal phase (LP) (early, mid, and late) separated by ovulation. The FP begins on the first day of the menses and continues, on average, for 9 days until ovulation, which lasts about 5 days. The LP begins after ovulation and lasts, on average, fourteen days until the next menses (Constantini et al. 2005). The estrogen–progesterone ratio is different during these three phases: (1) low estrogen and progesterone concentrations during the FP, (2) high estrogen and low progesterone concentrations during ovulation, (3) high estrogen and progesterone concentrations during the LP (Constantini et al. 2005).

Natural Ovarian Hormones and Substrate Metabolism During Endurance Exercise

Although the main function of ovarian hormones is to support reproduction, they also influence directly or indirectly other physiological systems, particularly energy metabolism at rest and during exercise where estrogen and progesterone may have antagonistic functions (Oosthuyse and Bosch 2010; Constantini et al. 2005).

As previously discussed (see section "Estrogen-induced sex differences in substrate metabolism"), studies in animals and humans on estrogen effect on substrate metabolism suggest that the hormonal fluctuations during the menstrual cycle could influence substrate metabolism in females.

In humans, most studies did not find any difference in substrate metabolism at rest between FP and LP (Heiling and Jensen 1992; Jensen et al. 1994; Magkos et al. 2006; Uranga et al. 2005; Piers et al. 1995; Horton et al. 2002). However, Hackney (1990) reported that the resting muscle glycogen content in *vastus lateralis* is higher in mid-LP than in mid-FP, suggesting a glycogen sparing effect during LP (Hackney 1990).

Conflicting results have been obtained when studying the effect of the menstrual cycle on CHO and fat metabolism during exercise in humans. In the late 1980s, Nicklas et al. reported higher muscle glycogen content in LP than FP after depletion exercise (Nicklas et al. 1989). Similarly, a muscle glycogen sparing effect during 60 min cycling at approximatively 70 % VO_{2max} was observed during LP compared with FP (Hackney 1999).

In regularly menstruating women during a 25 min cycling exercise performed at 90 % of the lactate thresholds, glucose Ra and Rd and CHO oxidation rates were lower and fat oxidation rates higher in LP than FP (Zderic et al. 2001). Similarly, women exhibited lower glucose Ra and Rd and lower total glycogen utilization in LP than FP during endurance exercise (cycling 90 min at 65 % VO_{2max}) (Devries et al. 2006). Thus, according to these studies, the higher E2 plasma levels in LP promote muscle glycogen storage and sparing during exercise (Devries et al. 2006; Oosthuyse and Bosch 2010). This is strengthened by the finding that E2 increases muscle glycogen synthase activity (Beckett et al. 2002). Glycogen sparing during the LP could be associated with and explained by enhanced reliance on lipid metabolism (Dombovy et al. 1987; Hackney 1999; Oosthuyse and Bosch 2010).

However, other studies did not find any difference in substrate metabolism between FP and LP during endurance exercise (Heiling and Jensen 1992; De Souza et al. 1990; Bailey et al. 2000; Horton et al. 2002; Horton et al. 2006; Suh et al. 2002, 2003; Kanaley et al. 1992). Similar RER were observed in FP and LP during maximal and submaximal exercises (De Souza et al. 1990) and the different menstrual cycle phases did not have any effect on substrate metabolism during a treadmill run performed at 70 % VO_{2max} until exhaustion (Bailey et al. 2000). Similarly, neither menstrual cycle phase nor menstrual status (amenorrheic vs eumenorrheic women) influenced CHO and fat oxidation rates during a 90 min run performed at 60 % VO_{2max} (Kanaley et al. 1992). However, pharmaceutically manipulated sex hormone concentrations may influence fuel utilization during exercise in eumenorrheic and oligomenorrheic women. In this population, high circulating sex steroid concentrations resulted in an enhanced fat oxidation and reduced CHO oxidation during endurance running (60 min at 65 % VO_{2max}) compared with low hormonal concentrations (Hackney et al. 2000).

Using stable isotopic tracers, no difference was found in whole-body substrate oxidation rates between FP and LP (Horton et al. 2006; Horton et al. 2002; Suh et al. 2002, 2003; Jacobs et al. 2005). Likewise, RER and glucose kinetics (Horton et al. 2002) as well as glycerol and FFA rates (Horton et al. 2006) were comparable between menstrual cycle phases during a 90 min cycling at 50 % VO_{2max}. Finally, similar substrate oxidation rates, glucose and lipid kinetics were observed in LP and FP during cycling at 45 % and 65 % VO_{2max} for 60 min (Suh et al. 2002, 2003; Jacobs et al. 2005).

The Estrogen–Progesterone Ratio

As noted earlier, the results of studies on the effect of the menstrual cycle on fuel metabolism during endurance exercise are contradictory. This could be partially explained by the complex balance between estrogen and progesterone concentrations and their fluctuations during the menstrual cycle. Some authors emphasized that estrogen inhibit gluconeogenesis (Matute and Kalkhoff 1973), favor glycogen storage, increase lipolysis and promote fat oxidation (Constantini et al. 2005). Progesterone antagonizes estrogen pro-lipolytic effects, but also shifts substrate metabolism toward fat utilization via its CHO-sparing effects (Constantini et al. 2005). Accordingly, D'Eon et al. (2002) hypothesized that the decreased glucose kinetics in women is most likely an estrogen-associated effect and progesterone seems to potentiate it.

However, more than the individual and isolated effects of estrogen and progesterone on substrate metabolism, their interaction seems to be critical. Indeed, in 2002, D'Eon et al. proposed that the estrogen–progesterone ratio needs to be sufficiently elevated to lead to metabolic changes. Jacobs et al. (2005) and Horton et al. (2006) emphasized that the magnitude of estrogen upregulation and particularly the increase in the estrogen–progesterone ratio are important factors in determining the final effect of these ovarian hormones on fat metabolism. This was later confirmed by Oosthuyse and Bosch (2010) who also suggested that intra- and inter-individual variations in ovarian hormones could partially explain the discrepancies between studies (Oosthuyse and Bosch 2010). Nevertheless, more work is needed to better understand the complex interactions between ovarian hormones and their effect on energy metabolism during prolonged exercise.

Non-Ovarian Hormones

Natural ovarian hormones not only directly influence substrate metabolism during endurance exercise, but also have some indirect effects through complex interactions with non-steroid hormones, such as insulin, catecholamine, growth hormone (GH), and cortisol (Bunt 1990; Matute and Kalkhoff 1973; Mc et al. 1958; Reinke et al. 1972; Sladek 1974; Bemben et al. 1992; Bonen et al. 1991). For instance, estrogen supplementation in rats increases sensitivity to catecholamine and hormone-sensitive lipase (HSL) activity (Benoit et al. 1982). Moreover, according to Bonen et al. (1991), the most significant effect of estrogen on substrate metabolism is through estrogen-mediated decrease of insulin sensitivity. Therefore, the effects of ovarian hormones on non-steroid hormones during the menstrual cycle may partially explain the substrate oxidation differences observed between FP and LP in some studies. Indeed, the increase in cortisol (Genazzani et al. 1975) and GH concentrations (Horton et al. 2002) as well as in sympathetic activity (Minson et al. 2000) associated with the reduction in insulin action (Escalante Pulido and Alpizar Salazar 1999) observed in LP could favor higher fat oxidation and lower CHO oxidation during endurance exercise.

Exercise Intensity

Exercise intensity is the main factor affecting substrate oxidation during exercise (Brooks and Mercier 1994). The menstrual cycle-dependent effects of female steroid hormones on fuel metabolism are also influenced by exercise intensity. For instance, the lower CHO and higher fat oxidation rates observed in mid-LP (compared with mid-FP) at low and moderate exercise intensities (10 min treadmill run at 35% and 60% VO_{2max}) disappear at higher exercise intensity (75% VO_{2max}) (Hackney et al. 1994). On the other hand, estrogen effect on hepatic glucose output is detected only when the exercise intensity is sufficiently elevated to increase the demand in glucose utilization above a certain level (Horton et al. 2002). Thus, at approximately 50% VO_{2max} (25.1 ml min^{-1} kg^{-1}), plasma glucose kinetics and CHO oxidation rates are lower in LP than FP. Conversely, no difference is observed when individuals cycle at 42% VO_{2max} (20.2 ml min^{-1} kg^{-1}) (Zderic et al. 2001). Likewise, glucose Ra is not different between menstrual cycle phases at 20.2 ml min^{-1} kg^{-1} (Horton et al. 2002). Conversely, it is significantly higher in early-FP than in mid-LP at 70% VO_{2max} (36.8 ml min^{-1} kg^{-1}) (Campbell et al. 2001) and at 65% VO_{2max} (25.4 ml min^{-1} kg^{-1}) (Devries et al. 2006). As highlighted by Oosthuyse and Bosch (2010), substrate metabolism differences during the menstrual cycle partially depend on the energy demand and higher intensity exercise leads to increased endogenous glucose production. Furthermore, the nutritional status also affects substrate oxidation rates and may contribute to regulating the crosstalk between ovarian hormones and exercise intensity/energy demands; see next section (Oosthuyse and Bosch 2010).

Nutritional Status

When investigating substrate metabolism during exercise, nutritional status is an important variable because fed conditions could blunt differences in substrate utilization between menstrual cycle phases; however, most studies are conducted after overnight fast, possibly due to protocol standardization (Zderic et al. 2001; Devries et al. 2006; Campbell et al. 2001).

Indeed, in women depleted in CHO, plasma glucose concentrations are maintained during submaximal bicycle exercise (90 min at 63% VO_{2max}) in FP, while they progressively decrease (70 and 90 min of exercise) in LP (Lavoie et al. 1987). Conversely, CHO loading can overcome glucose kinetic and muscle glycogen sparing differences in LP and FP (McLay et al. 2007). Similarly, lower CHO and higher fat oxidation rates in LP than in FP at rest and during exercise (cycle ergometer at 30, 50, and 70% VO_{2max}) are observed after a low CHO diet in comparison with a high CHO diet for 3 days (Wenz et al. 1997). According to Oosthuyse and Bosch (2010), glucose kinetics varies during the menstrual cycle when exercise is high enough to influence endogenous glucose production. Energy intake may modify this relationship. For instance, Campbell et al. (2001) showed that consumption of energy drinks during exercise masks differences in glucose Ra between FP and LP. The authors suggested that upon energy drink ingestion, glucose Ra is mostly determined by exogenous glucose absorption and this could blunt menstrual cycle-related differences (Campbell et al. 2001). Accordingly, no difference in substrate metabolism between menstrual cycle phases is observed when exercise is performed in postprandial conditions (Suh et al. 2002). Similarly, a study on the effects of menstrual cycle phases and diet (CHO loading compared with isoenergetic normal diet: 8.4 g kg^{-1} day^{-1} CHO vs. 5.2 g kg^{-1} day^{-1} CHO for 3 days) on muscle glycogen content and substrate oxidation rates during exercise (75 min cycling at 45–75 % VO$_{2max}$ followed by a 16 km time trial) showed lower resting glycogen concentrations in mid-FP than mid-LP. Conversely, substrate utilization during exercise was not affected by the menstrual cycle phases (McLay et al. 2007). Thus, CHO loading leads to similar substrate utilization during exercise, despite lower glycogen storage in mid-FP.

Discrepancies remain concerning the effect of menstrual cycle-related hormone fluctuations on substrate oxidation rates during endurance exercise. They could be explained by differences in the experimental protocols (mainly, exercise duration and intensity), but also by the many variables that can influence substrate metabolism during exercise (Jeukendrup 2003; Jeukendrup and Wallis 2005). Although some of them have been discussed here (exercise intensity, diet), studies on the effect of the prior physical activity level or weight status are still scarce.

Oral Contraceptive Effects on Substrate Metabolism During Endurance Exercise

Oral Contraceptive Formulations

Different contraceptive options are available to women and OC remain one of the most popular forms of birth control (de Melo et al. 2004). OC primary aim is to avoid pregnancy, but they can also be used to control menstrual cycle and premenstrual symptoms and to improve bone health (Bennell et al. 1999; Burrows and Peters 2007; Snow-Harter 1994). Three different OC types (monophasic, biphasic, and triphasic) that usually combine ethinyl estradiol (EE) and progestin are currently available. Monophasic OC provide constant synthetic steroid hormone concentrations and are easy to use. In triphasic OC, synthetic steroid hormone concentrations change three times to mimic the natural menstrual cycle. Biphasic OC (two different hormone concentrations) are less frequently prescribed and do not present any real advantage compared with monophasic and triphasic OC (Bennell et al. 1999; Burrows and Peters 2007). For women sensitive to estrogen, progestin-only OC are an option.

EE concentrations have drastically changed since OC introduction in the early 1960s. At the beginning, they were close to 150 µg and progestin components could reach 250 µg. Rapidly, EE concentrations decreased to 50 µg to offset the negative effects (insulin resistance and dyslipidemia). Today, low-dose (EE: 20–30 µg) OC are mostly prescribed (Benagiano et al. 2008). Recently, more natural compounds, such as estradiol and estradiol valerate have been introduced (Sitruk-Ware and Nath

2011), but studies on their effect on substrate metabolism during exercise are not available yet. Progestin concentrations are more variable and the compounds currently used in OC have different estrogenic, progestogenic, and androgenic effects (Constantini et al. 2005). New-generation progestin compounds have been developed in the last few years to minimize their side effects on insulin resistance, glucose intolerance, plasma cholesterol, and triglycerides. The effects of synthetic progestin compounds currently vary depending on their androgenicity. Norgestrel and levonorgestrel show the highest androgenic activities, while norethindrone is weaker (Constantini et al. 2005). Newer OC formulations with reduced EE and progestin doses and novel molecules with safer profiles are now available on the market (Shufelt and Bairey Merz 2009).

Synthetic Ovarian Hormone Effects on Substrate Metabolism During Endurance Exercise

Due to the specific hormone nature and concentrations, OC may affect substrate metabolism at rest and/or during exercise. Jensen and Levine (1998) did not find any difference in lipolysis and substrate oxidation rates at rest and during epinephrine infusion between eumenorrheic women (OC−) and women taking OC (OC+) (Jensen and Levine 1998). However, other authors observed substrate metabolism alterations in OC+. For instance, during 30 min treadmill exercise at 40 % VO_{2max}, OC+ women showed higher FFA and lower glucose plasma concentrations without any difference in RER compared with OC− women (Bonen et al. 1991). Likewise, OC+ women exhibited lower glucose levels and CHO oxidation rates during 90 min treadmill run at 50 % VO_{2max}, suggesting increased CHO sparing in OC+ women (Bemben et al. 1992).

Comparison of two OC with 35 μg EE and different progestin concentrations (low progestin concentrations: 500 μg; and high progestin concentrations: 1000 μg of norethisterone) showed no difference in metabolic parameters at rest. Conversely, RER was significantly lower in women using high progestin concentration than in women using low progestin concentration OC throughout the steady-state exercise test (20 min at 75 % VO_{2max}) (Redman et al. 2005). The authors proposed that high progestin level is associated with insulin resistance, glucose intolerance and reduced muscle glycogen utilization (Sutter-Dub and Vergnaud 1982; Picard et al. 2002; Campbell and Febbraio 2002). Moreover, progestin could increase fat oxidation rates by reducing the availability of glucose-6-phosphate for glycolysis (Redman et al. 2005). It should be noted that norethisterone binds to progesterone receptors but also to androgen receptors (with low affinity) and therefore exerts both progestogenic and androgenic effects (Redman et al. 2005).

Analysis of the effect of triphasic OC (4-month treatment) on lipid mobilization and utilization during endurance exercise (60 min cycling at 45 % VO_{2max} and at 65 % VO_{2max}) showed that in OC+ women, lipid mobilization increases during exercise without any change in fat oxidation rates (Casazza et al. 2004). The authors suggested that FFA re-esterification could explain these results (Jacobs et al. 2005). Using a similar experimental protocol, they also demonstrated that OC use decreases glucose flux without any change in CHO and fat oxidation rates during prolonged cycling (Suh et al. 2003). Similarly, Isacco and collaborators did not find any difference in RER, CHO and fat oxidation rates between OC users and nonusers during endurance exercise (45 min cycling at 65 % VO_{2max}) (Isacco et al. 2012b). More recently, they reported that OC use increases fat mobilization; however, this effect is blunted when lipolytic activity is stimulated by exercise (Isacco et al. 2014).

Due to their specific nature and concentrations, synthetic ovarian hormones contained in OC may influence substrate metabolism during exercise. Futures studies are necessary but it seems that OC use may increase lipolytic activity during endurance exercise without any substantial (or detectable) effect on substrate utilization (Casazza et al. 2004; Suh et al. 2003; Bonen et al. 1991; Isacco et al. 2012b; Isacco et al. 2014).

Oral Contraceptive Effects on Non-Ovarian Hormone Responses

Some specific non-ovarian hormone changes may be involved in the substrate metabolism differences observed in OC users and nonusers.

Growth Hormone (GH)

Like natural ovarian hormones, synthetic steroids can exert their effects directly or indirectly through non-steroid hormone actions. In the early 1990s, it was suggested that hormones contained in OC may affect plasma GH concentrations and thus substrate metabolism. Indeed, higher plasma GH concentrations were observed in OC+ than in OC− women during exercise (Bonen et al. 1991). Similarly, GH concentrations increase at 10 and 20 min of exercise in OC+ women (Bemben et al. 1992). GH concentrations are also higher during continuous (20 min at 60 % VO_{2max}) and intermittent cycling (higher than 80 % VO_{2max} for the same duration) in OC+ women (Bernardes and Radomski 1998). Finally, GH concentrations are higher from the 15th min of exercise (30 min cycling at 60 % VO_{2max}) in OC+ than in OC− women without any difference in glucose tolerance (Boisseau et al. 2001).

As GH reduces glucose uptake and favors lipolysis (Norrelund 2005), it was proposed that such differences in plasma GH concentrations in OC+ and OC− women may lead to opposite substrate metabolism activity (Bonen et al. 1991; Bemben et al. 1992; Boisseau et al. 2001). However, no or little effect of OC use was observed in substrate utilization, although higher GH concentrations have been associated with increased plasma FFA levels (Bonen et al. 1991) and reduced plasma glucose concentrations (Bonen et al. 1991; Bemben et al. 1992). Bonen and coworkers (1991) suggested that reduced GH efficiency, lower receptor sensitivity and/or transport bias in OC+ women could explain these results. Thus, the increase in plasma GH concentrations observed in OC users seems not to be associated with changes in GH activity.

On the other hand, according to Casazza et al. (2004), Isacco et al. (2014) did not find any difference in plasma GH concentrations between OC+ and OC− women, despite higher plasma glycerol and FFA concentrations in OC+ women, suggesting greater lipid mobilization during prolonged cycling (Isacco et al. 2014). The authors hypothesized that as GH requires 2–3 h to promote lipolysis, its effect is most likely negligible during the exercise trial (45 min) and the recovery period (2 h), and the difference in lipolytic activity between groups cannot be explained by OC effect on GH alone.

Atrial Natriuretic Peptide (ANP)

ANP has an important lipolytic action through a specific pathway (cyclic guanosine monophosphate—GMPc—and protein kinase G) that is independent from the signaling cascade regulated by catecholamines and insulin (cyclic adenosine monophosphate—AMPc—and protein kinase A) (Sengenes et al. 2005; Sengenes et al. 2003; Moro et al. 2004; Lafontan et al. 2005; Koppo et al. 2010). Studies in animals reported that E2 can affect plasma ANP concentrations. Specifically, combined administration of estradiol and progesterone has been shown to enhance ANP gene expression in a dose-dependent manner in ovariectomized female rats (Hong et al. 1992). Moreover, estradiol administration in follitropin-receptor knockout mice in which the ANP system is impaired increases ANP synthesis (Belo et al. 2008). In humans, ANP concentrations are higher in women than in men, mainly due to ovarian hormones (Clark et al. 1990). Similarly, three months of HRT increases plasma ANP concentrations in postmenopausal women, thus emphasizing the role of female steroids in plasma ANP level regulation (Maffei et al. 2001). As the biological activities of synthetic ovarian hormones in OC are more potent than those of natural hormones, OC could increase plasma ANP concentrations. Indeed, Davidson et al. reported greater ANP concentrations in OC+ than in OC− women (Davidson et al. 1988). Noradrenaline and ANP concentrations are higher also in women taking new-generation OC compared with nonusers, whereas plasma insulin, GH, and adrenaline levels are comparable between groups (Isacco et al. 2014). These hormonal responses, and particularly the higher ANP concentrations at baseline and throughout exercise, may in part explain the difference in lipid mobilization between groups (Isacco et al. 2014).

Nutritional Status

As already mentioned, nutrition is an important factor for fuel selection during endurance exercise. Most studies investigated OC effect either in fed or fast state (Bonen et al. 1991; Bemben et al. 1992; Suh et al. 2003; Jacobs et al. 2005; Casazza et al. 2004; Redman et al. 2005) and only one in both conditions (Isacco et al. 2012b).

Analysis of the effect of high CHO diet (80% CHO) and glucose ingestion (2 g kg^{-1}) on substrate oxidation rates during cycling (120 min at 57% VO$_{2max}$) showed that the high CHO diet and glucose ingestion favor CHO utilization. However, observed in fuel selection between OC+ and OC− women 2010). Some studies reported higher lipid mobilization in OC+ than ...n during exercise performed in postprandial conditions (Bonen et al. ...zza et al. 2004). However, these studies did not take into account the ... effects of food intake and daytime variations that may influence hormonal ...ses and energy metabolism. Thus, Isacco et al. investigated the interaction of ...use and nutritional status on substrate metabolism in women during prolonged ...ycling exercise (45 min at 65 % VO_{2max}). Fasting led to increased lipid mobilization and utilization compared with fed state, without any effect of the hormonal status (Isacco et al. 2012b). More recently, OC use has been shown to favor lipolysis in the postprandial state, but this effect is blunted when lipolytic activity is stimulated by exercise. Thus, it seems that exercise per se masks OC− induced greater postprandial lipid mobilization (Isacco et al. 2014). In conclusion, the nutritional status must be specified when interpreting OC effects on substrate metabolism and more studies are needed to clarify this interaction.

Maximal Lipid Oxidation Rate

Increased lipid oxidation favors body weight management and glycogen sparing, thus delaying fatigue during endurance exercise (Kelley 2005; Romijn et al. 1993). This is particularly important both for performance and health strategies. Higher lipid mobilization (Bonen et al. 1991; Casazza et al. 2004; Isacco et al. 2014; Jacobs et al. 2005) without any difference in fat oxidation rates during endurance exercise (Bemben et al. 1992; Isacco et al. 2012b) has been reported in OC+ compared with OC− women. Moreover, an exercise intensity that is specific to each individual ($Lipox_{max}$-FAT_{max}) elicits the maximal lipid oxidation rates (MLOR). This could be used to individualize training programs for people wishing to maximize their lipid utilization and/or to identify subjects with metabolic impairments (Perez-Martin et al. 2001; Achten et al. 2002). OC+ women have higher MLOR and $Lipox_{max}$ than OC− women (Isacco et al. 2015). Therefore, as the synthetic steroids currently used in OC formulations could affect MLOR and $Lipox_{max}$, the exercise intensity that elicits MLOR has to be targeted to highlight potential metabolic differences in OC+ and OC− women (Isacco et al. 2015). It is worth noting that lipid profile, anthropometric measures and body composition (total fat mass, fat mass localization, fat-free mass) could not explain the difference between groups that were matched for age and physical activity level. To explain the differences in $Lipox_{max}$ and MLOR between OC+ and OC− women, it has been hypothesized that EE has a more potent effect than E2. Moreover, the activities of natural and synthetic estrogen are mediated by the two major isoforms of estrogen receptors (ERα and ERβ) that elicit antagonist effects on metabolism. Increased glucose tolerance as well as lipid mobilization and utilization are associated with ERα activity, while ERβ stimulation leads to lipogenesis and insulin resistance (Oosthuyse and Bosch 2012). EE binds with high affinity to ERα and with a twofold lower affinity to ERβ. Conversely, natural estrogen display comparable binding affinities for both ERs (Tremollieres 2012).

Menopause Effects on Substrate Metabolism During Endurance Exercise

Menopause

Menopause signals the end of the fertile phase of a woman's lifespan and is defined retrospectively after 12 months of amenorrhea. The transition to menopause corresponds to a decrease in sex steroid hormones, and plasma estrogen reach similar levels as in men (i.e., 6–24 ng l^{-1}) (Simpson et al. 2002). Menopause changes also favor adiposity gain. The Study of Women's Health Across the Nation (SWAN), 800 women were followed for six years through the menopausal period, reported an average increase of 3.4 kg in fat mass and of 5.7 cm in waist circumference (Sowers et al. 2007). Estrogen and body fat mass changes in postmenopausal women might also have the potential to alter substrate metabolism during endurance exercise.

Sex Differences in Substrate Metabolism During Endurance Exercise in Older Individuals

The RER and fat oxidation rates adjusted for VO$_2$ are not different in 70-year-old men and 66-year-old (menopausal) women during a 30 min cycling bout at 45% VO$_{2max}$ (Toth et al. 1998). This indicates that the higher reliance on fat as substrate in premenopausal women than in men decreases after menopause, mainly due to the reduction in plasma E2 and, to a lesser extent, progesterone levels. However, during a 40-min cycling exercise at 50% VO$_{2max}$, RER is lower and fat oxidation rates (adjusted for fat-free mass) higher in obese postmenopausal women than in obese men (aged 57 ± 1 years) (Numao et al. 2009), despite similar E2 resting serum concentrations in both groups and higher plasma FFA levels in men. The exercise-induced higher increase in E2 plasma concentrations observed in premenopausal women compared with men (Horton et al. 1998) might still occur in postmenopausal obese women and this could explain the higher fat oxidation rates (Numao et al. 2009).

Menopause and Substrate Metabolism During Endurance Exercise: Comparison Between Premenopausal and Postmenopausal Women

As menopause leads to a significant decrease in estrogen circulating levels, it is not surprising that menopause is associated with lower whole-body fat oxidation rates at rest (Lovejoy et al. 2008). Moreover, postmenopausal women show lower fat oxidation rates (g min^{-1} kgFFM^{-1}) and energy expenditure (kcal min^{-1}) during a cycling exercise (45 min at 50% VO$_{2max}$) than premenopausal women. This could to reduce the capacity of substrate utilization by skeletal muscle (Abildgaard et al. 2013). The reduction in lean body mass seems to factor to explain the lower fat oxidation rates and energy expenditure in pausal women because they are closely correlated. Interestingly, different whole-body fat oxidation rates are not reflected in the mRNA expression at rest of factors involved in fat oxidation rates and energy expenditure regulation, such as CPT-I, citrate synthase (CS), PPARα, β-HAD, PGC-1, and pyruvate dehydrogenase kinase isozyme 4 (PDK4) (Abildgaard et al. 2013). Also, the activity of important oxidative enzymes (β-HAD and CS) is unchanged by the menopausal status. However, the same authors found that in postmenopausal women, exercise-induced adenosine monophosphate-activated protein kinase (AMPK) phosphorylation in skeletal muscle is lower than in premenopausal women. Although it was only a trend, this finding is compatible with earlier results showing that AMPK is activated by estrogen (D'Eon et al. 2005; D'Eon et al. 2008).

Menopause, Hormone Replacement Therapy and Substrate Metabolism During Endurance Exercise

HRT, also commonly known as hormone therapy (i.e., 0.625–1.250 mg day^{-1} of estrogen), is widely used for controlling menopausal symptoms and for preventing bone loss (Yasui et al. 2003).

Different studies showed that HRT increases exercise-induced fat oxidation rates in postmenopausal women due to its action on the concentration and activity of lipolytic hormones (Kohrt et al. 1998; O'Sullivan et al. 1998; Bjorntorp 1996). During endurance exercise, plasma levels of lipolytic hormones, such as cortisol or GH, are higher in postmenopausal HRT users than in nonusers (Kraemer et al. 1998; Johnson et al. 1997). However, in response to an acute running exercise (30 min on a treadmill) performed at 80% VO_{2max}, no difference in fat oxidation rates was observed between women taking (aged 53 ± 3 years) or not (aged 49 ± 3 years) HRT (Johnson et al. 2002). The higher exercise intensity of this protocol may probably explain the difference with the other studies, because lipid metabolism decreases with exercise intensity (Brooks and Mercier 1994). Thus, an exercise session performed at 80% of VO_{2max} (or greater) may blunt the difference in exercise-induced fat oxidation rates in women taking or not using HRT.

The route of estrogen replacement (oral or transdermal) also could affect energy metabolism and fuel selection (Lwin et al. 2008; O'Sullivan et al. 1998; dos Reis et al. 2003). In a crossover design study involving postmenopausal women (aged 57 ± 1 years), oral HRT was associated with decreased fat oxidation rates, increased body fat mass and decreased lean body mass at rest compared with transdermal HRT (both for 24 weeks) (O'Sullivan et al. 1998). In addition, 24-h indirect calorimetry measurements clearly showed a decrease in fat oxidation rates at rest in postmenopausal (aged 51 ± 4 years) women who received oral estrogen treatment (0.625 mg day^{-1} conjugated equine estrogen) for two months (Lwin et al. 2008). Oral estrogen could thus increase fat deposition by reducing fat oxidation, explaining why HRT generally causes weight/fat gain. Liver exposure to high concentrations of estrogen decreases the production of enzymes involved in fat oxidation (Weinstein et al. 1986; Gower et al. 2002) and increases enzymes involved in lipogenesis (Mandour et al. 1977). Data from studies in rodents also show that pharmacological doses of estrogen inhibit both mRNA and protein expression of CPT-I (Lwin et al. 2008) and may limit HSL activity (Gower et al. 2002). In contrast, transdermal estrogen administration does not affect fat oxidation rates (O'Sullivan et al. 1998; O'Sullivan and Ho 1995; dos Reis et al. 2003). Liver accounts for approximately 25% of whole-body resting metabolism (Konarzewski and Diamond 1995) and oxidizes more fat than skeletal muscle. Estrogen pass through the liver upon oral, but not transdermal administration, thus increasing GH and GH-binding protein levels and decreasing insulin-like growth factor 1 (IGF-1). This alters substrate metabolism and, indirectly, body composition (O'Sullivan et al. 1998; Hoffman et al. 1995) and could explain why fat oxidation rates increase in postmenopausal women who take transdermal estrogen and decrease in women taking oral estrogen (dos Reis et al. 2003). Unfortunately, all studies investigating the influence of the administration route have been conducted at rest and never during endurance exercise.

Recent data indicate that HRT does not really protect postmenopausal women against cardiovascular diseases and may even increase the risk of stroke (Boardman et al. 2015). Furthermore, HRT favors breast cancer development (Lupo et al. 2015), which led to a reduction in its use (Kocjan and Prelevic 2003). However, these results should be interpreted with caution, because in most of these studies women took conjugated estrogen rather than low E2 concentrations by transdermal administration. Thus, the type of estrogen used could also explain the different HRT effects on substrate metabolism.

In conclusion, more studies are required on HRT administration route and formulation (estrogen type and content) to precisely determine the risk–benefit ratio in postmenopausal women.

Conclusion

Sexual dimorphism in fuel metabolism during endurance exercise has been extensively studied in view of improving performance or health; however, data only on females are scarce. This is mainly due to the hormonal fluctuations throughout women's lifespan and thus to the difficulties in standardizing research protocols.

According to the current literature findings indicate that sex and menopause affect substrate metabolism during endurance exercise. However, results on the effects of the menstrual cycle and OC are less consistent. Methodological differences in exercise modalities (intensity, duration), ovarian hormone concentrations, OC type, diet, physical activity level, and weight status may partially explain these discrepancies. Moreover, the activities of natural and synthetic ovarian hormones are complex and tissue-specific.

In a society where physical activity promotion is becoming a health challenge, it is relevant to pursue research focused on women. Investigating the impact of sex, menstrual cycle, OC, and menopause (including HRT) on metabolic parameters during endurance exercise will lead to better performance management and health benefits for this population.

References

Abildgaard J, Pedersen AT, Green CJ, Harder-Lauridsen NM, Solomon TP, Thomsen C, et al. Menopause is associated with decreased whole body fat oxidation during exercise. Am J Physiol Endocrinol Metab. 2013;304(11):E1227–36.

Achten J, Gleeson M, Jeukendrup AE. Determination of the exercise intensity that elicits maximal fat oxidation. Med Sci Sports Exerc. 2002;34(1):92–7.

Bailey SP, Zacher CM, Mittleman KD. Effect of menstrual cycle phase on carbohydrate supplementation during prolonged exercise to fatigue. J Appl Physiol. 2000;88(2):690–7.

Beckett T, Tchernof A, Toth MJ. Effect of ovariectomy and estradiol replacement on skeletal muscle enzyme activity in female rats. Metabolism. 2002;51(11):1397–401.

Belo NO, Sairam MR, Dos Reis AM. Impairment of the natriuretic peptide system in follitropin receptor knockout mice and reversal by estradiol: implications for obesity-associated hypertension in menopause. Endocrinology. 2008;149(3):1399–406.

Bemben DA, Boileau RA, Bahr JM, Nelson RA, Misner JE. Effects of oral contraceptives on hormonal and metabolic responses during exercise. Med Sci Sports Exerc. 1992;24(4):434–41.

Benagiano G, Bastianelli C, Farris M. Hormonal contraception: present and future. Drugs Today (Barc). 2008;44(12):905–23.

Bennell K, White S, Crossley K. The oral contraceptive pill: a revolution for sportswomen? Br J Sports Med. 1999;33(4):231–8.

Benoit V, Valette A, Mercier L, Meignen JM, Boyer J. Potentiation of epinephrine-induced lipolysis in fat cells from estrogen-treated rats. Biochem Biophys Res Commun. 1982;109(4):1186–91.

Bernardes RP, Radomski MW. Growth hormone responses to continuous and intermittent exercise in females under oral contraceptive therapy. Eur J Appl Physiol Occup Physiol. 1998;79(1):24–9.

Berthon PM, Howlett RA, Heigenhauser GJ, Spriet LL. Human skeletal muscle carnitine palmitoyltransferase I activity determined in isolated intact mitochondria. J Appl Physiol (1985). 1998;85(1):148–53.

Bjorntorp P. The regulation of adipose tissue distribution in humans. Int J Obes Relat Metab Disord. 1996;20(4):291–302.

Blatchford FK, Knowlton RG, Schneider DA. Plasma FFA responses to prolonged walking in untrained men and women. Eur J Appl Physiol Occup Physiol. 1985;53(4):343–7.

Boardman HM, Hartley L, Eisinga A, Main C, Roque i Figuls M, Bonfill Cosp X, et al. Hormone therapy for preventing cardiovascular disease in post-menopausal women. Cochrane Database Syst Rev. 2015;3, CD002229.

Boisseau N, Rannou F, Delamarche P, Bentue-Ferrer D, Gratas-Delamarche A. Glucose tolerance during moderate prolonged exercise in women with oral contraceptives as compared to non-users. J Sports Med Phys Fitness. 2001;41(2):203–9.

Bonen A, Haynes FW, Graham TE. Substrate and hormonal responses to exercise in women using oral contraceptives. J Appl Physiol. 1991;70(5):1917–27.

Bordenave S, Metz L, Flavier S, Lambert K, Ghanassia E, Dupuy AM, et al. Training-induced improvement in lipid oxidation in type 2 diabetes mellitus is related to alterations in muscle mitochondrial activity. Effect of endurance training in type 2 diabetes. Diabetes Metab. 2008;34(2):162–8.

Brooks GA, Mercier J. Balance of carbohydrate and lipid utilization during exercise: the "crossover" concept. J Appl Physiol. 1994;76(6):2253–61.

Bunt JC. Metabolic actions of estradiol: significance for acute and chronic exercise responses. Med Sci Sports Exerc. 1990;22(3):286–90.

Burguera B, Proctor D, Dietz N, Guo Z, Joyner M, Jensen MD. Leg free fatty acid kinetics during exercise in men and women. Am J Physiol Endocrinol Metab. 2000;278(1):E113–7.

Burrows M, Peters CE. The influence of oral contraceptives on athletic performance in female athletes. Sports Med. 2007;37(7):557–74.

Campbell SE, Febbraio MA. Effect of ovarian hormones on mitochondrial enzyme activity in the fat oxidation pathway of skeletal muscle. Am J Physiol Endocrinol Metab. 2001;281(4):E803–8.

Campbell SE, Febbraio MA. Effect of the ovarian hormones on GLUT4 expression and contraction-stimulated glucose uptake. Am J Physiol Endocrinol Metab. 2002;282(5):E1139–46.

Campbell SE, Angus DJ, Febbraio MA. Glucose kinetics and exercise performance during phases of the menstrual cycle: effect of glucose ingestion. Am J Physiol Endocrinol Metab. 2001;281(4):E817–25.

Carter S, McKenzie S, Mourtzakis M, Mahoney DJ, Tarnopolsky MA. Short-term 17beta-estradiol decreases glucose R(a) but not whole body metabolism during endurance exercise. J Appl Physiol (1985). 2001a;90(1):139–46.

Carter SL, Rennie C, Tarnopolsky MA. Substrate utilization during endurance exercise in men and women after endurance training. Am J Physiol Endocrinol Metab. 2001b;280(6):E898–907.

Casazza GA, Jacobs KA, Suh SH, Miller BF, Horning MA, Brooks GA. Menstrual cycle phase and oral contraceptive effects on triglyceride mobilization during exercise. J Appl Physiol. 2004;97(1):302–9.

Clark BA, Elahi D, Epstein FH. The influence of gender, age, and the menstrual cycle on plasma atrial natriuretic peptide. J Clin Endocrinol Metab. 1990;70(2):349–52.

Constantini NW, Dubnov G, Lebrun CM. The menstrual cycle and sport performance. Clin Sports Med. 2005;24(2):e51–82. xiii–xiv.

Costill DL, Daniels J, Evans W, Fink W, Krahenbuhl G, Saltin B. Skeletal muscle enzymes and fiber composition in male and female track athletes. J Appl Physiol. 1976;40(2):149–54.

Davidson BJ, Rea CD, Valenzuela GJ. Atrial natriuretic peptide, plasma renin activity, and aldosterone in women on estrogen therapy and with premenstrual syndrome. Fertil Steril. 1988;50(5):743–6.

de Melo NR, Aldrighi JM, Faggion Jr D, Reyes VR, Souza JB, Fernandes CE, et al. A prospective open-label study to evaluate the effects of the oral contraceptive Harmonet (gestodene75/EE20) on body fat. Contraception. 2004;70(1):65–71.

De Souza MJ, Maguire MS, Rubin KR, Maresh CM. Effects of menstrual phase and amenorrhea on exercise performance in runners. Med Sci Sports Exerc. 1990;22(5):575–80.

D'Eon TM, Sharoff C, Chipkin SR, Grow D, Ruby BC, Braun B. Regulation of exercise carbohydrate metabolism by estrogen and progesterone in women. Am J Physiol Endocrinol Metab. 2002;283(5):E1046–55.

D'Eon TM, Souza SC, Aronovitz M, Obin MS, Fried SK, Greenberg AS. Estrogen regulation of adiposity and fuel partitioning. Evidence of genomic and non-genomic regulation of lipogenic and oxidative pathways. J Biol Chem. 2005;280(43):35983–91.

D'Eon TM, Rogers NH, Stancheva ZS, Greenberg AS. Estradiol and the estradiol metabolite, 2-hydroxyestradiol, activate AMP-activated protein kinase in C2C12 myotubes. Obesity (Silver Spring). 2008;16(6):1284–8.

Devries MC, Hamadeh MJ, Graham TE, Tarnopolsky MA. 17beta-estradiol supplementation decreases glucose rate of appearance and disappearance with no effect on glycogen utilization during moderate intensity exercise in men. J Clin Endocrinol Metab. 2005;90(11):6218–25.

Devries MC, Hamadeh MJ, Phillips SM, Tarnopolsky MA. Menstrual cycle phase and sex influence muscle glycogen utilization and glucose turnover during moderate-intensity endurance exercise. Am J Physiol Regul Integr Comp Physiol. 2006;291(4):R1120–8.

Devries MC, Lowther SA, Glover AW, Hamadeh MJ, Tarnopolsky MA. IMCL area density, but not IMCL utilization, is higher in women during moderate-intensity endurance exercise, compared with men. Am J Physiol Regul Integr Comp Physiol. 2007;293(6):R2336–42.

Dombovy ML, Bonekat HW, Williams TJ, Staats BA. Exercise performance and ventilatory response in the menstrual cycle. Med Sci Sports Exerc. 1987;19(2):111–7.

dos Reis CM, de Melo NR, Meirelles ES, Vezozzo DP, Halpern A. Body composition, visceral fat distribution and fat oxidation in postmenopausal women using oral or transdermal oestrogen. Maturitas. 2003;46(1):59–68.

Ellis GS, Lanza-Jacoby S, Gow A, Kendrick ZV. Effects of estradiol on lipoprotein lipase activity and lipid availability in exercised male rats. J Appl Physiol. 1994;77(1):209–15.

Esbjornsson-Liljedahl M, Sundberg CJ, Norman B, Jansson E. Metabolic response in type I and type II muscle fibers during a 30-s cycle sprint in men and women. J Appl Physiol (1985). 1999;87(4):1326–32.

Escalante Pulido JM, Alpizar Salazar M. Changes in insulin sensitivity, secretion and glucose effectiveness during menstrual cycle. Arch Med Res. 1999;30(1):19–22.

Froberg K, Pedersen PK. Sex differences in endurance capacity and metabolic response to prolonged, heavy exercise. Eur J Appl Physiol Occup Physiol. 1984;52(4):446–50.

Genazzani AR, Lemarchand-Beraud T, Aubert ML, Felber JP. Pattern of plasma ACTH, hGH, and cortisol during menstrual cycle. J Clin Endocrinol Metab. 1975;41(3):431–7.

Gower BA, Nagy TR, Blaylock ML, Wang C, Nyman L. Estradiol may limit lipid oxidation via Cpt 1 expression and hormonal mechanisms. Obes Res. 2002;10(3):167–72.

Hackney AC. Effects of the menstrual cycle on resting muscle glycogen content. Horm Metab Res. 1990;22(12):647.

Hackney AC. Influence of oestrogen on muscle glycogen utilization during exercise. Acta Physiol Scand. 1999;167(3):273–4.

Hackney AC, McCracken-Compton MA, Ainsworth B. Substrate responses to submaximal exercise in the midfollicular and midluteal phases of the menstrual cycle. Int J Sport Nutr. 1994;4(3):299–308.

Hackney AC, Muoio D, Meyer WR. The Effect of sex steroid hormones on substrate oxidation during prolonged submaximal exercise in women. Jpn J Physiol. 2000;50(5):489–94.

Hamadeh MJ, Devries MC, Tarnopolsky MA. Estrogen supplementation reduces whole body leucine and carbohydrate oxidation and increases lipid oxidation in men during endurance exercise. J Clin Endocrinol Metab. 2005;90(6):3592–9.

Hatta H, Atomi Y, Shinohara S, Yamamoto Y, Yamada S. The effects of ovarian hormones on glucose and fatty acid oxidation during exercise in female ovariectomized rats. Horm Metab Res. 1988;20(10):609–11.

Heiling VJ, Jensen MD. Free fatty acid metabolism in the follicular and luteal phases of the menstrual cycle. J Clin Endocrinol Metab. 1992;74(4):806–10.

Hoffman DM, O'Sullivan AJ, Freund J, Ho KK. Adults with growth hormone deficiency have abnormal body composition but normal energy metabolism. J Clin Endocrinol Metab. 1995;80(1):72–7.

Hong M, Yan Q, Tao B, Boersma A, Han KK, Vantyghem MC, et al. Estradiol, progesterone and testosterone exposures affect the atrial natriuretic peptide gene expression in vivo in rats. Biol Chem Hoppe Seyler. 1992;373(4):213–8.

Horton TJ, Pagliassotti MJ, Hobbs K, Hill JO. Fuel metabolism in men and women during and after long-duration exercise. J Appl Physiol. 1998;85(5):1823–32.

Horton TJ, Miller EK, Glueck D, Tench K. No effect of menstrual cycle phase on glucose kinetics and fuel oxidation during moderate-intensity exercise. Am J Physiol Endocrinol Metab. 2002;282(4):E752–62.

Horton TJ, Miller EK, Bourret K. No effect of menstrual cycle phase on glycerol or palmitate kinetics during 90 min of moderate exercise. J Appl Physiol (1985). 2006;100(3):917–25.

Isacco L, Duche P, Boisseau N. Influence of hormonal status on substrate utilization at rest and during exercise in the female population. Sports Med. 2012a;42(4):327–42.

Isacco L, Thivel D, Pelle AM, Zouhal H, Duclos M, Duche P, et al. Oral contraception and energy intake in women: impact on substrate oxidation during exercise. Appl Physiol Nutr Metab. 2012b;37(4):646–56.

Isacco L, Thivel D, Meddahi-Pelle A, Lemoine-Morel S, Duclos M, Boisseau N. Exercise per se masks oral contraceptive-induced postprandial lipid mobilization. Appl Physiol Nutr Metab. 2014;1–8.

Isacco L, Thivel D, Pereira B, Duclos M, Boisseau N. Maximal fat oxidation, but not aerobic capacity, is affected by oral contraceptive use in young healthy women. Eur J Appl Physiol. 2015;115(5):937–45.

Jacobs KA, Casazza GA, Suh SH, Horning MA, Brooks GA. Fatty acid reesterification but not oxidation is increased by oral contraceptive use in women. J Appl Physiol. 2005;98(5):1720–31.

Jensen MD, Levine J. Effects of oral contraceptives on free fatty acid metabolism in women. Metabolism. 1998;47(3):280–4.

Jensen MD, Martin ML, Cryer PE, Roust LR. Effects of estrogen on free fatty acid metabolism in humans. Am J Physiol. 1994;266(6 Pt 1):E914–20.

Jeukendrup AE. Modulation of carbohydrate and fat utilization by diet, exercise and environment. Biochem Soc Trans. 2003;31(Pt 6):1270–3.

Jeukendrup AE, Wallis GA. Measurement of substrate oxidation during exercise by means of gas exchange measurements. Int J Sports Med. 2005;26 Suppl 1:S28–37.

Johnson LG, Kraemer RR, Haltom R, Kraemer GR, Gaines HE, Castracane VD. Effects of estrogen replacement therapy on dehydroepiandrosterone, dehydroepiandrosterone sulfate, and cortisol responses to exercise in postmenopausal women. Fertil Steril. 1997;68(5):836–43.

Johnson LG, Kraemer RR, Kraemer GR, Haltom RW, Cordill AE, Welsch MA, et al. Substrate utilization during exercise in postmenopausal women on hormone replacement therapy. Eur J Appl Physiol. 2002;88(3):282–7.

Kanaley JA, Boileau RA, Bahr JA, Misner JE, Nelson RA. Substrate oxidation and GH responses to exercise are independent of menstrual phase and status. Med Sci Sports Exerc. 1992;24(8):873–80.

Kelley DE. Skeletal muscle fat oxidation: timing and flexibility are everything. J Clin Invest. 2005;115(7):1699–702.

Kendrick ZV, Steffen CA, Rumsey WL, Goldberg DI. Effect of estradiol on tissue glycogen metabolism in exercised oophorectomized rats. J Appl Physiol. 1987;63(2):492–6.

Kiens B, Roepstorff C, Glatz JF, Bonen A, Schjerling P, Knudsen J, et al. Lipid-binding proteins and lipoprotein lipase activity in human skeletal muscle: influence of physical activity and gender. J Appl Physiol (1985). 2004;97(4):1209–18.

Klein S, Coyle EF, Wolfe RR. Fat metabolism during low-intensity exercise in endurance-trained and untrained men. Am J Physiol. 1994;267(6 Pt 1):E934–40.

Kocjan T, Prelevic GM. Hormone replacement therapy update: who should we be prescribing this to now? Curr Opin Obstet Gynecol. 2003;15(6):459–64.

Kohrt WM, Ehsani AA, Birge Jr SJ. HRT preserves increases in bone mineral density and reductions in body fat after a supervised exercise program. J Appl Physiol. 1998;84(5):1506–12.

Konarzewski M, Diamond JM. Evolution of basal metabolic rate and organ masses in laboratory mice. Evolution. 1995;49:1239–48.

Koppo K, Larrouy D, Marques MA, Berlan M, Bajzova M, Polak J, et al. Lipid mobilization in subcutaneous adipose tissue during exercise in lean and obese humans. Roles of insulin and natriuretic peptides. Am J Physiol Endocrinol Metab. 2010;299(2):E258–65.

Kraemer RR, Johnson LG, Haltom R, Kraemer GR, Gaines H, Drapcho M, et al. Effects of hormone replacement on growth hormone and prolactin exercise responses in postmenopausal women. J Appl Physiol. 1998;84(2):703–8.

Lafontan M, Moro C, Sengenes C, Galitzky J, Crampes F, Berlan M. An unsuspected metabolic role for atrial natriuretic peptides: the control of lipolysis, lipid mobilization, and systemic nonesterified fatty acids levels in humans. Arterioscler Thromb Vasc Biol. 2005;25(10):2032–42.

Lambert EV, Hawley JA, Goedecke J, Noakes TD, Dennis SC. Nutritional strategies for promoting fat utilization and delaying the onset of fatigue during prolonged exercise. J Sports Sci. 1997;15(3):315–24.

Lavoie JM, Dionne N, Helie R, Brisson GR. Menstrual cycle phase dissociation of blood glucose homeostasis during exercise. J Appl Physiol (1985). 1987;62(3):1084–9.

Lebrun CM. The effect of the phase of the menstrual cycle and the birth control pill on athletic performance. Clin Sports Med. 1994;13(2):419–41.

Lovejoy JC, Champagne CM, de Jonge L, Xie H, Smith SR. Increased visceral fat and decreased energy expenditure during the menopausal transition. Int J Obes (Lond). 2008;32(6):949–58.

Lupo M, Dains JE, Madsen LT. Hormone replacement therapy: an increased risk of recurrence and mortality for breast cancer patients? J Adv Pract Oncol. 2015;6(4):322–30.

Lwin R, Darnell B, Oster R, Lawrence J, Foster J, Azziz R, et al. Effect of oral estrogen on substrate utilization in postmenopausal women. Fertil Steril. 2008;90(4):1275–8.

Maffei S, Del Ry S, Prontera C, Clerico A. Increase in circulating levels of cardiac natriuretic peptides after hormone replacement therapy in postmenopausal women. Clin Sci (Lond). 2001;101(5):447–53.

Magkos F, Patterson BW, Mittendorfer B. No effect of menstrual cycle phase on basal very-low-density lipoprotein triglyceride and apolipoprotein B-100 kinetics. Am J Physiol Endocrinol Metab. 2006;291(6):E1243–9.

Maher AC, Akhtar M, Vockley J, Tarnopolsky MA. Women have higher protein content of beta-oxidation enzymes in skeletal muscle than men. PLoS One. 2010;5(8), e12025.

Mandour T, Kissebah AH, Wynn V. Mechanism of oestrogen and progesterone effects on lipid and carbohydrate metabolism: alteration in the insulin: glucagon molar ratio and hepatic enzyme activity. Eur J Clin Invest. 1977;7(3):181–7.

Matute ML, Kalkhoff RK. Sex steroid influence on hepatic gluconeogenesis and glucogen formation. Endocrinology. 1973;92(3):762–8.

Mc KK, Coulomb B, Kaleita E, De Renzo EC. Some effects of in vivo administered estrogens on glucose metabolism and adrenal cortical secretion in vitro. Endocrinology. 1958;63(6):709–22.

McKenzie S, Phillips SM, Carter SL, Lowther S, Gibala MJ, Tarnopolsky MA. Endurance exercise training attenuates leucine oxidation and BCOAD activation during exercise in humans. Am J Physiol Endocrinol Metab. 2000;278(4):E580–7.

McLay RT, Thomson CD, Williams SM, Rehrer NJ. Carbohydrate loading and female endurance athletes: effect of menstrual-cycle phase. Int J Sport Nutr Exerc Metab. 2007;17(2):189–205.

Minson CT, Halliwill JR, Young TM, Joyner MJ. Sympathetic activity and baroreflex sensitivity in young women taking oral contraceptives. Circulation. 2000;102(13):1473–6.

Moro C, Crampes F, Sengenes C. Atrial natriuretic peptide contributes to the physiological control of lipid mobilization in humans. FASEB J. 2004;18:908–10.

Nicklas BJ, Hackney AC, Sharp RL. The menstrual cycle and exercise: performance, muscle glycogen, and substrate responses. Int J Sports Med. 1989;10(4):264–9.

Norrelund H. Consequences of growth hormone deficiency for intermediary metabolism and effects of replacement. Front Horm Res. 2005;33:103–20.

Numao S, Hayashi Y, Katayama Y, Matsuo T, Tanaka K. Sex differences in substrate oxidation during aerobic exercise in obese men and postmenopausal obese women. Metabolism. 2009;58(9):1312–9.

Oosthuyse T, Bosch AN. The effect of the menstrual cycle on exercise metabolism: implications for exercise performance in eumenorrhoeic women. Sports Med. 2010;40(3):207–27.

Oosthuyse T, Bosch AN. Oestrogen's regulation of fat metabolism during exercise and gender specific effects. Curr Opin Pharmacol. 2012;12(3):363–71.

O'Sullivan AJ, Ho KK. A comparison of the effects of oral and transdermal estrogen replacement on insulin sensitivity in postmenopausal women. J Clin Endocrinol Metab. 1995;80(6):1783–8.

O'Sullivan AJ, Crampton LJ, Freund J, Ho KK. The route of estrogen replacement therapy confers divergent effects on substrate oxidation and body composition in postmenopausal women. J Clin Invest. 1998;102(5):1035–40.

Perez-Martin A, Dumortier M, Raynaud E, Brun JF, Fedou C, Bringer J, et al. Balance of substrate oxidation during submaximal exercise in lean and obese people. Diabetes Metab. 2001;27(4 Pt 1):466–74.

Picard F, Wanatabe M, Schoonjans K, Lydon J, O'Malley BW, Auwerx J. Progesterone receptor knockout mice have an improved glucose homeostasis secondary to beta -cell proliferation. Proc Natl Acad Sci U S A. 2002;99(24):15644–8.

Piers LS, Diggavi SN, Rijskamp J, van Raaij JM, Shetty PS, Hautvast JG. Resting metabolic rate and thermic effect of a meal in the follicular and luteal phases of the menstrual cycle in well-nourished Indian women. Am J Clin Nutr. 1995;61(2):296–302.

Redman LM, Scroop GC, Westlander G, Norman RJ. Effect of a synthetic progestin on the exercise status of sedentary young women. J Clin Endocrinol Metab. 2005;90(7):3830–7.

Reilly T. The menstrual cycle and human performance: an overview. Biol Rhythm Res. 2000;31(1):29–40.

Reinke U, Ansah B, Voigt KD. Effect of the menstrual cycle on carbohydrate and lipid metabolism in normal females. Acta Endocrinol (Copenh). 1972;69(4):762–8.

Roepstorff C, Steffensen CH, Madsen M, Stallknecht B, Kanstrup IL, Richter EA, et al. Gender differences in substrate utilization during submaximal exercise in endurance-trained subjects. Am J Physiol Endocrinol Metab. 2002;282(2):E435–47.

Roepstorff C, Donsmark M, Thiele M, Vistisen B, Stewart G, Vissing K, et al. Sex differences in hormone-sensitive lipase expression, activity, and phosphorylation in skeletal muscle at rest and during exercise. Am J Physiol Endocrinol Metab. 2006;291(5):E1106–14.

Romijn JA, Coyle EF, Sidossis LS, Gastaldelli A, Horowitz JF, Endert E, et al. Regulation of endogenous fat and carbohydrate metabolism in relation to exercise intensity and duration. Am J Physiol. 1993;265(3 Pt 1):E380–91.

Romijn JA, Coyle EF, Sidossis LS, Rosenblatt J, Wolfe RR. Substrate metabolism during different exercise intensities in endurance-trained women. J Appl Physiol. 2000;88(5):1707–14.

Ruby BC, Robergs RA, Waters DL, Burge M, Mermier C, Stolarczyk L. Effects of estradiol on substrate turnover during exercise in amenorrheic females. Med Sci Sports Exerc. 1997;29(9):1160–9.

Sengenes C, Bouloumie A, Hauner H, Berlan M, Busse R, Lafontan M, et al. Involvement of a cGMP-dependent pathway in the natriuretic peptide-mediated hormone-sensitive lipase phosphorylation in human adipocytes. J Biol Chem. 2003;278(49):48617–26.

Sengenes C, Moro C, Galitzky J, Berlan M, Lafontan M. Natriuretic peptides: a new lipolytic pathway in human fat cells. Med Sci (Paris). 2005;21 Spec No:29–33.

Shufelt CL, Bairey Merz CN. Contraceptive hormone use and cardiovascular disease. J Am Coll Cardiol. 2009;53(3):221–31.

Simpson ER, Clyne C, Rubin G, Boon WC, Robertson K, Britt K, et al. Aromatase--a brief overview. Annu Rev Physiol. 2002;64:93–127.

Sitruk-Ware R, Nath A. Metabolic effects of contraceptive steroids. Rev Endocr Metab Disord. 2011;12(2):63–75.

Sladek CD. Gluconeogenesis and hepatic glycogen formation in relation to the rat estrous cycle. Horm Metab Res. 1974;6(3):217–21.

Snow-Harter CM. Bone health and prevention of osteoporosis in active and athletic women. Clin Sports Med. 1994;13(2):389–404.

Sowers M, Zheng H, Tomey K, Karvonen-Gutierrez C, Jannausch M, Li X, et al. Changes in body composition in women over six years at midlife: ovarian and chronological aging. J Clin Endocrinol Metab. 2007;92(3):895–901.

Steffensen CH, Roepstorff C, Madsen M, Kiens B. Myocellular triacylglycerol breakdown in females but not in males during exercise. Am J Physiol Endocrinol Metab. 2002;282(3):E634–42.

Suh SH, Casazza GA, Horning MA, Miller BF, Brooks GA. Luteal and follicular glucose fluxes during rest and exercise in 3-h postabsorptive women. J Appl Physiol. 2002;93(1):42–50.

Suh SH, Casazza GA, Horning MA, Miller BF, Brooks GA. Effects of oral contraceptives on glucose flux and substrate oxidation rates during rest and exercise. J Appl Physiol. 2003;94(1):285–94.

Sutter-Dub MT, Vergnaud MT. Progesterone and glucose metabolism in the female rat adipocyte: effect on hexokinase activity. J Endocrinol. 1982;95(3):369–75.

Tarnopolsky MA. Sex differences in exercise metabolism and the role of 17-beta estradiol. Med Sci Sports Exerc. 2008;40(4):648–54.

Tarnopolsky LJ, MacDougall JD, Atkinson SA, Tarnopolsky MA, Sutton JR. Gender differences in substrate for endurance exercise. J Appl Physiol. 1990;68(1):302–8.

Tarnopolsky MA, Atkinson SA, Phillips SM, MacDougall JD. Carbohydrate loading and metabolism during exercise in men and women. J Appl Physiol (1985). 1995;78(4):1360–8.

Tarnopolsky MA, Zawada C, Richmond LB, Carter S, Shearer J, Graham T, et al. Gender differences in carbohydrate loading are related to energy intake. J Appl Physiol (1985). 2001;91(1):225–30.

Tarnopolsky MA, Rennie CD, Robertshaw HA, Fedak-Tarnopolsky SN, Devries MC, Hamadeh MJ. Influence of endurance exercise training and sex on intramyocellular lipid and mitochondrial ultrastructure, substrate use, and mitochondrial enzyme activity. Am J Physiol Regul Integr Comp Physiol. 2007;292(3):R1271–8.

Toth MJ, Gardner AW, Arciero PJ, Calles-Escandon J, Poehlman ET. Gender differences in fat oxidation and sympathetic nervous system activity at rest and during submaximal exercise in older individuals. Clin Sci (Lond). 1998;95(1):59–66.

Tremblay J, Peronnet F, Massicotte D, Lavoie C. Carbohydrate supplementation and sex differences in fuel selection during exercise. Med Sci Sports Exerc. 2010;42(7):1314–23.

Tremollieres F. Oral combined contraception: is there any difference between ethinyl-estradiol and estradiol? Gynecol Obstet Fertil. 2012;40(2):109–15.

Uranga AP, Levine J, Jensen M. Isotope tracer measures of meal fatty acid metabolism: reproducibility and effects of the menstrual cycle. Am J Physiol Endocrinol Metab. 2005;288(3):E547–55.

Vieira-Potter VJ, Zidon TM, Padilla J. Exercise and estrogen make fat cells "Fit". Exerc Sport Sci Rev. 2015;43(3):172–8.

Weinstein I, Cook GA, Heimberg M. Regulation by oestrogen of carnitine palmitoyltransferase in hepatic mitochondria. Biochem J. 1986;237(2):593–6.

Wenz M, Berend JZ, Lynch NA, Chappell S, Hackney AC. Substrate oxidation at rest and during exercise: effects of menstrual cycle phase and diet composition. J Physiol Pharmacol. 1997;48(4):851–60.

White LJ, Ferguson MA, McCoy SC, Kim H. Intramyocellular lipid changes in men and women during aerobic exercise: a (1)H-magnetic resonance spectroscopy study. J Clin Endocrinol Metab. 2003;88(12):5638–43.

Wolfe RR, Peters EJ, Klein S, Holland OB, Rosenblatt J, Gary Jr H. Effect of short-term fasting on lipolytic responsiveness in normal and obese human subjects. Am J Physiol. 1987;252(2 Pt 1):E189–96.

Yasui T, Uemura H, Takikawa M, Irahara M. Hormone replacement therapy in postmenopausal women. J Med Invest. 2003;50(3-4):136–45.

Zderic TW, Coggan AR, Ruby BC. Glucose kinetics and substrate oxidation during exercise in the follicular and luteal phases. J Appl Physiol. 2001;90(2):447–53.

Zehnder M, Ith M, Kreis R, Saris W, Boutellier U, Boesch C. Gender-specific usage of intramyocellular lipids and glycogen during exercise. Med Sci Sports Exerc. 2005;37(9):1517–24.

Chapter 4
Sex Hormone Effects on the Nervous System and their Impact on Muscle Strength and Motor Performance in Women

Matthew S. Tenan

Introduction

Understanding the integration of the nervous system and the endocrine system can be daunting. Both systems, by definition, have the ability to enact effects in the local tissues as well as have far-reaching effects across the human body. Furthermore, both systems are largely governed by homeostatic mechanisms which are consistently dynamic, moving either towards or away from the given homeostatic setpoint. This chapter attempts to tackle the complex interactions of these two systems. First, the neurological effects of sex hormones and their metabolites are examined at a basic level to determine if it is reasonable to expect that they change human behavior on a larger scale. Since sex hormones do not change in isolation (e.g., the menstrual cycle results in predictable changes in multiple hormones), I explore how the menstrual cycle modifies the motor nervous system in vivo. Next, the effect of the menstrual cycle on human motor behavior is considered. Finally, a number of caveats relating to the interpretation of present scientific knowledge in the area are addressed. By the end of this chapter, the reader should firmly grasp the nonreproductive effects of sex hormones on the nervous system at a mechanistic level; however, they will also be acutely aware that translating and/or leveraging the effects of sex hormones to alter motor behavior remains an extremely challenging task.

M.S. Tenan, Ph.D. (✉)
United States Army Research Laboratory, 459 Mulberry Poinot Road,
Aberdeen Proving Ground, Adelphi, MD 21005, USA
e-mail: matthew.s.tenan.civ@mail.mil

Sex Hormones, Their Metabolites, and a Dynamic Ecosystem

While "female sex hormones" are classically conceived as two classes of hormones, estrogens and progesterones, this may not fully reflect the dynamic biochemical metabolism of sex hormones as a whole. A more complex view, where primary sex hormones (testosterone, estradiol, and progesterone) are considered to simply be metabolic derivatives of cholesterol with numerous intermediaries is a more encompassing, but still insufficient perspective (see Fig. 4.1).

It is not enough to acknowledge that sex hormones are chemically related, the metabolic intermediaries between the primary sex hormones need to be recognized as hormones which may actively alter muscular strength or function. In both human and animal models, the production and clearance rates of these hormones are poorly understood and appear to be different between biologic compartments (e.g., brain areas, plasma, fat, peripheral nerve, and tendon) (Wang et al., 1997; Bixo et al., 1997; Morfin et al., 1992) and change across the lifespan (Payne and Jaffe, 1975). The intermingled web of transitory sex hormones is difficult to untangle and isolate, but it is further complicated when one recognizes that the precursor cholesterol molecule exists in both a sulfonated and unsulfonated form, creating a parallel web of sex hormones and intermediaries that have distinctly different biologic properties. Indeed, the metabolism between sulfonated sex hormone intermediaries may be slowed by as much as 40% compared to their non-sulfonated counterparts in humans (Neunzig et al., 2014). A slower conversion rate may create a longer time period in

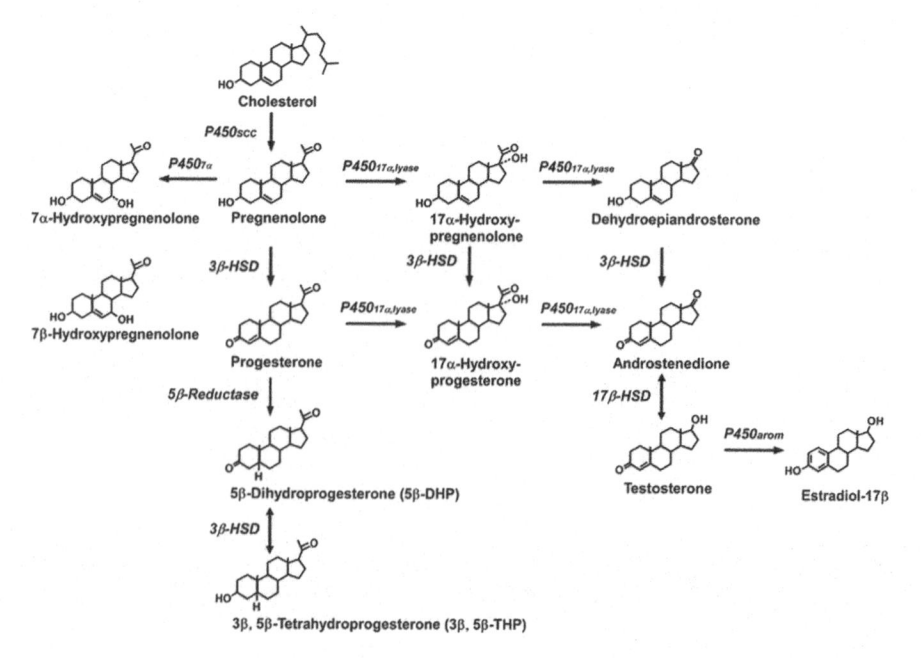

Fig. 4.1 The general metabolic pathway for sex hormones in the brain (Tsutsui, 2011). Image reproduced with the author's permission

which sex hormones and their intermediaries can enact changes on the muscle tissue or nervous system. It should not be assumed that sulfonated and unsulfonated hormones exist in equal quantities, and it has been shown that their appearance is highly tissue dependent in humans (Morfin et al., 1992; Bixo et al., 1997) and life-cycle dependent (Leowattana, 2004). While there is no direct correlation between serum and brain levels of sex hormones in women, there is a general trend towards higher brain estradiol levels in the preoptic area, hypothalamus and substantia nigra of women with high serum estradiol. There does not appear to be a similar trend for testosterone and there is substantial variation across brain areas for both testosterone and estradiol (Bixo et al., 1997). The quantity of sulfonated and unsulfonated DHEA and pregnenolone in tendons and peripheral nerves also have substantial variance across the population; however, limited data suggest that unsulfonated pregnenolone and sulfonated DHEA predominate in peripheral nerves of women while muscle and tendon contain both sulfonated and unsulfonated types of pregnenolone and DHEA without any variant being dominant (Morfin et al., 1992). Finally, serum and cerebral spinal fluid levels of both sulfonated and unsulfonated forms of DHEA decrease after 18–25 years of age (Leowattana, 2004; Guazzo et al., 1996).

It is necessary to be mindful of this highly complex and dynamic ecosystem when addressing whether sex hormones, the menstrual cycle and hormonal contraceptives alter motor function in women. Our failure to fully comprehend the entire sex hormone ecosystem does not prohibit us from drawing conclusions on the effect of sex hormones on the nervous system, but it does urge a cautious interpretation of existing applied research.

Do Sex Hormones and/or the Menstrual Cycle Affect the Nervous System?

Sex hormones are among a larger class of hormones called neurosteroids, indicating that they exert their action at the level of the brain and are often times synthesized within the central nervous system itself (Stoffel-Wagner, 2001). Sex hormones in the plasma can also easily traverse the blood-brain barrier due to their high lipid solubility (Stoffel-Wagner, 2001) and other unknown mechanisms (Wang et al., 1997). Thus, there are at least two ways in which sex hormones and their metabolites may be introduced to the nervous system to enact effects on the motor system. This section explores the ways in which sex hormones and their metabolites exert inhibitory or excitatory effects on the nervous system and how they specifically alter the human motor nervous system.

General Effects on the Nervous System

Sex hormones and their intermediary metabolites have been shown to have profound effects on the nervous system at the cellular level. The general mechanisms of action for the most potent hormones will be discussed. To aid in the comprehension of the effects, their overall actions will be simplified as either net excitatory or inhibitory to the nervous system. For example, a molecule may be a gamma-Aminobutyric acid (GABA) receptor antagonist (blocker), but since GABA's effects are largely neural-inhibitory in nature, the net effect of a GABA antagonist is as an excitatory agent on the nervous system.

Pregnenolone is a first-order precursor to progesterone which has been shown to both enhance the action of GABA as well as directly activate the $GABA_A$ receptor in bovine preparations (Callachan et al., 1987). It is capable of both prolonging the temporal influx of chloride ions through the receptor's channel as well as directly opening the channel when pregnenolone levels are further elevated. Thus, unsulfonated pregnenolone has inhibitory effects on the nervous system. In contrast, pregnenolone-sulfate is a GABA receptor antagonist in rodent cell cultures (Mienville and Vicini, 1989). Pregnenolone-sulfate decreases the frequency which the chloride channels open on the GABA receptor, decreasing the ability to inhibit neuron discharge (Mienville and Vicini, 1989) and creating net excitatory effects on the nervous system. The effects of pregnenolone and pregnenolone-sulfate create an interesting dichotomy for two chemically similar hormones that have extremely potent, but opposing, effects on the GABA receptor. Both of these hormones oscillate across the menstrual cycle (Wang et al., 1996), but they also are synthesized locally and have differing levels based on the tissue and location (Takase et al., 1999; Morfin et al., 1992).

Progesterone is also a neurosteroid which can be synthesized within the nervous system as well as be introduced from plasma via the blood–brain barrier (Wang et al., 1997). Progesterone has a net inhibitory effect on the nervous system (Smith et al., 1987). While not as robust as pregnenolone, progesterone is able to increase the inhibitory response of the $GABA_A$ receptor up to 80% in the presence of GABA (Smith, 1989). This net inhibitory effect has been shown in the rodent model where progesterone decreases cerebellum neuron discharge during treadmill locomotion (Smith et al., 1989).

Estradiol appears to play a broad role in both the development and maintenance of the central nervous system (McEwen and Alves, 1999). This is evidenced by the wide array of brain structures which contain various densities of estrogen receptor isoforms (McEwen and Alves, 1999). The long-term and developmental effects of estradiol have largely overshadowed the short-term transitory effects of estradiol which are the focus of this chapter and book as a whole. Recent work in rodents has indicated that estrogen receptors on GABA releasing (GABAergic) neurons may be the primary way in which estradiol creates a net excitatory effect on the nervous system (Schultz et al., 2009). Activation of estrogen receptor α on GABAergic neurons attenuates the release of GABA. This mechanism explains how estradiol rapidly affects neurotransmitter pathways for both dopamine (Becker, 1990; Xiao et al., 2003) and glutamate (Smith et al., 1988) in rodent models. This excitatory effect has been shown in vivo whereby estradiol administration increases neuronal discharge of the rat cerebellum during treadmill walking (Smith et al., 1989).

DHEA and DHEA-sulfate [DHEA(S)] have been shown to target multiple neuronal receptors (Spivak, 1994; Monnet et al., 1995; Mellon and Griffin, 2002) and modulate a number of neurotransmitter systems (Rhodes et al., 1996; Wolf and Kirschbaum, 1999; Murray and Gillies, 1997; Meyer et al., 2002) in animal models.

Levels of DHEA(S) arising from the human adrenal cortex or adrenal gland (in fetal humans) fluctuate wildly across the human lifespan (Peretti and Forest, 1978); however, there is evidence that DHEA(S) produced in the nervous system are unrelated to their counterparts in the periphery of animal models (Baulieu, 1996; Baulieu and Robel, 1998). Therefore, differential levels of peripheral DHEA(S) or the use of nutritional supplements purporting to affect DHEA(S) should have little effect on the nervous system. DHEA(S) has been shown to produce a net excitatory effect on the rodent nervous system primarily through its action on GABA and glutamate releasing neurons (Wolf and Kirschbaum, 1999; Meyer et al., 2002; Dong et al., 2007), though also through actions on acetylcholine (Rhodes et al., 1996) and dopamine (Murray and Gillies, 1997).

Sex hormones and their metabolites have clear effects on nervous system function; however, the net result of these many neuro-excitatory and inhibitory hormones is less certain. That the levels of these hormones change dynamically throughout the day, across the menstrual cycle, and vary across different regions of the nervous system further complicates the process of determining their effect on human performance. At the clinical level, it is typically more feasible to track how performance is modified as a function of external biological processes. Therefore, the remainder of this chapter will consider the holistic effect of the menstrual cycle on parameters of neuromotor athletic performance.

Sex Hormone/Menstrual Cycle Effects on Motor Function in Humans

There are two primary ways to examine the excitation of the motor system across the menstrual cycle: (1) direct stimulation of nervous tissue or (2) recording of single motor unit activity during voluntary contractions. When the motor cortex is directly stimulated magnetically (transcranial magnetic stimulation or TMS), this stimulates the orderly recruitment of motor units by isolating the corticospinal tract (Bawa and Lemon, 1993), the primary tract involved with voluntary movement. TMS allows us to noninvasively examine the excitatory/inhibitory environment of the entire tract, from brain to muscle cell depolarization. Corticospinal tract excitability is highest and inhibition is lowest in the late follicular phase compared to early follicular and mid luteal menstrual phases (Smith et al., 2002). Stimulation of a peripheral nerve with electricity (H-reflex) activates a component of the stretch reflex and enables us to examine the changes at the level of the spine. Early research suggests that H-reflexes, and thus spinal excitability, do not change across the menstrual cycle (Hoffman et al., 2008). The summation of the stimulation research indicates that the corticospinal tract is altered at the level of the brain by the menstrual cycle and that movement generation may be facilitated in the late follicular phase of the menstrual cycle. Recording of single motor unit discharges during voluntary exercise allows us to understand how the nervous system as a whole is able to generate movement. Preliminary results examining motor unit activity during the menstrual cycle indicate

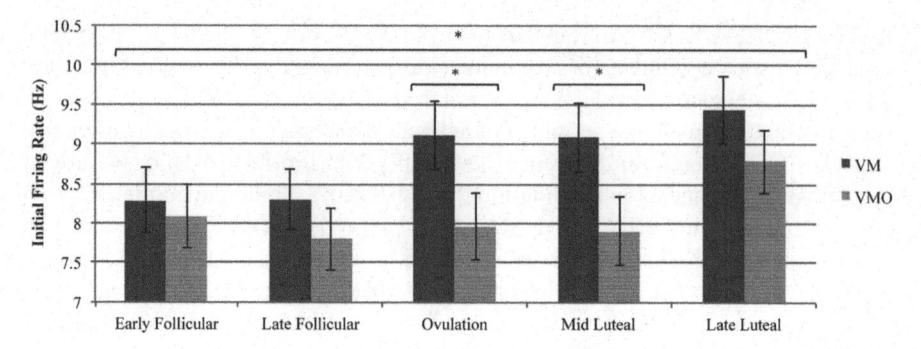

Fig. 4.2 Changes in motor unit discharge rate of the vastus medialis (VM) and vastus medialis oblique (VMO) across five phases of the menstrual cycle. While both muscles increase in discharge rate across the cycle, the timing of increases are different (Tenan et al., 2013)

that discharge rates increase for some muscles (see Fig. 4.2), but not others, after ovulation (Tenan et al., 2013). The menstrual cycle creates evident modulations in motor activity which are observable via both stimulation and direct evaluation of motor neuron (motor unit) discharge. The following sections will explore how these modulations in the nervous system appear to manifest themselves as behavioral changes in muscle strength, endurance, and movement quality.

Do Sex Hormones/Menstrual Cycle Affect Muscle Strength?

The potential effect of sex hormones and the menstrual cycle on muscular strength has been an area of high interest and controversy for many years; however, a clear pattern is starting to emerge. There is an apparent diurnal effect of menstrual phase on muscular strength (Birch and Reilly, 2002). During morning testing, maximal strength is lower in the luteal phase compared to the follicular phase, but testing in the afternoon suggests strength is augmented in the luteal phase. This diurnal effect may have confounded the numerous studies which did not control for time of day or simply kept time of day constant within participants. Research which focuses on the effect of whole menstrual phases has a tendency to show changes in maximal force (Phillips et al., 1996; Sarwar et al., 1996; Tenan et al., 2015; Birch and Reilly, 2002); whereas, studies focused on specific hormones seldom see a clear effect (Elliott et al., 2003; Greeves et al., 1997), though there are notable exceptions to this generalization (Janse de Jonge et al., 2001; Kubo et al., 2009). The reasons for this discrepancy may be due to participant intraindividual variability, the timing of testing (within-day variability as well as between consecutive days) as well as intraindividual differences in tissue-specific sex hormone levels.

Generally, maximal force generation increases throughout the follicular phase; after ovulation, the ability to generate force decreases between 8 and 23 % until returning to early follicular levels just prior to menses (Phillips et al., 1996; Sarwar et al., 1996; Tenan et al., 2015). The biphasic pattern of maximal force generation appears to be relatively uniform with research support for both the upper extremity (Phillips et al., 1996; Sarwar et al., 1996), lower extremity (Sarwar et al., 1996; Tenan et al., 2015) and whole body exercise (Birch and Reilly, 2002). The increase in force generating ability may be a result of increased corticospinal tract excitability (Smith et al., 2002). The decrease in maximal force after ovulation corresponds to the increase in motor unit discharge at lower force levels (Tenan et al., 2013); this suggests that maximal forces may be lower in the luteal phase because maximal motor unit discharge is insufficient to generate the same level of force obtained in the follicular phase. For power-oriented athletes, it may be reasonable to check ovulatory status via urinary excretion of luteinizing hormone or basal body temperature tracking to determine if their athletic performance appears to be affected post-ovulation. Simple counting of days from menses to determine ovulation does not appear to be effective to examine strength changes (Dibrezzo et al., 1988; Tourville et al., 2016). While athlete monitoring to determine performance variability is advised, the clinician/coach should approach this training tactic with caution since the evidence is conflicting and there may be substantial intraindividual variability.

Do Sex Hormones/Menstrual Cycle Affect Motor Performance?

The effect of sex hormones or the menstrual cycle on motor performance can be broadly classified into two categories: fine motor skill and gross motor skill. The neurologic pathways which characterize the two categories greatly overlap. Both incorporate levels of descending motor drive, integration of sensory information and the actual feedback from sensory nerve endings in the muscle and joints as well as visual and auditory inputs. The present context is primarily concerned with changes in the behavioral outcome (e.g., dexterity goes up or down) as opposed trying to determine precisely why the behavioral outcome changes (e.g., differences in descending motor drive from the cortex, differential activation from the cerebellum, and differential perceptual visual inputs).

Although the number of studies examining fine motor skill across the menstrual is small, they have generally all indicated that fine motor skill is increased in the mid luteal phase of the menstrual cycle compared to the follicular phases (Hampson and Kimura, 1988; Šimić et al., 2010; Zimmerman and Parlee, 1973; Zoghi et al., 2015). Moreover, functional asymmetries (e.g., fine motor skill differences between left and right hand) appear to be decreased during the mid luteal phase (Bayer and Hausmann, 2012). In contrast, the quality of a gross motor task in both a normal and fatigued state appears to be lower in the mid luteal phase (Tenan et al., 2015). The reason for this discrepancy is unclear. From a sporting perspective, the application of this work is also unclear since the majority of events incorporate both gross- and fine-motor control. Hormonal contraceptives may also exert effects on motor task performance. Limited cross sectional research has suggested that oral hormonal contraceptives may decrease variability across the menstrual cycle, but taking oral hormonal contraceptives also create systematic differences in vocal singing qualities and decreased steadiness in marksmanship (La et al., 2012; La et al., 2007; Hudgens et al., 1988) compared to women not on hormonal contraception. Before the "bench" science can be translated to the "real-world" more applied research is necessary. The translation of basic research into applied research is further complicated by menstrual cycle irregularities and hormonal manipulation via contraceptive methods.

Caveats: The "Normal Menstrual Cycle" and Hormonal Contraception

The occurrence of amenorrhea (absence of menses) and oligomenorrhea (light or infrequent menses) have clear and evident physical manifestations which suggest an underlying hormonal disturbance. Less well characterized are the subtle menstrual cycle disturbances such as luteal phase defects or anovulation which also profoundly affect the hormonal profile of women in childbearing years. More than 50% of regularly exercising women exhibit some form of menstrual disturbance and half of them display no clinical abnormalities (i.e., appearance of normal menses but actually anovulatory or luteal phase defect) (De Souza et al., 2010). How menstrual cycle disturbances alter the nervous system is largely unknown. There are two perspectives from which menstrual disturbances can be viewed: (1) a lack of hormonal variation results in decreased motor performance variance or (2) a lack of expected hormonal variation causes an increase in performance variation. Perspective #1 is relatively easy to understand; if hormones do not cycle normally, then the effects of these hormones are unlikely to be observed. Perspective #2 is more counterintuitive; the normally cycling sex hormones, and resulting metabolites, have far reaching effects and the time-synchronization and balance of hormones may be important to modulate motor performance. For instance, it is possible that the neuro-inhibitory effects of progesterone arising from ovulation are effected primarily at the peripheral level; this will not mitigate the neuro-inhibitory effects of progesterone in the central nervous system which is produced endogenously. It is also possible that the effects of sex hormones are tightly regulated and a decrease in circulating progesterone from ovulation simply results in an increase in progesterone produced by the nervous system locally. Both of these perspectives may be incorrect, but they relay the present lack of information regarding how disturbed menstrual patterns affect the nervous system. The sobering prevalence statistics about menstrual abnormalities suggest caution when assuming that an athlete, not on hormonal contraception, has a normal sex hormone profile.

Hormonal contraception can now be delivered systemically (oral contraceptive, injection, etc.) or locally (intrauterine device or ring). It is nearly completely unknown how these synthetic sex hormone analogues alter neurotransmitter function

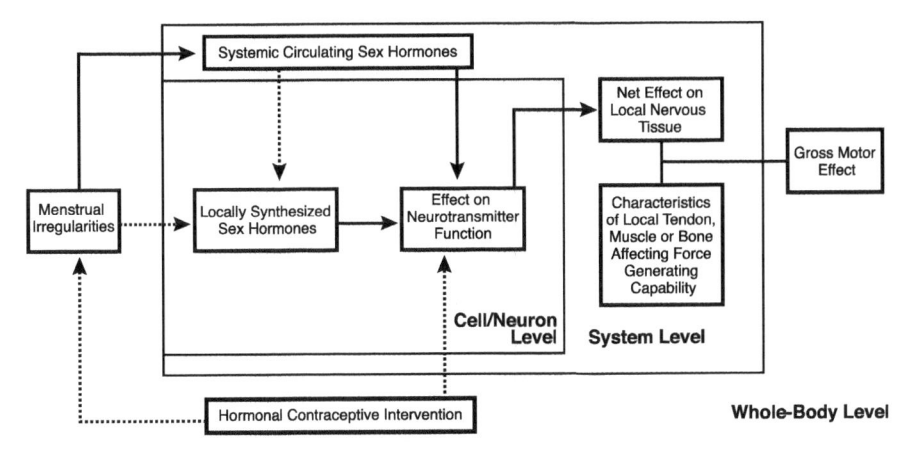

Fig. 4.3 General flow chart depicting how sex hormones modify motor behavior from the cellular to the whole-body level. *Solid lines* indicate known effects and *dashed lines* indicate possible or probable effects

(Pletzer and Kerschbaum, 2014). It is possible that they are neurologically inert and that their only neurologic effects are mediated by their effective decrease on endogenous production of bioactive sex hormones. However, it seems unlikely that the synthetic hormones, and their resulting metabolites, have no bioactive component on neurotransmitter systems when the endogenous analogues have profound effects. Devices delivering contraceptive hormones locally result in a decreased distribution of the synthetic hormones (van den Heuvel et al., 2005), which may minimize any possible effects of synthetic hormones traversing the blood-brain barrier. It is also unknown if the use of hormonal contraceptives affect the production of sex hormones in the nervous system the way they do in the reproductive system. There is presently a lack of both basic and applied research showing either neurologic benefit or detriment as a result of hormonal contraceptive use (Fig. 4.3).

Conclusions

Where does the field of study go from here? There is irrefutable evidence that sex hormones and their metabolites alter the nervous system at a cellular level. It is also clear that many of these hormones can be produced within the nervous system itself and that the production of sex hormones from reproductive organs may only account for small change in the level of hormones in the nervous system. Moreover, the amount of sex hormones in nervous tissue is not uniformly distributed, and it is unknown how menstrual cycle irregularities and hormonal contraception affect the nervous system. All of this information points toward the idea that sex hormones may profoundly increase or decrease human performance but that (1) capturing these effects and leveraging them for athletic or rehabilitation gains is difficult, (2) intraindividual variability is likely extremely high, and (3) the complete underlying mechanisms which result in gains or losses is astronomically complex. Clinicians and researchers should be immediately wary of news outlets or individuals making blanket statements and claims such as "women shouldn't exercise before their period to avoid injury" or "athletic performance is decreased by taking birth control." Claims of this nature extend beyond what is scientifically known at this time and are typically made by individuals with ulterior motives and/or conflicts of interest (i.e., a potentially biased perspective).

With the above warning in place, it is sensible for the coach or clinician to understand the menstrual status of their patient or client as this does have the potential to affect performance. Systematically track objective performance variation, the patient/client's perception of performance variation and menstrual status. At the individual level, this information may be valuable in understanding the variability often observed in athletic performance or across an injury rehabilitation protocol.

References

Baulieu E. Neurosteroids: of the nervous system, by the nervous system, for the nervous system. Recent Prog Horm Res. 1996;52:1–32.

Baulieu E-E, Robel P. Dehydroepiandrosterone (DHEA) and dehydroepiandrosterone sulfate (DHEAS) as neuroactive neurosteroids. Proc Natl Acad Sci U S A. 1998;95:4089–91.

Bawa P, Lemon RN. Recruitment of motor units in response to transcranial magnetic stimulation in man. J Physiol. 1993;471:445–64.

Bayer U, Hausmann M. Menstrual cycle-related changes of functional cerebral asymmetries in fine motor coordination. Brain Cogn. 2012;79:34–8.

Becker JB. Direct effect of 17 beta-estradiol on striatum: sex differences in dopamine release. Synapse. 1990;5:157–64.

Birch K, Reilly T. The diurnal rhythm in isometric muscular performance differs with eumenorrheic menstrual cycle phase. Chronobiol Int. 2002;19:731–42.

Bixo M, Andersson A, Winblad B, Purdy RH, Bäckström T. Progesterone, 5α-pregnane-3, 20-dione and 3α-hydroxy-5α-pregnane-20-one in specific regions of the human female brain in different endocrine states. Brain Res. 1997;764:173–8.

Callachan H, Cottrell GA, Hather NY, Lambert JJ, Nooney JM, Peters JA. Modulation of the GABAA receptor by progesterone metabolites. Proc R Soc Lond B Biol Sci. 1987;231:359–69.

De Souza M, Toombs R, Scheid J, O'Donnell E, West S, Williams N. High prevalence of subtle and severe menstrual disturbances in exercising women: confirmation using daily hormone measures. Hum Reprod. 2010;25:491–503.

Dibrezzo R, Fort IL, Brown B. Dynamic strength and work variations during three stages of the menstrual cycle. J Orthop Sports Phys Ther. 1988;10:113–6.

Dong L-Y, Cheng Z-X, Fu Y-M, Wang Z-M, Zhu Y-H, Sun J-L, Dong Y, Zheng P. Neurosteroid dehydroepiandrosterone sulfate enhances spontaneous glutamate release in rat prelimbic cortex through activation of dopamine D1 and sigma-1 receptor. Neuropharmacology. 2007;52:966–74.

Elliott KJ, Cable NT, Reilly T, Diver MJ. Effect of menstrual cycle phase on the concentration of bioavailable 17-beta oestradiol and testosterone and muscle strength. Clin Sci (Lond). 2003;105:663–9.

Greeves JP, Cable NT, Luckas MJ, Reilly T, Biljan MM. Effects of acute changes in oestrogen on muscle function of the first dorsal interosseus muscle in humans. J Physiol. 1997;500(Pt 1):265–70.

Guazzo E, Kirkpatrick P, Goodyer I, Shiers H, Herbert J. Cortisol, dehydroepiandrosterone (DHEA), and DHEA sulfate in the cerebrospinal fluid of man: relation to blood levels and the effects of age. J Clin Endocrinol Metab. 1996;81:3951–60.

Hampson E, Kimura D. Reciprocal effects of hormonal fluctuations on human motor and perceptual-spatial skills. Behav Neurosci. 1988;102:456–9.

Hoffman M, Harter RA, Hayes BT, Wojtys EM, Murtaugh P. The interrelationships among sex hormone concentrations, motoneuron excitability, and anterior tibial displacement in women and men. J Athl Train. 2008;43:364–72.

Hudgens GA, Fatkin LT, Billingsley PA, Mazurczak J. Hand steadiness: effects of sex, menstrual phase, oral contraceptives, practice, and handgun weight. Hum Factors. 1988;30:51–60.

Janse De Jonge XA, Boot CR, Thom JM, Ruell PA, Thompson MW. The influence of menstrual cycle phase on skeletal muscle contractile characteristics in humans. J Physiol. 2001;530:161–6.

Kubo K, Miyamoto M, Tanaka S, Maki A, Tsunoda N, Kanehisa H. Muscle and tendon properties during menstrual cycle. Int J Sports Med. 2009;30:139–43.

La FM, Ledger WL, Davidson JW, Howard DM, Jones GL. The effects of a third generation combined oral contraceptive pill on the classical singing voice. J Voice. 2007;21:754–61.

La FM, Sundberg J, Howard DM, Sa-Couto P, Freitas A. Effects of the menstrual cycle and oral contraception on singers' pitch control. J Speech Lang Hear Res. 2012;55:247–61.

Leowattana W. DHEAS as a new diagnostic tool. Clin Chim Acta. 2004;341:1–15.

McEwen BS, Alves SE. Estrogen actions in the central nervous system. Endocr Rev. 1999;20: 279–307.

Mellon SH, Griffin LD. Neurosteroids: biochemistry and clinical significance. Trends Endocrinol Metab. 2002;13:35–43.

Meyer DA, Carta M, Partridge LD, Covey DF, Valenzuela CF. Neurosteroids enhance spontaneous glutamate release in Hippocampal neurons. Possible role of metabotropic sigma1-like receptors. J Biol Chem. 2002;277:28725–32.

Mienville J-M, Vicini S. Pregnenolone sulfate antagonizes GABA A receptor-mediated currents via a reduction of channel opening frequency. Brain Res. 1989;489:190–4.

Monnet FP, Mahé V, Robel P, Baulieu E-E. Neurosteroids, via sigma receptors, modulate the [3H] norepinephrine release evoked by N-methyl-D-aspartate in the rat hippocampus. Proc Natl Acad Sci U S A. 1995;92:3774–8.

Morfin R, Young J, Corpechot C, Egestad B, Sjövall J, Baulieu E-E. Neurosteroids: pregnenolone in human sciatic nerves. Proc Natl Acad Sci U S A. 1992;89:6790–3.

Murray H, Gillies G. Differential effects of neuroactive steroids on somatostatin and dopamine secretion from primary hypothalamic cell cultures. J Neuroendocrinol. 1997;9:287–95.

Neunzig J, Sánchez-Guijo A, Mosa A, Hartmann M, Geyer J, Wudy S, Bernhardt R. A steroidogenic pathway for sulfonated steroids: the metabolism of pregnenolone sulfate. J Steroid Biochem Mol Biol. 2014;144:324–33.

Payne AH, Jaffe RB. Androgen formation from pregnenolone sulfate by fetal, neonatal, prepubertal and adult human testes. J Clin Endocrinol Metab. 1975;40:102–7.

Peretti ED, Forest MG. Pattern of plasma dehydroepiandrosterone sulfate levels in humans from birth to adulthood: Evidence for testicular production*. J Clin Endocrinol Metab. 1978;47:572–7.

Phillips SK, Sanderson AG, Birch K, Bruce SA, Woledge RC. Changes in maximal voluntary force of human adductor pollicis muscle during the menstrual cycle. J Physiol. 1996;496(Pt 2):551–7.

Pletzer B, Kerschbaum HH. 50 years of hormonal contraception—time to find out, what it does to our brain. Front Neurosci. 2014;8:1–6.

Rhodes ME, Li P-K, Flood JF, Johnson DA. Enhancement of hippocampal acetylcholine release by the neurosteroid dehydroepiandrosterone sulfate: an in vivo microdialysis study. Brain Res. 1996;733:284–6.

Sarwar R, Niclos BB, Rutherford OM. Changes in muscle strength, relaxation rate and fatiguability during the human menstrual cycle. J Physiol. 1996;493(Pt 1):267–72.

Schultz KN, Von Esenwein SA, Hu M, Bennett AL, Kennedy RT, Musatov S, Toran-Allerand CD, Kaplitt MG, Young LJ, Becker JB. Viral vector-mediated overexpression of estrogen receptor-alpha in striatum enhances the estradiol-induced motor activity in female rats and estradiol-modulated GABA release. J Neurosci. 2009;29:1897–903.

Šimić N, Tokić A, Peričić M. Performance of fine motor and spatial tasks during the menstrual cycle. Arh Hig Rada Toksikol. 2010;61:407–14.

Smith SS. Progesterone enhances inhibitory responses of cerebellar Purkinje cells mediated by the GABA A receptor subtype. Brain Res Bull. 1989;23:317–22.

Smith SS, Waterhouse BD, Chapin JK, Woodward DJ. Progesterone alters GABA and glutamate responsiveness: a possible mechanism for its anxiolytic action. Brain Res. 1987;400:353–9.

Smith SS, Waterhouse BD, Woodward DJ. Locally applied estrogens potentiate glutamate-evoked excitation of cerebellar Purkinje cells. Brain Res. 1988;475:272–82.

Smith SS, Woodward DJ, Chapin JK. Sex steroids modulate motor-correlated increases in cerebellar discharge. Brain Res. 1989;476:307–16.

Smith MJ, Adams LF, Schmidt PJ, Rubinow DR, Wassermann EM. Effects of ovarian hormones on human cortical excitability. Ann Neurol. 2002;51:599–603.

Spivak CE. Desensitization and noncompetitive blockade of GABAA receptors in ventral midbrain neurons by a neurosteroid dehydroepiandrosterone sulfate. Synapse. 1994;16:113–22.

Stoffel-Wagner B. Neurosteroid metabolism in the human brain. Eur J Endocrinol. 2001;145:669–79.

Takase M, Ukena K, Yamazaki T, Kominami S, Tsutsui K. Pregnenolone, pregnenolone sulfate, and cytochrome P450 side-chain cleavage enzyme in the amphibian brain and their seasonal changes. Endocrinology. 1999;140:1936–44.

Tenan MS, Peng Y-L, Hackney AC, Griffin L. Menstrual cycle mediates vastus medialis and vastus medialis oblique muscle activity. Med Sci Sports Exerc. 2013;45:2151–7.

Tenan M, Hackney AC, Griffin L. Maximal force and tremor changes across the menstrual cycle. Eur J Appl Physiol. 2015;116(1):153–60.

Tourville TW, Shultz SJ, Vacek PM, Knudsen EJ, Bernstein IM, Tourville KJ, Hardy DM, Johnson RJ, Slauterbeck JR, Beynnon BD. Evaluation of an algorithm to predict menstrual-cycle phase at the time of injury. J Athl Train. 2016;51:47–56.

Tsutsui K. Neurosteroid biosynthesis and function in the brain of domestic birds. Front Endocrinol. 2011;2:37.

van den Heuvel MW, van Bragt AJM, Alnabawy AKM, Kaptein MCJ. Comparison of ethinylestradiol pharmacokinetics in three hormonal contraceptive formulations: the vaginal ring, the transdermal patch and an oral contraceptive. Contraception. 2005;72:168–74.

Wang M, Seippel L, Purdy RH, Bäckström T. Relationship between symptom severity and steroid variation in women with premenstrual syndrome: study on serum pregnenolone, pregnenolone sulfate, 5 alpha-pregnane-3, 20-dione and 3 alpha-hydroxy-5 alpha-pregnan-20-one. J Clin Endocrinol Metab. 1996;81:1076–82.

Wang M-D, Wahlström G, Bäckström T. The regional brain distribution of the neurosteroids pregnenolone and pregnenolone sulfate following intravenous infusion. J Steroid Biochem Mol Biol. 1997;62:299–306.

Wolf OT, Kirschbaum C. Actions of dehydroepiandrosterone and its sulfate in the central nervous system: effects on cognition and emotion in animals and humans. Brain Res Rev. 1999;30:264–88.

Xiao L, Jackson LR, Becker JB. The effect of estradiol in the striatum is blocked by ICI 182,780 but not tamoxifen: pharmacological and behavioral evidence. Neuroendocrinology. 2003;77:239–45.

Zimmerman E, Parlee MB. Behavioral changes associated with the menstrual cycle: an experimental Investigation1. J Appl Soc Psychol. 1973;3:335–44.

Zoghi M, Vaseghi B, Bastani A, Jaberzadeh S, Galea MP. The effects of Sex hormonal fluctuations during menstrual cycle on cortical excitability and manual dexterity (a pilot study). PLoS One. 2015;10, e0136081.

Chapter 5
Estrogen and Menopause: Muscle Damage, Repair and Function in Females

Peter M. Tiidus

Over the last 20–25 years, science has come to appreciate the wide ranging and physiologically significant effects that estrogen has on skeletal muscle. Paradoxically, these important effects are often most discernable when they are lost, as happens following menopause in aging women. The acute and rapid reduction in muscle strength and mass, the ability of muscle to effect post-injury repair and post-atrophy recovery of mass, the metabolic and mitochondrial function alterations that all accompany menopause are greatly influenced by the steep drop in estrogen levels following menarche in aging women (Spangenburg et al. 2012; Tiidus et al. 2013).

This chapter primarily examines the effects of estrogen on the skeletal muscle damage and repair mechanisms and also touches upon related physiological mechanisms associated with muscle mass and recovery from atrophy as well as muscle strength related issues. It also summarizes the potential health implications of post-menopause hormone replacement and how it may counteract the negative effects of estrogen loss on skeletal muscle function. While the focus of the chapter is on the influence of estrogen and its postmenopausal loss on muscle function in older females, animal studies which related to these issues are also cited as they often add corroboration and provide further evidence of for physiological mechanisms associated with the effects of estrogen on skeletal muscle function, that are discerned from human studies.

P.M. Tiidus, B.Sc., M.Sc., Ph.D. (✉)
Faculty of Applied Health Sciences, Brock University, 1812 Sir Isaac Brock Way,
St. Catharines, ON, Canada L2S3A1
e-mail: peter.tiidus@brocku.ca

© Springer International Publishing Switzerland 2017
A.C. Hackney (ed.), *Sex Hormones, Exercise and Women*,
DOI 10.1007/978-3-319-44558-8_5

Muscle Damage

Some of the first studies that implicated estrogen in mitigating indices of exercise induced muscle damage did so using rodents. In comparing male and female rats as well as ovariectomized female rats, with or without estrogen replacement, studies from the Bar laboratory in the 1980s and 1990s consistently found that estrogen attenuated muscle creatine kinase enzyme efflux following exercise or in vitro muscle contractions (Amelink et al. 1988, 1990). Measures of muscle creatine kinase and other specific enzyme efflux and blood levels of these enzymes is a commonly used semi-quantitative indicator of muscle membrane stability and in particular of muscle membrane damage and repair (Warren and Palubinskas 2008). It was postulated that estrogen acted to directly stabilize muscle membranes by influencing membrane fluidity and decreasing susceptibility to damage (Tiidus 1995). Subsequent research in our laboratory confirmed that estrogen reduced indices of muscle damage through non-receptor mediated mechanisms which could include membrane stabilization (Enns et al. 2008; Iqbal et al. 2008). Female rats also demonstrate a more stable muscle calcium homeostasis following exercise than male rats, suggesting greater membrane stability and less susceptibility to exercise induced membrane disruption in females relative to male animals (Sonobe et al. 2010).

Studies which examined the effects of hormone replacement in older women have also demonstrated that the presence of estrogen will essentially eliminate a post-exercise rise in blood creatine kinase in those women who are long term users of hormone replacement while the same muscular exercise induced two to threefold increases in blood creatine kinase in those postmenopausal women who were not estrogen replaced (Dieli-Conwright et al. 2009a, 2009b). This implies that estrogen in the form of hormone replacement will also provide protection against exercise induced muscle damage in postmenopausal women.

Komulainen et al. (1999) reported sex based differences in damage to muscle structural proteins (desmin, actin, dystrophin), fiber swelling and necrosis following downhill running with male rodents exhibiting significantly more and earlier onset of post-exercise damage than females. The early post-exercise loss of the sub-membrane protein dystrophin which occurred in male but not female animals suggested that the higher estrogen levels in the females helped stabilize muscle membranes and diminish exercise induced muscle disruption. Other markers of muscle damage such as activation of muscle lysosomal and calcium activated proteases have also been demonstrated to be elevated following exercise in male and ovariectomized female rats, while normal female rats and ovariectomized female rats with estrogen replacement show little or no post-exercise increases in muscle protease activities (Komulainen et al. 1999; Enns and Tiidus 2008; Enns et al. 2008; Tiidus 2003). Markers of muscle oxidative damage following exercise or ischemia–reperfusion injury are also reduced by estrogen (Persky et al. 2000; Stupka and Tiidus 2001). This should be expected as estrogen has been reported to exhibit antioxidant properties (Tiidus 1995).

Taken together these findings from animal studies suggest that estrogen can have significant influence in the amelioration of exercise induced muscle damage. This can be of particular importance for postmenopausal women who may be more susceptible to exercise induced muscle disruption as a result of their decline in circulating estrogen. Hormone replacement in postmenopausal females can restore circulating estrogen levels and therefore potentially restore the protective effects of estrogen on exercise induced muscle damage. Dieli-Conwright et al. (2009a, 2009b) compared the effects of eccentric muscle exercise in postmenopausal women who were or were not using hormone replacement. They measured markers of muscle damage such as serum creatine kinase activities and found significant attenuation of these indices of damage in following exercise in those women using hormone replacement relative to those that were not, suggesting that the loss of estrogen in aging women made them more susceptible to exercise induced muscle disruption.

Exposure to estrogen will also induce increased basal heat shock protein expression in skeletal muscles (Bombardier et al. 2009). Heat shock proteins (HSP) such as HSP70 are expressed when cells are stressed and serve to protect proteins and membranes from damage and to assist in protein assembly (Noble et al. 2008). Ovariectomized female rats with estrogen replacement will express significantly more muscle HSP70 relative to those animals without estrogen. Exercise will typically increase HSP70 expression in male rats and ovariectomized female rats to levels achieved in unexercised normal female rats or ovariectomized females with estrogen replaced (Bombardier et al. 2009, 2013). Hence, it is possible that the increased expression of HSP70 exhibited in muscles exposed to estrogen may also act to limit exercise induced muscle disruption and help maintain membrane integrity.

Muscle Inflammation

Muscle damage is followed by a well-documented sequence of events including increased muscle inflammation and leukocyte infiltration, subsequent activation and proliferation of muscle satellite cells and repair signaling, collagen synthesis and consequent muscle repair (Tidball 2005). Estrogen has been reported to influence all of the above steps in the reaction to and consequent repair of skeletal muscle following injury (Tiidus et al. 2013). The first step in this process is the initiation of muscle inflammatory responses and infiltration of muscle by neutrophils and macrophages (Tiidus 1998).

The presence of estrogen has been repeatedly demonstrated to attenuate post-exercise and post-ischemia/reperfusion injury muscle neutrophil and macrophage infiltration in rodent models (Tiidus and Bombardier 1999; Tiidus et al. 2001; Stupka and Tiidus 2001; Iqbal et al. 2008). The provision of estrogen to male rats (Tiidus et al. 2001) or to ovariectomized female rats (Iqbal et al. 2008) will significantly reduce post-exercise muscle leukocyte (neutrophils and macrophages) infiltration relative to their unsupplemented cohorts. While the mechanisms by which estrogen may be able to attenuate post-exercise muscle leukocyte infiltration are not fully known, it has been hypothesized that the potential membrane stabilizing effects of estrogen may attenuate some of the generation of and signaling by neutrophil and macrophage chemoattractants generated by exercise and subsequent muscle disruption and thereby reduce the adhesion and infiltration of these leukocytes into muscle following exercise (Tiidus 2003).

Indirect support for such a hypothesis has been shown in a study which used an estrogen receptor blocker to demonstrate involvement or non-involvement of estrogen receptors in exercise related muscular events (Enns et al. 2008). Blocking estrogen receptors had no significant effect on the ability of estrogen to attenuate post-exercise muscle leukocyte infiltration in white vastus muscle (see Fig. 5.1) (Enns et al. 2008). This suggested that the mechanisms by which estrogen was able to attenuate post-exercise leukocyte infiltration was a non-receptor mediated process, hence the possibility that mechanisms associated with its possible direct effects on muscle membranes should be further investigated (Enns et al. 2008). Hormone replacement therapy in older females typically provides both estrogen and progesterone. However, animal based studies have demonstrated that most of the anti-inflammatory effects of female sex hormones are mediated through estrogen with progesterone having relatively little influence on factors such as post-exercise muscle leukocyte infiltration (Iqbal et al. 2008)

The physiological consequences of the attenuation of muscle inflammatory responses following exercise, particularly the attenuation of muscle neutrophil and macrophage infiltration are not certain. Inflammation and leukocyte infiltration are important obligatory responses to muscle damage which facilitate the breakdown, removal and clearance of damaged components of the muscle, which is required to precede muscle repair (Tiidus 1998; Tidball 2005). Leukocyte and particularly macrophage infiltration has also been demonstrated to be important in signaling the activation of aspects of muscle repair such as muscle satellite cell proliferation (Hawke and Gerry 2001). However, inflammation and neutrophil infiltration following exercise have also been shown to induce further disruption and damage to components of muscle in conjunction with the removal of muscle damage debris (Tiidus 1998). Ideally, a fine balance of inflammation and repair signaling needs to be maintained in order to optimize muscle recovery. These seemingly paradoxical effects, of estrogen whereby it is able to achieve both a reduction in inflammation and an augmentation of muscle repair indices will be discussed in the next section.

Human studies have also demonstrated a reduction in inflammatory markers in postmenopausal females using hormone replacement containing estrogen (Tiidus et al. 2013). Dieli-Conwright et al. (2009a, 2009b) examined two groups of postmenopausal females who were either taking hormone replacement or not before and after a bout of eccentric quadriceps muscle contractions designed to induce muscle disruption and soreness. They found that following eccentric muscle exercise, postmenopausal women who were taking hormone replacement expressed little change in muscle mRNA levels of inflammation related cytokines and interleukins such as tumor necrosis factor alpha (TNF-α), interleukin-6 (IL-6), IL-8, and IL-15 while those women not on hormone replacement expressed five to tenfold increases in the messenger RNA (mRNA) of these inflammation and muscle turnover related mediators. The provision of estrogen to young males also results

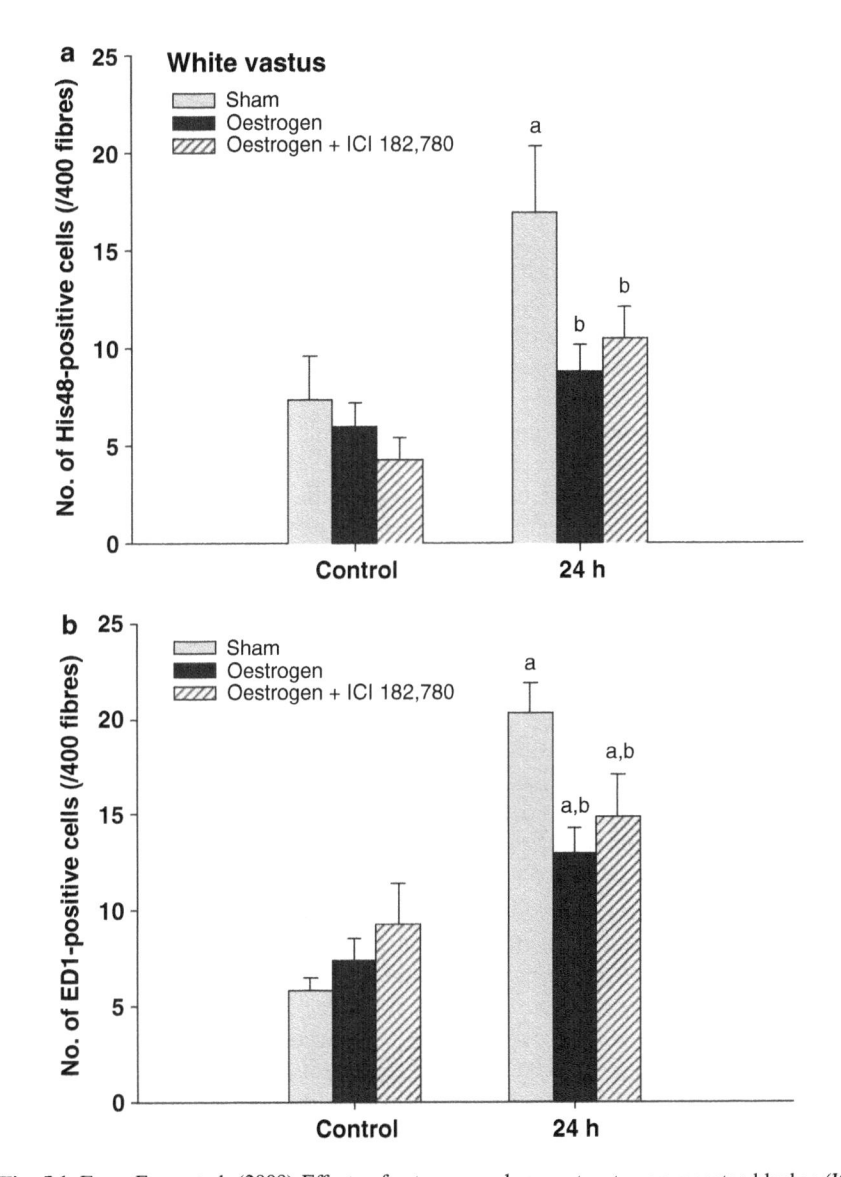

Fig. 5.1 From Enns et al. (2008) Effects of estrogen replacement, estrogen receptor blocker (ICI 182,780) and their combination on (**a**) neutrophil (His48 positive) and (**b**) macrophage (ED-1 positive) infiltration of skeletal muscle 24 h after downhill running exercise in ovariectomized female rats

in attenuated post-exercise muscle neutrophil infiltration (MacNeil et al. 2011). Thus studies in humans have corroborated animal results demonstrating that estrogen will attenuate indices of post-exercise muscle inflammatory response. It is possible that the smaller inflammatory responses engendered by estrogen could result in a reduction in inflammation induced secondary muscle damage and thereby attenuate the damaging effects of exercise and injury on overall muscle damage (Tiidus 1995; Enns and Tiidus 2010).

Muscle Satellite Cells and Muscle Repair

Estrogen has also been found to facilitate post-exercise muscle repair, particularly by enhancing the activation and proliferation of muscle satellite cells (Enns and Tiidus 2008). Adult muscle cells are post-mitotic and hence rely on muscle satellite cells, which are myogenic precursor cells, in order to hypertrophy and to effect repair (Hawke and Gerry 2001). Satellite cells are normally quiescent and reside in the periphery of muscle cells under the basal lamina. When stimulated by exercise or muscle damage, satellite cells become activated, proliferate and can ultimately fuse with and/or donate their nuclei to muscle cells in order to optimize protein synthesis in response to hypertrophic or damage/repair signaling (Hawke and Gerry 2001). Muscle hypertrophy and muscle repair cannot occur to any great extent without activation and proliferation of satellite cells, and the rate of repair and hypertrophy is directly correlated to the degree of muscle satellite cell activation and proliferation (Yin et al. 2013).

Studies have repeatedly demonstrated that supplementation of ovariectomized female rodentsas well as male rodents with estrogen, will augment post-exercise muscle satellite cell activation and proliferation (Tiidus et al. 2005; Enns and Tiidus 2008; Enns et al. 2008; Mangan et al. 2014). Other animal models have also demonstrated positive effects of estrogen exposure on muscle satellite cell activation and proliferation (e.g. McFarland et al. 2013). Figure 5.2 illustrates such an effect in muscles of ovariectomized female rats with or without estrogen replacement sampled at 72 h following downhill running exercise (Enns and Tiidus 2008).

These findings suggest that estrogen exposure would enhance muscle repair and/or hypertrophy related mechanisms consequent to damaging exercise.

The mechanisms of how estrogen communicates with muscle satellite cells have not yet been fully elucidated. Nevertheless, it has been demonstrated that estrogen receptors in muscle appear to be critical to this effect. Both estrogen receptor-α and -β have been shown to be present in animal and human muscles, with greater receptor concentration typically found in type I than type II muscle fibers (Lemoine et al. 2003; Wiik et al. 2005). Blocking estrogen receptors not only completely negates the augmentation effect of estrogen on post-exercise muscle satellite cell activation and proliferation, it also completely eliminates the ability of muscle satellite cells to respond at all to the exercise/damage stimuli (Enns et al. 2008). Results vary as to whether estrogen receptor-α or -β are the most critical to this effect (Thomas et al. 2010; Velders et al. 2012). Additionally, it appears that estrogen dependent muscle satellite cell activation occurs via estrogen receptor communication with the phosphatidylinositide 3-kinase (PI3K) signaling pathway (Mangan et al. 2014). Similar to the effect of blocking estrogen receptors, blocking the PI3K signaling pathway will not only negate the augmentation effect of estrogen on post-exercise satellite

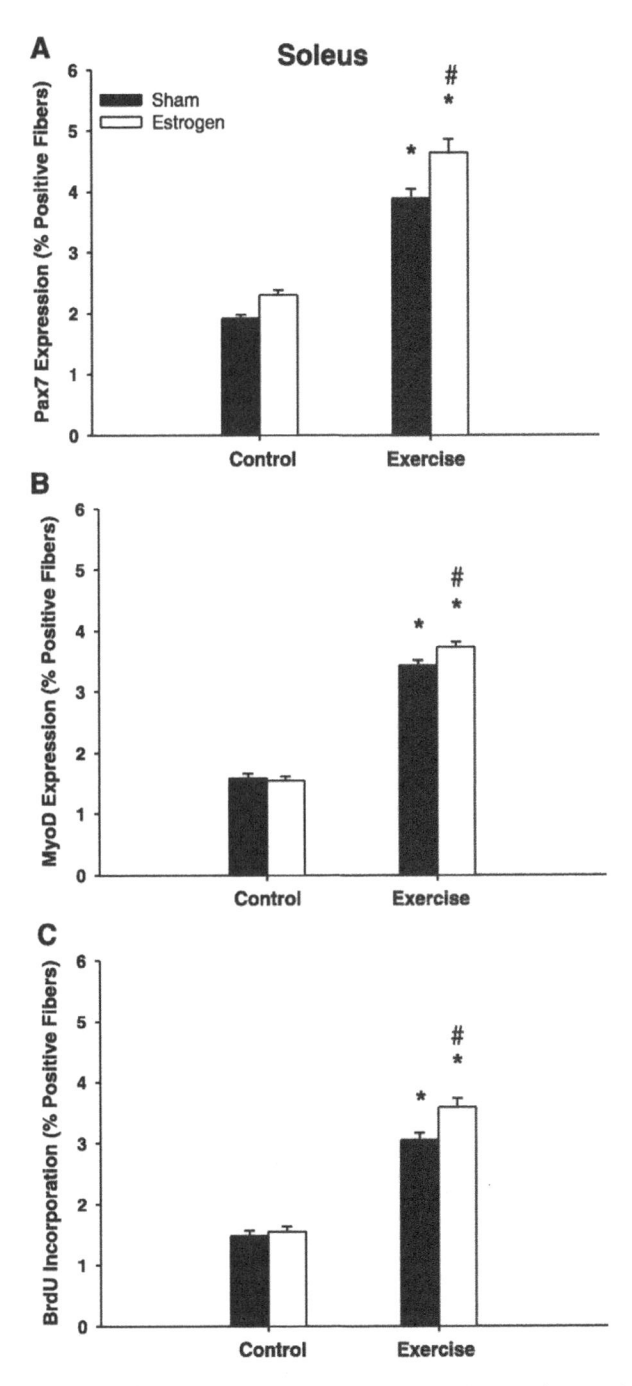

Fig. 5.2 From Enns and Tiidus (2008). Effects of estrogen supplementation on relative numbers of myofibers expressing total (Pax7; **A**), activated (MyoD; **B**), and proliferating (BrdU; **C**) satellite cell markers in rat soleus muscle 72 h following downhill running. Values are means ± SE; $n=11$ rats per group. *$P<0.05$ compared with control. #$P<0.05$ compared with sham

cell activation, it will also completely eliminate any positive muscle satellite cell response to exercise (Mangan et al. 2014).

Most of the studies examining the effects of estrogen on post-exercise muscle satellite cell activity and muscle repair have been conducted in animal models. While it has yet to be demonstrated that these specific benefits of estrogen on muscle repair mechanisms and satellite cell proliferation also operate in humans, particularly in postmenopausal females, other evidence, discussed later in this chapter illustrate the benefits of estrogen on muscle mass and strength in older females, both of which rely in part on enhanced muscle satellite cell activation and proliferation. Hence, it is likely that the positive effects of estrogen on muscle satellite cell activity seen in animal models are also functional in aging female humans.

Muscle Mass and Recovery from Atrophy

Several rodent studies have demonstrated that skeletal muscle mass recovery following disuse atrophy is attenuated without the presence of estrogen (McClung et al. 2006; Brown et al. 2005; Sitnick et al. 2006). For example, McClung et al. (2006) induced atrophy of hind-limb muscles of ovariectomized and intact rats by unweighting. When weight bearing was reinitiated after 10 days of atrophy, the muscles of the ovariectomized rats took twice as long (14 days) to recover pre-atrophy mass as those animals with normal estrogen levels (7 days). Nonfunctional collagen formation or fibrosis was also significantly increased the recovering muscles of ovariectomized rats relative to the normal animals, which may have inhibited recovery (McClung et al. 2006).

The potential implications for older postmenopausal females of slower recovery from muscle loss such as might occur following inactivity due to injury or surgery, suggest that loss of estrogen might contribute to a higher incidence and degree of functional decline related to greater muscle mass and strength loss and inhibited recovery. If hormone replacement were able to reverse these negative effects of estrogen loss on post-atrophy recovery of muscle mass, its potential to reduce and reverse loss of muscle function and reduced mobility in elderly females could potentially be highly significant.

The effects of estrogen on muscle mass in postmenopausal females and its use in combination with resistance training in this population has, in most cases, demonstrated positive results (Enns and Tiidus 2010). A milestone study examining postmenopausal twins where one twin in each pair was taking hormone replacement and the other was not (Ronkainen et al. 2009) found greater overall muscle mass, less fat mass and greater thigh muscle cross-sectional areas for those twins taking hormone replacement relative to those twins who were not. Other studies have also reported beneficial effects of hormone replacement on muscle mass in sedentary postmenopausal females as well as enhanced effects of resistance training on muscle mass gain relative to those older females not taking hormone replacement (Sipila et al. 2001; Taafe et al. 2005).

Postmenopausal hormone replacement also significantly augments a pro-anabolic signaling environment in skeletal muscle of older females (Tiidus et al. 2013, Sipila et al. 2015). The anabolic PI3K/Akt (a serine/threonine kinase also known as protein kinase B [PKB]) signaling pathway has been implicated in animal studies as a means by which estrogen enhances muscle satellite cell activation and proliferation following exercise (Mangan et al. 2014). Human studies have also demonstrated the up-regulation of this pathway by estrogen which consequently may provide an enhanced muscle anabolic signal for postmenopausal women taking hormone replacement (Sipila et al. 2015). Dieli-Conwright et al. (2009a, 2009b) have also reported that postmenopausal women taking hormone replacement have significantly higher resting muscle mRNA levels of muscle a number of positive regulators of muscle hypertrophy such as myogenic differentiation protein D (MyoD), Myogenic factor protein (Myf5) and myogenin and lower levels of negative muscle hypertrophy regulators such as myostatin than cohorts not taking estrogen replacement. Furthermore, although a single bout of resistance training enhances these pro-anabolic signaling pathways in all women, these exercise effects on muscle anabolic signaling are greatly augmented in those postmenopausal women who are taking hormone replacement (Dieli-Conwright et al. 2009a, 2009b). These results suggest that in the presence of estrogen, muscle in postmenopausal females is chronically exposed to greater pro-anabolic signaling and this signaling is further enhanced by exercise, particularly when estrogen is present (Dieli-Conwright et al. 2009a, 2009b).

In summary, these findings suggest that estrogen in the form of hormone replacement will have significant positive effects in postmenopausal females for the maintenance of muscle mass, the recovery of muscle mass following atrophy and the enhancement of exercise induced muscle hypertrophy. These benefits have important implications for health and functional longevity in aging females.

Muscle Strength

In addition to enhanced muscle size and the consequent increase in contractile proteins, it appears that additional effects of estrogen on other specific muscle contractile mechanisms can act to further enhance muscle force production (Tiidus et al. 2013; Pollanen et al. 2015). Skelton et al. (1999) found that women taking hormone replacement exhibited increased adductor pollicis muscle strength relative to a matched group not taking hormone replacement. In a follow up to the previously described postmenopausal female twin study which demonstrated greater lower body muscle power in the hormone replaced twin (Ronkainen et al. 2009), Qaisar et al. (2013) reported that force relative to cross-sectional area in single muscle fibers was 25 % greater in the twin taking hormone replacement relative to the non-hormone replaced twin. In addition, a recent meta-analysis of literature comparing strength measures in postmenopausal hormone replaced vs non-replaced women concluded that significant strength enhancement due to estrogen was evident in these populations (Greising et al. 2009). Postmenopausal women performing extended strength training while on hormone replacement also tend to increase muscle strength to a greater extent than matched cohorts not on hormone replacement (Taafe et al. 2005; Perry et al. 2005).

Animal studies have also reported similar effects of estrogen removal and replacement on muscle strength. For example, ovariecomy in mice results in a 25 % loss in tetanic muscle force and this loss of force is restored by estrogen replacement (Moran et al. 2007). It has been suggested that these effects of estrogen in enhancing muscle contraction may be related to increases in strong binding of myosin heads to actin during active contraction (Lowe et al. 2010). These suggestions have been directly verified by measures of active muscle stiffness during contraction (Greising et al. 2011). The mechanisms of how estrogen might be able to directly influence myosin binding and thus enhance muscle force production are currently under active investigation. Possible mechanisms for this effect include the antioxidant properties of estrogen acting to maintain myosin structure during contraction (Lowe et al. 2010; Tiidus et al. 2013) and the possibility that estrogen could enhance myosin phosphorylation (Lai et al. 2016).

Myosin regulatory light chain phosphorylation induces potentiation of muscle force by increasing calcium sensitivity and myosin structure to allow for increased strong binding during contraction (Vandenboom et al. 2013). Recently estrogen has been shown to enhance myosin regulatory light chain phosphorylation in cultured muscle cells (Lai et al. 2016). In addition, older postmenopausal females, who lacked estrogen had 50 % less contraction induced myosin phosphorylation than age matched males (Miller et al. 2013), suggesting that estrogen may be able to enhance myosin phosphorylation and thereby increase muscle force potentiation.

The implications for effects of estrogen muscle strength in older females, as with its effects on muscle mass, also suggest that loss of estrogen could further exacerbate strength and muscle function loss in postmenopausal females.

Hormone Replacement, Health, and Exercise in Older Women

The above noted multifaceted beneficial effects of estrogen on muscle mass, strength and repair mechanisms suggest that estrogen in the form of hormone replacement could have significant benefits for muscle function and consequent mobility, functionality and independent living in postmenopausal women. Concerns regarding health issues with hormone replacement, primarily founded on results of the Women's Health Initiative (WHI) have contributed to a decline in hormone replacement prescriptions provided by physicians in subsequent years (Hondis et al. 2012).

Subsequent research has demonstrated that the health concerns related to hormone replacement suggested by the WHI study may have been overstated (Tiidus et al. 2013; Gurney et al. 2014). The average age of the women in the WHI study was 61 years, and therefore, most of the women had been postmenopausal for many years before initiating hormone replacement (Hondis et al. 2012). These were the cohorts who had significantly increased risks of coronary disease in the WHI study, while reanalysis of the WHI data demonstrated that younger women who started hormone replacement proximal to menopause onset actually decreased risk of heart disease and other health risks (LaCroix et al. 2011). Two meta-analyses of more recent studies have also demonstrated that beginning hormone replacement proximal to menopause results in significantly decreased risk of overall mortality and cardiovascular risk factors in postmenopausal women, relative to women who were not hormone replaced (Schierbeck et al. 2012; Salpeter et al. 2009). Another comprehensive review of the related literature also concluded that hormone replacement is "generally safe and beneficial for women under 60 years of age" (Rozenberg et al. 2013).

A further example of the beneficial health effects of estrogen in postmenopausal women is a 10 year trial which followed 1000 recently postmenopausal women and concluded that those on hormone replacement had significantly reduced overall mortality and cardiovascular incidents without increased risk of cancer or other health threats, relative to the cohort not taking hormone replacement (Schierbeck et al. 2012). These studies all suggest that a "window of opportunity" exists where estrogen, as hormone replacement, if begun proximal to menopause will provide significant health benefits for most women and that it can be safely used for at least 10 years post-menopause (Schierbeck et al. 2012; Gurney et al. 2014). However, for women with pre-existing heart disease or those over 70 years of age use of hormone replacement may still be contraindicated (LaCroix et al. 2011; Rozenberg et al. 2013).

In addition to these health benefits, estrogen and hormone replacement in postmenopausal women has also been shown to maintain bone mass, reduce abdominal obesity, maintain insulin sensitivity, maintain mitochondrial and metabolic function, and enhance cognitive and neuro-regenerative functions (Spangenburg et al. 2012; Tiidus et al. 2013).

Rodent studies have also found that a delay in starting estrogen replacement, following ovariectomy will negate the cardiovascular and neuro-regenerative benefits provided by estrogen in these tissues (Suzuki et al 2007). More specifically related to the topics covered in this chapter, Mangan et al. (2015) recently reported that the previously described effects of estrogen in enhancing post-exercise muscle satellite cell activation and proliferation were also lost if estrogen replacement were delayed by 11 weeks (equivalent to several years delay following menopause in humans) following ovariectomy in rats.

Hence, it appears that in addition to its beneficial effects on muscle mass, strength and regeneration, estrogen has significant health benefits for most, older women if replacement is started proximal to menopause. However a significant delay in postmenopausal estrogen replacement following menopause will negate beneficial effects that estrogen has on muscle and neural recovery from injury and also negate health benefits associated with estrogen replacement (Suzuki et al. 2007; Mangan et al. 2015; Gurney et al. 2014).

Summary

In summary, the use of hormone replacement in postmenopausal women could be recommended as means to mitigate loss of muscle force, mass, and function and to enhance muscle recovery following atrophy (as seen following immobilization with surgery or injury) in older women. Estrogen replacement could potentially help mitigate age related declines in mobility and muscle strength and functionality that lead to frailty in older women. It is likely that regular vigorous resistance and aerobic exercise can also deliver many of the same benefits as estrogen to muscle and metabolic health and function in aging women (Tiidus et al. 2013). However, a number of studies have suggested that the effects of regular exercise on muscle mass in older women are further enhanced when they are on hormone replacement (Taafe et al. 2005). In addition, the majority of older women do not regularly participate in resistance or aerobic exercise training. Therefore, timely postmenopausal return of estrogen in the form of hormone replacement could be an important prophylactic in helping mitigate age-related loss of muscle mass and function in aging females.

References

Amelink GJ, Kamp HH, Bar PR. Creatine kinase isoenzyme profiles after exercise in the rat: sex-linked differences in leakage of CK-MM. Pflugers Arch. 1988;412:417–21.

Amelink GJ, Koot RW, Erich WB, Van Gijn J, Bar PR. Sex-linked variation in creatine kinase release, and its dependence on oestradiol, can be demonstrated in an in vitro rat skeletal muscle preparation. Acta Physiol Scand. 1990;138:115–24.

Bombardier E, Vigna C, Iqbal S, Tiidus PM, Tupling AR. Effects of ovarian sex hormones and downhill running on fiber type-specific Hsp70 expression in rat soleus. J Appl Physiol. 2009;106:2009–15.

Bombardier E, Vigna C, Bloemberg D, Quadrilatero J, Tiidus PM, Tupling AR. The role of estrogen receptor-α in estrogen-mediated regulation of basal and exercise-induced Hsp70 and Hsp27 expression in rat soleus. Can J Physiol Pharmacol. 2013;91:823–9.

Brown M, Foley AM, Ferreira JA. Ovariectomy, hindlimb unweighting and recovery effects on skeletal muscle in adult rats. Aviat Space Environ Med. 2005;76:1012–8.

Dieli-Conwright CM, Specktor TM, Rice JC, Sattler FR, Schroder ET. Influence of hormone replacement therapy on eccentric exercise induced myogenic gene expression in postmenopausal women. J Appl Physiol. 2009a;107:1381–8.

Dieli-Conwright CM, Specktor TM, Rice JC, Schroder ET. Hormone therapy attenuates exercise-induced muscle damage in postmenopausal women. J Appl Physiol. 2009b;107:853–8.

Enns DL, Tiidus PM. Estrogen influences satellite cell activation and proliferation following downhill running in rats. J Appl Physiol. 2008;104:347–53.

Enns DL, Tiidus PM. The influence of estrogen on skeletal muscle: sex matters. Sports Med. 2010;40:41–58.

Enns DL, Iqbal S, Tiidus PM. Oestrogen receptors mediate oestrogen-induced increases in post-exercise rat skeletal muscle satellite cells. Acta Physiol. 2008;194:81–93.

Greising SM, Baltgalvis KA, Lowe DA, Warren GL. Hormone therapy and skeletal muscle strength: a meta-analysis. J Gerontol A Biol Sci Med Sci. 2009;64:1071–81.

Greising SM, Baltgalvis KA, Kosir AM, Moran AL, Warren GL, Lowe DA. Estradiol's beneficial effect on murine muscle function is independent of muscle activity. J Appl Physiol. 2011;110: 109–15.

Gurney EP, Nachtagall MJ, Nachtagall LE, Naftolin F. The women's health initiative trial and related studies: 10 years later: a clinician's view. J Steroid Biochem Mol Biol. 2014;142:4–11.

Hawke TJ, Gerry DJ. Myogenic satellite cells: physiology to molecular biology. J Appl Physiol. 2001;91:534–51.

Hondis HN, Collins P, Mack WJ, Schierbeck LL. The timing hypothesis for coronary heart disease prevention and hormone therapy: past, present and future in perspective. Climeractic. 2012;15: 217–28.

Iqbal S, Thomas A, Bunyan K, Tiidus PM. Progesterone and estrogen influence post-exercise skeletal muscle leukocyte infiltration in overiectomized female rats. Appl Physiol Nutr Metabol. 2008;33:1207–12.

Komulainen J, Koskinen S, Kalliokoski R, Takala T, Vihko V. Gender differences in skeletal muscle damage after eccentrically biased downhill running in rats. Acta Physiol Scand. 1999;165:57–63.

LaCroix AZ, Chiebowski RT, Manson JE, Aragaki AK, Johnson KC, Martin L, Margolis KL, Stefanick ML, Brzyski R, Curb JD, Howard BV, Lewis CE, Wactawski-Wende J. Health outcomes after stopping conjugated equine estrogens among postmenopausal women with prior historectomy. JAMA. 2011;305:1305–14.

Lai S, Collins BC, Colson BA, Kararigas G, Lowe DA. Estradiol modulates myosin regulatory light chain phosphorylation and contractility in skeletal muscle of female mice. Am J Physiol Endocrinol Metab. 2016;310(9):E724–33.

Lemoine S, Granier P, Tiffoche C. Effect of endurance training on oestrogen receptor alpha expression in different rat skeletal muscle type. Acta Physiol Scand. 2003;174:283–9.

Lowe DA, Baltgalvis KA, Greising SM. Mechanisms behind estrogen's beneficial effect on muscle strength in females. Exerc Sport Sci Rev. 2010;38:61–7.

MacNeil LG, Baker SK, Stevic I, Tarnopolsky MA. 17β-estradiol attenuates exercise-induced neutrophil infiltration in men. Am J Physiol Regul Integr Comp Physiol. 2011;300:R1443–51.

Mangan G, Bombardier E, Mitchell A, Quadrilatero J, Tiidus PM. Oestrogen-dependent satellite cell activation and proliferation following a running exercise occurs via the PI3K signalling pathway and not IGF-1. Acta Physiol. 2014;212:75–85.

Mangan G, Iqbal S, Hubbard A, Hamilton V, Bombardier E, Tiidus PM. Delay in post-ovariectomy estrogen-replacement negates estrogen-induced augmentation of post-exercise satellite cell proliferation. Can J Physiol Pharmacol. 2015;93:945–51.

McClung JM, Davis JM, Wilson MA, Goldsmith EC, Carson JA. Estrogen status and skeletal muscle recovery from disuse atrophy. J Appl Physiol. 2006;100:2012–3.

McFarland DC, Pesall JE, Coy CS, Velleman SG. Effects of 17β-estradiol on turkey myogenic satellite cell proliferation, differentiation, and expression of glypican-1, MyoD and myogenin. Comp Biochem Physiol A Mol Integr Physiol. 2013;164:556–71.

Miller MS, Bedrin NG, Callahan DM, Previs MJ, Jennings ME, Ades PA, Maughan DA, Palmer BM, Toth MJ. Age-related slowing of myosin actin cross-bridge kinetics is sex specific and predicts decrements in whole skeletal muscle performance in humans. J Appl Physiol. 2013;115:1004–14.

Moran AL, Nelson SA, Landisch RM, Warren GL, Lowe DA. Estradiol replacement reverses ovariectomy-induced muscle contractile and myosin dysfunction in mature female mice. J Appl Physiol. 2007;102:1387–93.

Noble EG, Milne KJ, Melling CWJ. Heat shock proteins and exercise: a primer. Appl Physiol Nutr Metab. 2008;33:1050–65.

Perry SK, Radke A, Bombardier E, Tiidus PM. Hormone replacement and strength training positively influence balance during gait in post-menopausal females: a pilot study. J Sports Sci Med. 2005;4:372–82.

Persky AM, Green PS, Stubley L, Howell CO, Zaulyanov L, Baseau GA, Simpkins JW. Protective effect of estrogens against oxidative damage to heart and skeletal muscle in vivo and in vitro. Proc Soc Exp Biol Med. 2000;223:59–66.

Pollanen E, Kangas R, Horttanainen M, Niskala P, Kaprio J, Butler-Browne G, Mouly V, Sipila S, Kovanen V. Intramuscular sex steroid hormones are associated with skeletal muscle strength and power in women with different hormonal status. Aging Cell. 2015;14:236–48.

Qaisar R, Renaud G, Hedstrom Y, Pollanen E, Ronkainen P, Kaprio J, Alen M, Sipila S, Artemenko K, Bergquist J, Kovanen V. Hormone replacement therapy improves contractile function and myonuclear organization of single muscle fibres from postmenopausal monozygotic female twin pairs. J Physiol. 2013;591:2333–44.

Ronkainen PHA, Kovanen V, Alen M, Pollanen E, Palonen EM, Ankarberg-Lindgren C, Hamalainen E, Trupeinen U, Kujula UM, Puolakka J, Kaprio J, Sipila S. Postmenopausal hormone replacement therapy modifies skeletal muscle composition and function: a study with monozygotic twin pairs. J Appl Physiol. 2009;107:25–33.

Rozenberg S, Vandromme J, Antoine C. Postmenopausal hormone therapy: risks and benefits. Nat Rev Endocrinol. 2013;9:216–27.

Salpeter SR, Cheng J, Thabene L, Buckley EE, Salpeter NS. Bayesian meta-analysis of hormone therapy and mortality in younger postmenopausal women. Am J Med. 2009;122:1016–22.

Schierbeck LL, Rejnmark L, Torteng CL, Stigren L, Eiken P, Mosekilde L, Kober L, Jensen JEB. Effect of hormone replacement therapy on cardiovascular events in recently postmenopausal women: randomized trial. Br Med J. 2012;345, e6409.

Sipila S, Taafe DR, Cheng S, Puolakka J, Toivanen J, Suominen H. Effects of hormone replacement therapy and high-impact physical exercise on skeletal muscle in post-menopausal women: a randomized placebo-controlled study. Clin Sci. 2001;101:147–57.

Sipila S, Finni T, Kovanen V. Estrogen influences on neuromuscular function in postmenopausal women. Calcif Tissue Int. 2015;96:222–33.

Sitnick M, Foley AM, Brown M, Spangenburg EE. Ovariectomy prevents the recovery of atrophied gastrocnemius skeletal muscle mass. J Appl Physiol. 2006;100:286–93.

Skelton DA, Phillips SK, Bruce AS, Naylot CH, Woledge RC. Hormone replacement therapy increases isometric muscle strength of adductor pollicis in post-menopausal women. Clin Sci. 1999;96:257–364.

Sonobe T, Inagaki T, Sudo M, Poole DC, Kano Y. Sex differences in intracellular Ca^{2+} accumulation following eccentric contractions of rat skeletal muscle in vivo. Am J Physiol Regul Integr Comp Physiol. 2010;299:R1006–12.

Spangenburg EE, Geiger PC, Leinwand LA, Lowe DA. Regulation of physiological and metabolic function of muscle by female sex steroids. Med Sci Sports Exerc. 2012;44:1653–62.

Stupka N, Tiidus PM. Effects of ovariectomy and estrogen on ischemia-reperfusion injury in hindlimbs of female rats. J Appl Physiol. 2001;91:1828–35.

Suzuki S, Brown CM, Dela-Cruz CD, Yang E, Bridwell DA, Wise PM. Timing of estrogen therapy after ovariectomy dictates the efficacy of its neuroprotective and anti-inflammatory actions. Proc Natl Acad Sci U S A. 2007;104:6013–8.

Taafe DR, Siplia S, Cheng S, Puolakka J, Toivanen J, Suominen H. The effect of hormone replacement therapy and/or exercise n skeletal muscle attenuation in postmenopausal women: a yearlong intervention. Clin Physiol Funct Imaging. 2005;25:297–304.

Thomas A, Bunyan K, Tiidus PM. Oestrogen receptor-alpha activation augments post-exercise muscle myoblast proliferation. Acta Physiol. 2010;198:81–9.

Tidball JG. Inflammatory processes in muscle injury and repair. Am J Physiol Regul Integr Comp Physiol. 2005;288:R345–53.

Tiidus PM. Can estrogens diminish exercise induced muscle damage? Can J Appl Physiol. 1995;20:26–38.

Tiidus PM. Radical species in inflammation and overtraining. Can J Physiol Pharmacol. 1998;76:533–8.

Tiidus PM. Influence of estrogen and gender on muscle damage, inflammation and repair. Exerc Sport Sci Rev. 2003;31:40–4.

Tiidus PM, Bombardier E. Oestrogen attenuates myeloperoxidase activity in skeletal muscle of male rats. Acta Physiol Scand. 1999;166:85–90.

Tiidus PM, Holden D, Bombardier E, Zajchowski S, Enns D, Belcastro A. Estrogen effect on post-exercise skeletal muscle neutrophil infiltration and calpain activity. Can J Physiol Pharmacol. 2001;79:400–6.

Tiidus PM, Deller M, Liu XL. Estrogen influence on myogenic satellite cells following downhill running in male rats; a preliminary study. Acta Physiol Scand. 2005;184:67–72.

Tiidus PM, Lowe DA, Brown M. Estrogen replacement and skeletal muscle: mechanisms and population health. J Appl Physiol. 2013;115:569–78.

Vandenboom R, Gittings W, Smith IC, Grange RW, Stull JT. Myosin phosphorylation and force potentiation in skeletal muscle: evidence from animal models. J Muscle Res Cell Motil. 2013;34:317–32.

Velders M, Schleipen B, Fritzemeier KH, Zierau O, Diel P. Selective estrogen receptor-beta activation stimulates skeletal muscle growth and regeneration. FASEB J. 2012;26:1909–20.

Warren GL, Palubinskas LE. Human and animal experimental muscle injury models. In: Tiidus PM, editor. Muscle damage and repair. Champaign IL: Human Kinetics; 2008. p. 13–36.

Wiik A, Gustafsson T, Esbjornsson M, Johansson O, Ekman M, Sundberg CJ, Jansson E. Expression of oestrogen receptor α and β is higher in skeletal muscle of highly endurance-trained than moderately active men. Acta Physiol Scand. 2005;184:105–12.

Yin H, Price F, Rudnicki MA. Satellite cells and the muscle stem cell niche. Physiol Rev. 2013;93:23–67.

Chapter 6
Nutritional Strategies and Sex Hormone Interactions in Women

Nancy J. Rehrer, Rebecca T. McLay-Cooke and Stacy T. Sims

Introduction

There are a number of nutrients, foods and supplements the manipulation of which has the potential to augment health and/or exercise performance and/or recovery. The focus of this chapter is to address those dietary manipulations that have particular relevance for women. By and large these are related to differences imposed by female sex hormone fluctuations and decreases with age, or in response to stressors, including exercise training load and energy balance. This chapter begins by addressing those elements of the diet known to have the largest effect on and be altered by exercise, beginning with energy supply and macronutrient intakes, particularly carbohydrate and protein. The varying impact of manipulation will be highlighted with respect to timing of intake relative to exercise. This is followed by a discussion of fluid and electrolyte handling and application to thermal regulation, exercise tolerance and exercise associated hyponatraemia. Hereafter, oestrogen as an antioxidant is discussed and a number of more minor nutrients are highlighted that, due to specific action of oestrogen, or lack thereof, may warrant increased consumption.

N.J. Rehrer, B.A., M.Sc., Ph.D. (✉)
School of Physical Education Sport & Exercise Sciences, University of Otago,
46 Union St West, PO Box 56, Dunedin 9054, Otago, New Zealand
e-mail: nancy.rehrer@otago.ac.nz

R.T. McLay-Cooke, B.Ph.Ed., B.Sc., M.Sc.
Department of Human Nutrition, University of Otago, Dunedin 9054, Otago, New Zealand

S.T. Sims, B.A., M.Sc., Ph.D.
Health, Sport and Human Performance, University of Waikato, 52 Miro Street,
Adams Centre for High Performance, Mount Maunganui 3116, New Zealand

© Springer International Publishing Switzerland 2017
A.C. Hackney (ed.), *Sex Hormones, Exercise and Women*,
DOI 10.1007/978-3-319-44558-8_6

Energy and Macronutrients

Traditionally high/er carbohydrate diets have been recommended for athletes engaging in endurance and high intensity intermittent exercise (Jeukendrup 2011; Broad and Cox 2008). This recommendation has been established on the basis that both forms of exercise, either as a result of the duration or dominance of carbohydrate as a substrate, put a drain on body carbohydrate stores. Based on research conducted primarily in males, it has been assumed that these recommendations would translate equally well for the female population performing similar activity. Evidence from metabolic studies conducted in animal and human populations indicate that both oestrogen and progesterone have varying effects on carbohydrate, lipid and protein metabolism. Specifically, the female sex hormones appear to have an influence on insulin-stimulated and contraction-stimulated glucose uptake (Hansen et al. 1996; Latour et al. 2001; Campbell and Febbraio 2002; Van Pelt et al. 2003), glycogen storage (Nicklas et al. 1989; Hackney 1990; McLay et al. 2007), plasma glucose availability during exercise (Campbell et al. 2001; Zderic et al. 2001; Devries et al. 2006), whole body glucose kinetics (D'Eon et al. 2002), lipolysis (Casazza et al. 2004), cellular capacity for fatty acid oxidation (Campbell and Febbraio 2001) and protein catabolism (Lamont et al. 1987; Lariviere et al. 1994; Kriengsinyos et al. 2004). Further, it is highly conceivable that the ingestion of specific nutrients before, during and after exercise has the potential to affect the impact of the ovarian hormones on metabolism, raising the possibility that sex-specific or even hormonal-status specific dietary guidelines for exercising females may be warranted.

The following sections are limited to describing nutritional strategies where research has been conducted using exercising females and variation in ovarian hormones (e.g., menstrual cycle phase or oral contraceptive use) has been incorporated. To date, this research is limited to manipulation of carbohydrate and protein intake and predominantly in relation to endurance exercise. Research investigating low-carbohydrate, high-fat diets (acute and chronic adaptation and fat adaptation with carbohydrate restoration) has almost exclusively been conducted using male participants (Burke 2015). As a consequence, the research in this area that incorporates fluctuations in ovarian hormones is non-existent.

Habitual Diet

Few studies have actually tested the impact of modifying the habitual diet of female athletes prior to exercise. Those that have been conducted have used a variety of protocols, performance tests and female participants in various states of hormonal influence, making it difficult to discern consistent results. Increasing the daily carbohydrate content (up to 8 g/kg body weight per day) of the habitual diet of well-trained eumenorrhoeic female cyclists in the week preceding cycling exercise to fatigue has been shown to both improve performance (O'Keeffe et al. 1989) and to also have no effect (Reznik

Dolins et al. 2003). The application of these results is limited as the research was either conducted in only one phase of the menstrual cycle (Reznik Dolins et al. 2003) or did not include any control of menstrual cycle phase (O'Keeffe et al. 1989).

Recently, an empirical estimate of the protein requirements of female endurance athletes undertaking training of moderate intensity and duration (1.5 h day^{-1}) during the midfollicular phase of the menstrual cycle was determined using nitrogen balance (Houltham and Rowlands 2014). Estimated mean protein requirement was 1.63 g kg^{-1} day^{-1}, which is similar to previous estimates for men, but somewhat higher compared to previous non-empirical estimates for endurance training women (1.2–1.4 g kg^{-1} day^{-1}). This appears to be the first study of its kind to incorporate and control for the potential effects of menstrual cycle phase.

Nutrient Intake in the Days Before Exercise

Results of early research suggested menstrual cycle phase might influence muscle glycogen concentration (Nicklas et al. 1989), which in turn, has the potential to affect subsequent exercise capacity or performance of eumenorrhoeic female athletes (Nicklas et al. 1989). Carbohydrate loading is a performance-enhancement strategy often used by endurance athletes before competition to increase muscle glycogen stores in an effort to improve performance in events lasting longer than 90 min (Sedlock 2008). Recent 'modified' versions of the approach involve combining a high dietary carbohydrate intake and exercise taper for several days prior to competition (Sedlock 2008). Only a small number of studies have attempted to elucidate this relationship by investigating the impact of a modified carbohydrate loading regime prior to exercise in females under a variety of hormonal influences. Carbohydrate loading (8.4–9 g kg body weight^{-1} day^{-1}) has been shown to increase muscle glycogen concentration in the midfollicular phase of the menstrual cycle (Paul et al. 2001; Tarnopolsky et al. 2001; McLay et al. 2007). In contrast, following carbohydrate loading during the midluteal phase, muscle glycogen concentration has remained unchanged (McLay et al. 2007) or shown only a modest increase (13%) (Walker et al. 2000) compared to what is generally reported for male athletes (18–47%) (Sherman et al. 1981; Rauch et al. 1995; Hawley et al. 1997; Burke et al. 2000; Tarnopolsky et al. 2001; Rauch et al. 2005) or female athletes during the follicular phase (17–31%) (Paul et al. 2001; McLay et al. 2007; Tarnopolsky et al. 2001).

The impact of carbohydrate loading on the muscle glycogen content of oral contraceptive users is even less clear. Endurance trained female athletes taking a triphasic oral contraceptive (ethinyl oestradiol/levonorgestrel) showed increased muscle glycogen concentration following carbohydrate loading in both the midfollicular and midluteal phases (James et al. 2001). However, unlike a normal natural menstrual cycle where resting levels of both oestradiol and progesterone are higher during the midluteal than midfollicular phase, James et al. (2001) reported no difference in the levels of ovarian hormones between phases at the time muscle glycogen content was measured. This lack of difference in hormone profiles between phases raises the possibility that the midluteal phase could actually be interpreted in the same way as the midfollicular phase results from this study, potentially adding to the evidence that carbohydrate loading in the midfollicular phase increases resting muscle glycogen content (Hackney 1990; Paul et al. 2001; McLay et al. 2007; Tarnopolsky et al. 2001). At this time it is unknown what effect carbohydrate loading may have on muscle glycogen concentration in female athletes taking an oral contraceptive with a different chemical composition.

Although the lower level of muscle glycogen storage in the midfollicular phase of the menstrual cycle appears to be overcome by carbohydrate loading, this has not necessarily always translated into improved time trial performance (Paul et al. 2001; McLay et al. 2007). In contrast, cycle time to exhaustion at 80% VO_2max, measured during the midluteal phase of the menstrual cycle, increased (approximately 9 min) in response to the small CHO loading induced improvement in muscle glycogen concentration (Walker et al. 2000), whereas time trial performance was not improved following carbohydrate loading in the midluteal phase (McLay et al. 2007).

As with research conducted using male participants, there are a number of factors that can influence performance outcomes in studies investigating carbohydrate loading. These include the training status of the participants; the, often, small sample sizes used; the pre-loading glycogen depletion; the type of exercise performance test that is employed (e.g., time trial versus exercise to exhaustion); and the duration and intensity of the exercise undertaken prior to or as part of the performance assessment (Sedlock 2008; Correia-Oliveira et al. 2013). An additional factor to consider in research investigating the effect of menstrual cycle phase on performance outcomes is the magnitude and relative proportions of the fluctuations of the ovarian hormones. It has been proposed that a metabolic response to changes in the ovarian hormones (and the associated potential performance effects) occur only when the oestrogen to progesterone ratio (E/P) is elevated sufficiently in the luteal compared to follicular phase and the magnitude of the increase in oestrogen between the follicular and luteal phases is in the order of at least twofold or more (D'Eon et al. 2002; Oosthuyse and Bosch 2010). It is likely the effect of carbohydrate loading on performance in female athletes is also impacted by this particular hormone milieu.

Achieving the high intakes of CHO (≥ 8 g kg body weight^{-1} day^{-1}) needed for carbohydrate loading can be difficult for women whose habitual energy intakes are <2000 kcal day^{-1} (8400 kJ day^{-1}) (Tarnopolsky et al. 1995; Wismann and Willoughby 2006; Sedlock 2008), as this dose amounts to ingesting more than 90% of total energy intake as carbohydrate for a 60 kg woman. Therefore, women who attempt to carbohydrate load should pay particular attention to consuming sufficient total energy to achieve the necessary relative carbohydrate intake, especially during the follicular phase of the menstrual cycle.

Nutrient Intake in the Hours Before Exercise

Menstrual cycle phase appears to influence glucose kinetics during exercise due to the ability of oestrogen to impede gluconeogenesis (Matute and Kalkhoff 1973; Lavoie et al. 1987). Glucose rate of appearance in the luteal phase is reduced compared to the follicular phase when the energy demands of exercise are high enough to exert pressure on endogenous glucose production (>50% VO_2max) (Campbell et al. 2001; Zderic et al. 2001). The influence of menstrual cycle phase on glucose kinetics is evident in females who exercise in a fasted state but is negated by feeding in the pre-exercise period, as this reduces the demand on endogenous glucose production (Suh et al. 2002; Oosthuyse and Bosch 2010). Eumenorrhoeic female athletes should, therefore, follow the recommendation to consume a pre-exercise meal or snack containing carbohydrate 3–4 h before beginning endurance exercise, especially during the luteal phase of the menstrual cycle.

Exogenous ovarian hormones appear to exert greater effects on glucose flux during exercise than endogenous hormones, as decreases in glucose rate of appearance and disappearance can be observed in recently fed women taking a triphasic oral contraceptive compared to before oral contraceptive use (Suh et al. 2003). Findings from studies investigating oral contraceptive use and substrate utilisation may vary due to the use of different types of oral contraceptive agents, monophasic vs. triphasic and different oral contraceptive formulations, and varied definitions of oral contraceptive phase (Rechichi et al. 2009). As well as the acute effects, oral contraceptive use may have effects on glucose kinetics that persist into the inactive phase (Suh et al. 2003). Female athletes using a triphasic oral contraceptive should, therefore, ensure carbohydrate is consumed prior to exercise during both the active and inactive phases.

Nutrient Intake During Exercise

Carbohydrate ingestion has a positive influence during endurance exercise (Temesi et al. 2011; Cermak and van Loon 2013). However, the majority of research has been conducted using trained male participants and the findings generalised and applied to female athletes. The performance of moderately trained females can be improved with carbohydrate supplementation during endurance exercise compared to a placebo (Sun et al. 2015; Campbell et al. 2001; Bailey et al. 2000). When exogenous glucose is provided during exercise to ovulatory females, the influence of the menstrual cycle phase on glucose kinetics is minimised as the demand for endogenous glucose production is reduced (Campbell et al. 2001). Further, menstrual cycle phase appears to have little impact on performance under these conditions (Campbell et al. 2001; Bailey et al. 2000), although amino acid catabolism was reduced when carbohydrate supplementation was provided during exercise (Bailey et al. 2000). Also of interest is the finding that provision of a carbohydrate-electrolyte beverage during endurance exercise in the heat attenuates immune disturbances compared to a placebo beverage, especially in the luteal phase of the menstrual cycle (Hashimoto et al. 2014). During the follicular phase in endurance-trained women the highest rates of exogenous carbohydrate oxidation and greatest endogenous carbohydrate sparing were observed when carbohydrate was ingested at a rate of 1.0 g min^{-1} (60 g h^{-1}) with no further increases when the rate was increased to 1.5 g min^{-1} (90 g h^{-1}) (Wallis et al. 2007). In light of the limited data available it would seem prudent to recommend eumenorrhoeic female endurance athletes ingest carbohydrate at a rate of 60 g h^{-1} during exercise to offset menstrual cycle effects on glucose kinetics/exercise metabolism, and to limit potential immune disturbances in the heat and protein catabolism.

Nutrient Intake and Recovery from Exercise

Little is known on how extensively fluctuations in ovarian hormones may actually impact on post-exercise needs for recovery of energy stores or structural repair in exercising females. As with the influence of ovarian hormones on exercise metabolism, the impact on recovery may also be secondary to factors such as nutritional status/energy availability, exercise intensity and overall energy demand of exercise (Hausswirth and Le Meur 2011).

Following depleting exercise undertaken 4 days prior, muscle glycogen repletion has been shown to be reduced in the follicular phase compared to the luteal phase in moderately trained eumenorrhoeic women consuming a diet containing 56 % of energy intake from carbohydrate (Nicklas et al. 1989), suggesting a potential impairment in muscle glycogen resynthesis in the follicular phase. However, muscle glycogen repletion during the follicular phase of the menstrual cycle has been shown to occur in similar proportions to males following carbohydrate consumed in the hours after depleting exercise using both untrained (Kuipers et al. 1989) and endurance-trained (Tarnopolsky et al. 1997) participants. Further, post-exercise supplementation (1.2 g kg^{-1} of carbohydrate, 0.1 g kg^{-1} of protein and 0.02 g kg^{-1} of fat), following four training sessions across a week during the follicular phase, improved time to exhaustion during a subsequent bout of endurance exercise (Roy et al. 2002). These effects have not been tested during different phases of the menstrual cycle or in women taking oral contraceptives.

Eumenorrhoeic women should aim to consume carbohydrate as soon as possible following glycogen-depleting exercise, particularly during the follicular phase of the menstrual cycle, in order to maximise glycogen replenishment. This may be especially important if the next training session or event is likely to occur in <8 h.

Protein catabolism appears to be increased in the luteal phase compared with the follicular phase at rest (Lariviere et al. 1994; Kriengsinyos et al. 2004) and compared to the early follicular phase during prolonged exercise (Lamont et al. 1987; Bailey et al. 2000). It appears progesterone is responsible for the increased catabolism of protein in the luteal phase (Kriengsinyos et al. 2004). Oestrogen may have a role to play in reducing protein oxidation; however, this has only been observed in oestrogen supplemented men (Hamadeh et al. 2005a) and has not been examined across the menstrual cycle. It is possible the energy–protein ratio in the luteal phase of the menstrual cycle may also be an important determinant of the extent of protein catabolism in this phase (Oosthuyse and Bosch 2010).

The protein requirements for female endurance training women were recently estimated to be 1.63 g kg^{-1} day^{-1} (Houltham and Rowlands 2014). However, as this research was conducted in the follicular phase where the hormonal environment is potentially less catabolic, this may represent the minimal protein requirement across the menstrual cycle for women engaged in endurance training.

Research into the role of dietary protein ingested after exercise on recovery processes and subsequent performance in females is lacking. There is some evidence from research conducted in males that the consumption of protein, and the simultaneous ingestion of carbohydrate and protein, offer protection against exercise-induced muscle damage (Howatson and van Someren 2008). In contrast to research in males, high protein feeding immediately after and for 2 days following a 2.5 h high-intensity ride did not improve subsequent exercise performance in trained female cyclists (Rowlands and Wadsworth 2011). This research was undertaken in the follicular phase, and as noted previously, during this phase protein catabolism may be less than encountered in the luteal phase and this may have influenced the results of this study. Although not systematically tested across different phases of the menstrual cycle, exercise-induced muscle damage has been shown to negatively affect functional performance for several days in female athletes tested in the luteal phase (Keane et al. 2015). The pattern and magnitude of exercise-induced muscle damage showed differences compared to previous research in male athletes and is in contrast to animal research in which females have been shown to experience less damage than males.

In order to offset the potential increased protein catabolism and to protect against exercise-induced muscle damage, eumenorrhoeic women should focus on consuming protein, possibly coupled with carbohydrate, during the post-exercise recovery period in the luteal phase of the menstrual cycle. Endurance training women should endeavour to consume a diet containing around 1.6 g kg^{-1} day^{-1}, and possibly more, during the luteal phase.

Summary

Although speculative and open to adjustment and revision as more information becomes available, some broad recommendations regarding the manipulation of energy and macronutrient intake in relation to sex hormone interactions can be garnered from the currently available research. These recommendations are summarised in Table 6.1.

The research knowledge necessary to support potential gender-specific or hormone-status specific dietary guidelines is vast and as yet the field is barely in its infancy. Small steps have been taken with regard to endurance exercise but this is by no means complete. Additional avenues that may warrant exploration include the effect of a carbohydrate mouth rinse and fat adaptation with carbohydrate restoration. A broader scope beyond endurance exercise is needed and future research directions should include the impact of fluctuations in ovarian hormones on macronutrient-based nutritional strategies associated with ultra-endurance exercise, strength-based activities and high-intensity intermittent (team sport) exercise. For future studies investigating menstrual cycle phase variation, consideration should be given to the increase in oestrogen relative to progesterone in the luteal phase and the absolute magnitude of increase in oestrogen between any two menstrual phases.

Table 6.1 Potential macronutrient manipulations recommended for female athletes in relation to fluctuations in ovarian hormones

	Nutritional strategy	Target	Recommendation	Rationale
Habitual diet	Protein Requirement	Eumenorrhoeic, endurance training	Protein intake: ≥ 1.6 g kg^{-1} day^{-1}	Only assessed in the FP. A higher intake may be required in the LP due to increased protein catabolism at rest and during exercise.
Days before exercise	Modified CHO Loading	Eumenorrhoeic—FP[a], endurance	Increase energy intake by up to 30 % to achieve CHO intake >8 g kg^{-1} day^{-1} on CHO loading days.	To overcome lower muscle glycogen storage in FP.
Hours before exercise	Pre-Exercise Feeding	Eumenorrhoeic—LP[a], endurance Triphasic OC—active and inactive phases	High CHO meal or snack 3–4 h before exercise	To reduce demand on endogenous glucose production which can be suppressed in the luteal phase and under OC influence
During exercise	Exogenous source of CHO	Eumenorrhoeic, endurance	CHO intake: 60 g h^{-1} during prolonged exercise	To reduce demand on endogenous glucose production. Limit potential immune disturbance and protein catabolism.
Recovery after exercise	CHO Protein + CHO	Eumenorrhoeic—FP[a], endurance Eumenorrhoeic—LP[a], endurance, activities that induce muscle damage	Ingestion of CHO as soon as practical following prolonged glycogen-depleting exercise Co-ingestion of protein and CHO during the recovery period	To overcome potential reduced muscle glycogen resynthesis in FP. To offset increase in protein catabolism and protect against EIMD in the LP.

CHO carbohydrate, *EIMD* exercise-induced muscle damage, *FP* follicular phase, *LP* luteal phase, *OC* oral contraceptive
[a]Particular attention needed to adhere to the recommendation in this phase though benefits are likely in other phases too

Oral contraceptive use is prevalent in athletes (Rechichi et al. 2009) but data evaluating macronutrient manipulation and the effects of oral contraceptives is virtually non-existent and this needs to be addressed. What is becoming evident is that many researchers are now at least acknowledging the potential for menstrual cycle driven effects on metabolism and subsequent performance with numerous studies testing female participants during the mid-follicular phase. Unfortunately, by choosing this more subdued hormonal environment relative to the late follicular or luteal phases, interesting and informative interactions may be missed.

Fluids and Electrolytes

Thermoregulation and Body Fluids

It has been established that women and men differ in their thermoregulatory responses to exercise heat stress largely due to females having a reduced sudomotor function (Gagnon and Kenny 2012; 2011), thus decreasing evaporative heat loss capacity with the resultant increase in physiological strain (Moran et al. 1999; Kawahata 1960; Mack and Nadel 2010). Women and men display similar rates of heat dissipation at low requirements for heat loss; however, sex differences in sudomotor function have been demonstrated beyond a certain requirement for heat loss (Gagnon and Kenny 2012). On the other hand, when males and females display similar heat loss for a given heat production, females may display a higher change in body temperature due to physical characteristics (Mee et al. 2015; Gagnon et al. 2008). These results suggest that women may become hyperthermic in a shorter time period than men, consequently, women have been more frequently diagnosed as heat intolerant compared with males (Druyan et al. 2012; Charkoudian and Stachenfeld 2011), potentially putting them at greater risk of experiencing a heat-related illness.

Due to central and peripheral effects of female sex hormones and oral contraceptives on fluid balance and thermoregulation, women may be at a further disadvantage when exercising in warm conditions. Plasma volume (PV) is highest during the preovulatory phase of the menstrual cycle, when oestrogen levels are increasing. However, PV falls by as much as 8 % during the midluteal phase when both oestrogen and progesterone levels are elevated. Progesterone and oestrogen function in body fluid regulation by modifying sodium and water distribution rather than retention (Oian et al. 1987; Stachenfeld and Keefe 2002; Stachenfeld et al. 1999, 2001a; Bisson et al. 1992; Kang et al. 2001). Increased progesterone is associated with increased resting core and skin temperatures as well as changes in the threshold temperatures for sweating and active cutaneous vasodilation (Charkoudian and Johnson 1999; Charkoudian et al. 1999; Kolka and Stephenson 1997a, b; Stephens et al. 2002; Stephenson and Kolka 1999) These effects appear to result from a central thermoregulatory effect of progesterone (Kolka and Stephenson 1997a, b), which may also account for core temperature being elevated throughout the 28-day OC cycle relative to that in the natural menstrual cycle (Stachenfeld et al. 2000). Oestrogen also functions in vasodilation via modulation of prostacyclin and nitric oxide release (Charkoudian and Johnson 1997; Charkoudian et al. 1999; Hiroshoren 2002; Houghton et al. 2005). Moreover, plasma volume has been found to differ significantly in the two phases at higher ambient temperatures, as oestrogen enhances aldosterone-mediated sodium absorption in the renal tubules and increases nitric oxide-mediated vasodilation (Houghton et al. 2005; Kang et al. 2001; Salazar and Llinas 1996).

Charkoudian and Johnson (1999) reported that oral contraceptive use shifts baseline core temperature and the threshold for the active vasodilator system to higher internal temperatures via effects on the central thermoregulatory function. Further, it was reported that this shift in active vasodilation results in 43% lower skin blood flow for a given level of internal temperature during passive heating in the high hormone vs. low hormone phases of the oral contraceptive cycle; consistent with the theory that it is the progestational activity which dominates the effects of oestrogen on the central thermoregulatory mechanisms (Charkoudian and Johnson 1997). Further, Houghton and colleagues found that the nitric-oxide dependent portion of active vasodilation was greater in women taking an oral contraceptive with a lower vs. higher level of progestational bioactivity, with the higher level of progestation bioactivity associated with less relative nitric oxide contribution to reflex cutaneous vasodilation. Furthermore, it is suggested that the synthetic oestrogen and progestins found in oral contraceptive pills have similar influences on the cutaneous vascular response to heat stress. Charkoudian and Johnson (1999) investigated the effect of oral contraceptives on cutaneous vascular control during heat stress, expecting to find an inhibition of the active cutaneous vasodilator system. They determined that oral contraceptives inhibit skin blood flow in response to body heating and that they cause the function of the cutaneous active vasodilator system to be shifted to higher internal temperatures, similar to that observed in the midluteal phase of the menstrual cycle. Moreover, central influences of oestrogen and progesterone on hypothalamic thermoregulatory centres have been reported (Stephenson and Kolka 1988; Stephenson et al. 1989; Stephenson and Kolka 1999; Stachenfeld et al. 2000). Increases in the threshold for cutaneous vasodilation and sweating during heat stress in the luteal phase have been attributed to an increase in the hypothalamic thermoregulatory set-point temperature, thus, the heat dissipation effector functions are not initiated until this higher set-point temperature is reached.

Plasma volume maintenance can be important for exercise performance, especially in the heat (Berger et al. 2006). Fluid balance is often not achieved as a result of an inability to take on sufficient fluids or limits to gastric emptying, preventing the rate of ingestion and absorption from matching sweat rate (Maughan et al. 1997, 2007). In these situations plasma volume can decrease considerably. Therefore, an increased plasma volume can have positive implications for those exercising in thermally challenging environments in which large sweat losses occur. One method of inducing hyperhydration and hypervolaemia—originally developed to help offset effects of plasma volume loss in microgravity (Greenleaf et al. 1997; Fortney et al. 1984)—is 'sodium loading'. A sodium concentrated beverage composed of sodium citrate and sodium chloride (164 mmol $Na^+ \cdot L^{-1}$), with moderate osmolality (253 mOsm kg^{-1}), has been shown to be effective in inducing hyperhydration and hypervolaemia at rest in both phases of the menstrual cycle, although attenuated in the high hormonal state, irrespective of pill usage (Sims et al. 2007a). This sodium-loading strategy has also been found to be effective in aerobically trained men in warm conditions (Greenleaf et al. 1997, 1998a, b; Sims et al. 2007b). Moreover, earlier studies (Frey et al. 1991) demonstrated that ingested saline solutions between 0.9 and 1.07 % expanded plasma volume over a 4-h post ingestion time period. Frey and colleagues (Frey et al. 1991) determined that the 1.07 % saline solution elicited the greatest plasma volume expansion and urine concentration over the 4-h post-ingestion period; however, the addition of 1 % glucose did not improve the effectiveness of plasma volume expansion, but did increase diuresis. Thus, the authors concluded that a slightly hypertonic saline-only solution provided the most effective means of plasma volume expansion.

Electrolyte Handling and Imbalances

Menstrual cycle hormones affect fluid dynamics by altering capillary permeability, vasomotor function, the central set-point control of renal hormones and plasma osmolality (Charkoudian and Stachenfeld 2011). The elevation in plasma progesterone concentration during the luteal phase inhibits aldosterone-dependent sodium reabsorption in the kidneys due to progesterone competing with aldosterone for the mineralocorticoid receptor. Moreover, Eijsvogels and colleagues (2013) determined that women demonstrate a post-exercise increase in plasma volume concomitant with a decreased plasma sodium concentration as compared to age-and fitness-matched men; suggesting that the control of fluid balance is regulated differently between the sexes during prolonged exercise.

Both oestrogens and progestogens can influence neural and hormonal control of thirst, fluid intake, sodium appetite and sodium regulation. Moreover, there are sex differences in the activity and stimulus of the cell bodies of the periventricular nuclei and the supra-optic nuclei (located in the anterior hypothalamus), where arginine vasopressin is synthesised (Ishunina and Swaab 1999; Sar and Stumpf 1980). Stachenfeld and colleagues demonstrated an oestrogen associated shift to an earlier threshold in the osmotic sensitivity of thirst and release of arginine vasopressin, indicating a smaller increase in plasma osmolality is required to trigger arginine vasopressin release and thirst in the brain. This shift persists during OC use (Stachenfeld and Keefe 2002; Stachenfeld et al. 2001b; Verney 1947)).

Exercise-associated hyponatraemia (EAH) refers to a clinically relevant reduction in the serum, plasma or blood sodium concentration during or up to 24 h after physical activity [99]. This can be a result of solute (primarily sodium) loss and/or excess fluid load (Hew-Butler et al. 2015). Women are at greater risk for EAH and this risk has been primarily attributed to their lower body weight and size, excess water ingestion and longer racing times relative to men (Almond et al. 2005). While these factors may contribute to the greater incidence of hyponatraemia in women, it is likely that the differential effects of female sex hormones on sodium handling play a role.

Menopause, Ageing and Hydration

Independent of menopause, ageing in itself has important effects on fluid balance. Ageing is associated with a higher baseline plasma osmolality, coupled with an age-related blunting of thirst sensation during exercise (and water deprivation); the usual thirst mechanism that occurs with a drop in fluid volume (dehydration) is impaired (Stachenfeld et al. 1998). Older women are slower to excrete water (as compared to younger, premenopausal women) increasing the risk of hyponatraemia (Rosner et al. 2013; Stachenfeld 2014). Moreover, rehydration is a slower process with ageing, primarily due to slower kidney function and hormonal responses to sodium and water flux. Oestrogen-based hormone replacement therapy results in an increased basal plasma osmolality, plasma volume expansion, and an earlier osmotic threshold for arginine vasopressin release (e.g., 280 vs. 285 mOsmol kg^{-1} H$_2$O), but a reduction in urine output, resulting in greater overall fluid retention. This overall fluid retention is, however, not due to increased free-water retention, but rather increased sodium retention—the synthetic oestrogens inducing a reduction in sodium excretion (Stachenfeld et al. 1998, 2001b), eliciting a slight reduction in the hyponatraemic risk.

Summary

Drinking fluids with a higher sodium concentration than in regular sports drinks, before exercise, can elicit a transient hypervolaemic response that is partly preserved (relative to a low-sodium beverage) in exercise and is associated with improved physiological status and exercise capacity in warm conditions in female athletes. In women susceptible to EAH, more fluid is retained and more sodium lost when both oestradiol and progesterone are elevated. As women are at greater risk of EAH, knowledge of the hormonal status of women who develop it may prove helpful in the prevention of EAH. Moreover, during long-lasting exercise special care should be taken to monitor fluid and electrolytes in women susceptible to hyponatraemia when both oestrogen and progesterone are elevated, such as during pregnancy, while taking oral contraceptives, during the luteal phase of the menstrual cycle, and in perimenopausal athletes.

Oestrogen and Antioxidants

Oestrogen has wide-ranging metabolic effects impacting on immune and tissue integrity, energy stores and repair. Most recently its role as a potent antioxidant has been touted with evidence provided from research with numerous animal models and in humans. Differences between men and women in inflammatory disease states, coronary heart and cardiovascular disease, and quite possibly longevity, have been suggested to be attributed to differences in antioxidant capacity (Vina et al. 2005) (see Fig. 6.1).

Fig. 6.1 Theoretical relationship between oestrogen ROS and longevity of females (Adapted from Vina et al. (2005))

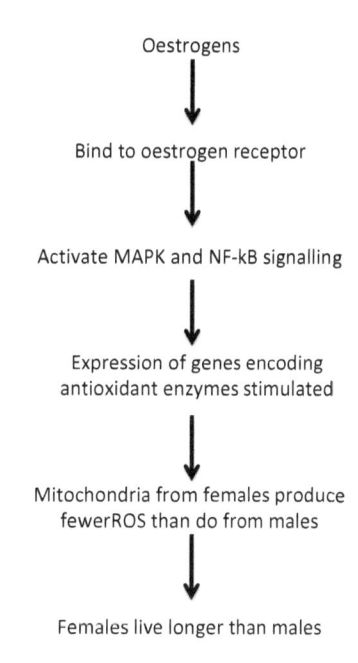

Oestrogens
↓
Bind to oestrogen receptor
↓
Activate MAPK and NF-kB signalling
↓
Expression of genes encoding antioxidant enzymes stimulated
↓
Mitochondria from females produce fewerROS than do from males
↓
Females live longer than males

Reactive oxygen species (ROS), although integral in the immune response and signalling pathways, can result in lipid peroxidation, cellular and mitochondrial membrane and DNA damage as well as protein and low-density lipoprotein (LDL) oxidation (Kehrer 1993). Exercise with a high rate of flux through the electron transport chain and/or increased hypoxanthine production and catabolism increases ROS production (Sjödin et al. 1990). Females have higher immune responses and lower oxidation and inflammation than male mammals, but this is reduced in ovariectomised females (Baeza et al. 2011), and reinstated with oestradiol supplementation (Stupka and Tiidus 2001) as in menopausal women reinstated with oestrogens and progestins (Tranquilli et al. 1995). Most human studies have been done in postmenopausal women, with and without hormone replacement therapy or in amenorrhoeic in contrast to eumenorrhoeic (Ayres et al. 1998) (Massafra et al. 1996). With the increase in lipid peroxidation and associated potential membrane damage with lack of oestrogen in females a case might be made for increased vitamin E supplementation in postmenopausal or amenorrhoeic women engaged in strenuous exercise regimens. However, Akova et al. (2001) observed a greater effect of endogenous oestrogen level on post exercise damage than vitamin E, with no synergistic effect.

Differences across the menstrual cycle are less well studied and findings not all consistent especially regarding the responses of varying measures of oxidative stress and antioxidant systems (See Fig. 6.2 for an overview of major endogenous antioxidant systems.).

Chung et al. (1999) observed subtle differences in total glutathione and oxidation thereof in response to exercise between the luteal and follicular phases of the menstrual cycle and concluded that there was a nominal menstrual cycle effect on

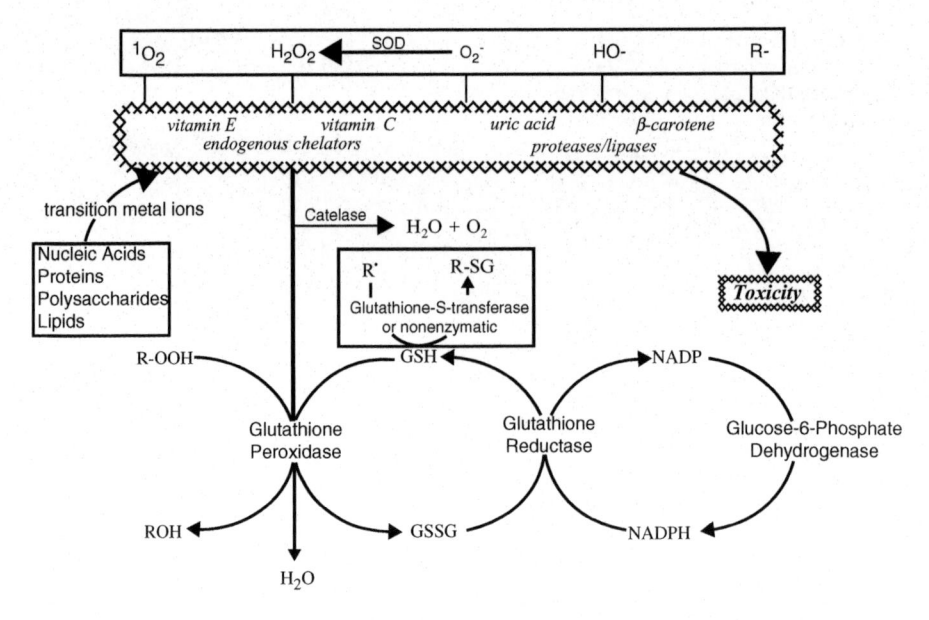

Fig. 6.2 Overview of endogenous antioxidant systems [from (Kehrer 1993)]

this endogenous antioxidant system. Joo et al. (2004) also noted an inverse correlation between superoxide dismutase activity and oestrogen concentration but reduced thiobarbituric acid reactive substances (Tbars) (indicating lipid peroxidation) in response to exercise in the late follicular compared to midluteal phases, and total superoxide dismutase activity greatest after exercise in the luteal phase.

More recently, however, Cornelli et al. (2013) monitored oxidative stress (hydroperoxides) every 3 days over the menstrual cycle and found that the greatest oxidative stress was at the oestrogen peak, decreasing through the progestin (luteal) phase until the end of the cycle. They concluded that oestrogen itself was not an antioxidant, but rather prooxidant, like exercise, such that, in response, antioxidant systems were upregulated. There is, however, considerable conflicting evidence, supporting oestrogen's role as an antioxidant. The varying models, species, methodologies and timing of measurement may explain some of the contradiction in findings and interpretation thereof.

If Cornelli et al.'s (2013) findings and conclusions are upheld, it may be that supplementing premenopausal women with antioxidants may not only be ineffective, but counterproductive.

Research conducted analysing vitamin C (ascorbic acid) and its oxidised state (dehydroascorbic acid) across the menstrual cycle demonstrated that ascorbic acid concentration and total antioxidant plasma status were greatest during ovulation when oestrogen peaks and in the midluteal phase, with dehydroascorbic acid greatest at menstruation and the midfollicular phases (Michos et al. 2006). From this study it is concluded that in eumenorrhoeic women antioxidant responses are modulated in concert with oestrogen and may offer protection in times of particular need.

Whether vitamin C and/or vitamin E supplementation could offer protection from damaging levels of oxidative stress and inflammatory responses, particularly after increased or unaccustomed exercise or other situations of ischaemia/reperfusion, in postmenopausal women is open to conjecture. However, in a study of more than 34,000 postmenopausal women only dietary vitamin E was associated with reduced coronary disease (proposed to be related to LDL oxidation) but isolated vitamin supplementation was not (Kushi et al. 1996).

Furthermore, antioxidant vitamin supplementation can reduce adaptations to endurance training as well as hinder the cellular adaptation to become more oxidant resistant, including upregulation of endogenous antioxidant systems (For review see Petrnelij and Coombes (2011)). There are, however, conflicting results, probably due to varying levels of supplementation, training status, exercise type, load and measure of oxidation status. It can be tentatively concluded that high doses of individual antioxidant vitamins, in most well-nourished (non-deficient) individuals, will not enhance physical performance, and although they may reduce exercise related oxidation there is no clear evidence that this confers any recovery or health advantage (Peternelj and Coombes 2011).

An interesting finding was made in a study comparing antioxidant capacity and muscle enzyme leakage after exhausting exercise on low and high CHO diets across the menstrual cycle (Klapcinska et al. 2002). A number of antioxidant enzyme systems were improved on the low CHO diet supported by reduced membrane leakage of creatine kinase into plasma, with no significant menstrual cycle phase effects. The authors attributed the improvement in antioxidant function to the greater vitamin E, selenium and haem iron consumed on the low CHO diet (Klapcinska et al. 2002), although changes in the fatty acid composition of the diet or other nutrients cannot be discounted.

The limited available data suggest that further research is warranted to assess positive or negative effects of antioxidant vitamin supplementation in a systematic manner, particularly in women during specific phases of the menstrual cycle while heavily training, and in those with low circulating sex hormones.

Soy and Isoflavones

Soy is the predominant dietary source of isoflavones, one of several classes of phytoestrogens (oestrogen mimickers derived from plants which can bind to oestrogen receptors) (Cederroth and Nef 2009). Although some have found beneficial metabolic effects (including lower body mass index (BMI), higher high density lipoproteins (HDL), lower low density lipoproteins (LDL), lower blood glucose and insulin) in postmenopausal women who consume soy or soy-based purified phytoestrogens, this is not universally observed (Cederroth and Nef 2009). Furthermore there has been some concern that due to its oestrogen-like functionality, it may be promote breast cancer, thus those at risk or diagnosed have been advised to avoid phytoestrogens. In premenopausal women soy phytoestrogens (45 mg isoflavones) have been observed to decrease FSH and LH and a greater concentration of oestrogen has been observed in the follicular phase with 1 month of daily supplementation (Cassidy et al. 1994). However, the follicular phase and menstrual cycle was lengthened and the progestin peak delayed. This is somewhat at odds with earlier concerns regarding phytoestrogens and cancer propagation, and may infer a reduced risk of cancer due to less total time over a woman's life in the luteal phase. Additionally, cholesterol was observed to be lowered in these premenopausal women consuming phytoestrogens (Cassidy et al. 1994). There may be different longer term effects than those observed over the short term, as some adaptation may occur. In support of this is a study in which 100 mg of soy isoflavones were given for 1 year and no alteration in menstrual cycle length or hormone levels was observed (Maskarinec et al. 2002).

In a crossover study with young, eumenorrhoeic women receiving soy (52 mg isoflavones) or placebo "cookies" daily for one menstrual cycle, in addition to greater progesterone concentration 3 days before ovulation, the ratio of a marker of bone resorption/bone formation was higher at the midluteal phase (Zittermann et al. 2004). Whether this response would be observed with longer-term dietary intakes in young women and if this would have long-term negative consequences in terms of bone health is unknown. In contrast, in postmenopausal women a positive correlation has been observed between mineral bone density and phytoestrogen intake; however, this correlation was not observed in premenopausal women (Mei et al. 2001).

In a study with teenage swimmers, all with normal menstrual cycles, supplementation (26 days) with *Lippia citriodora* (lemon verbena) extract, in a beverage which also contained vitamins C and E, was observed to increase glutathione peroxidase and reductase activities in red blood cells, and superoxide dismutase activity in lymphocytes, to a greater extent after exercise than with just a beverage with vitamins C and E. This extract contains two phytoestrogens which have the potential to bind with oestrogen receptors. 17-β-oestradiol and testosterone were observed to be lower and sex hormone-binding globulin to be greater with the extract, in the basal condition as well as after exercise (Mestre-Alfaro et al. 2011). Although this phytoestrogen containing extract enhances antioxidant systems, it is questionable whether this group of young, regularly training and competing women would benefit from or be negatively impacted by the reduction in circulating, free, sex-hormones.

In support of phytoestrogens having antioxidant functionality, similar to oestrogen, a study in which daily consumption of soy milk (113–207 mg/day isoflavones for one menstrual cycle reduced lipid peroxidation in premenopausal women, with a greater effect in older women with lower doses (Nhan et al. 2005).

Another source of isoflavones is red clover. Results with supplementation with this source of isoflavone extract have been inconsistent. In one study 86 mg isoflavones were consumed per day, for three menstrual cycles, by premenopausal women and no alterations in cholesterol or cholesterol subtractions or other blood parameters were observed (Blakesmith et al. 2003). In another study, a similar amount of red clover isoflavones was consumed by premenopausal as well as postmenopausal women for 1 month (Campbell et al. 2004). They did, however, observe an increase in HDL cholesterol with supplementation, but this was only significant in postmenopausal women.

Although there have been some positive effects observed, particularly in postmenopausal women who use phytoestrogens as an alternative to hormone replacement therapy, long term risk and health benefits are unclear (Moreira et al. 2014; Patisaul and Jefferson 2010). Even less is known as to whether phytoestrogen supplementation enhances or reduces exercise training adaptations, including ROS signalling and endogenous antioxidant systems in this growing segment of the population.

Fish Oil

It has been proposed that enhancement of endothelial nitric oxide (NO) production and down-regulation of acute phase cytokines by oestrogen and fish oil may play a role in deterring the development or progression of Alzheimer's disease (McCarty 1999). The omega 3 fatty acids in fish have been proposed to reduce inflammation via inhibitory effects on Interleukin-1 (IL-1) and Interleukin-6 (IL-6) and may have a positive effect on endothelial NO production. Oestrogen can also increase endothelial NO formation and has an inhibitory effect on IL-6, both reducing inflammation. It has been suggested that some of the other negative effects of menopause may also be attributed to this increased inflammation (McCarty 1999). This being the case fish oil supplementation may be particularly beneficial in postmenopausal women.

A case has also been made for fish oil supplementation in premenopausal women who have premenstrual symptoms (PMS). It has been suggested that more rigid red blood cells result from linoleic acid insufficiency, or altered metabolism, thereby reducing prostaglandin E1 (PGE1) synthesis, which could make red blood cells less deformable. This could result in greater intracapillary pressures needed for blood flow, resulting in fluid movement into the extravascular compartment (Simpson 1988). If this could account for some of the PMS symptoms, then it is reasoned that by enhancing PGE1 synthesis through precursor fatty acids (e.g., found in fish oil or evening primrose oil) then the red blood cells would be more able to move through the capillaries at lower pressures and reduce fluid filtration and retention.

In a recent double blind, crossover study daily fish oil tablet (80 mg eicosapentaenoic acid and 120 mg docosahexaenoic acid) consumption for 3 months reduced premenstrual pain and ibuprofen use (Rahbar et al. 2012). Others have found similar results in combination with B-12 supplementation (Deutch et al. 2000). In a review of efficacy of treatment for dysmenorrhoea the use of fish oil was concluded to be "possibly effective", strength of recommendation "B" (Morrow and Naumburg 2009).

Although the strength of evidence is moderate, enhancing dietary intakes of fish or other sources of omega 3-rich foods or supplements have little to no known negative effects and may prove efficacious, for those with PMS and in postmenopausal or amenorrhoeic women. One cautionary note regarding fish or fish oil supplements, where the source of the fish and purity is unclear, is the possibility that mercury levels could pose health risks if consumed on a regular basis. However, it appears that supplements may not pose more of a risk of mercury toxicity than regular fish consumption (Foran et al. 2003; Hightower and Moore 2003).

Vitamin D/Calcium

Vitamin D and calcium are important for fertility (Stumpf and Denny 1989) and vitamin D is positively correlated with FSH concentration (Jukic et al. 2015). Decreasing calcium concentration and increases in parathyroid hormone have been theorised to play a role in premenstrual syndrome and supplementation may decrease symptoms (Thys-Jacobs 2000) and low vitamin D in the luteal phase may be involved (Thys-Jacobs et al. 2007). However, oestrogen plays a role in calcium regulation (Pitkin et al. 1978) and simply supplementing with calcium and or vitamin D will unlikely compensate for the lack of oestrogen in amenorrhoeic athletes (Baer et al. 1992), or postmenopausal women. The decreasing bone mineral density in athletes without menstrual cycles and the increase in bone density after resumption of menstruation (Drinkwater et al. 1986) are evidence hereof.

Branched Chain Amino Acids (BCAA)

There appears to be an effect of oestrogen on BCAA metabolism, such that the breakdown of these to keto-acids (leading to further catabolism for energy or gluconeogenesis) is inhibited and, thus, these amino acids are preserved for protein synthesis (Obayashi et al. 2004; Shimomura et al. 2001; Kobayashi et al. 1997). As the majority of this work has been conducted in animals it is unclear to what extent this applies to women, and if so, is there a menstrual cycle effect such that when oestrogen is low should protein intakes be increased, particularly when total energy and protein intakes are low and energy expenditure is high, such as often the case in endurance female athletes. In males, supplementing with oestrogen improved nitrogen balance during endurance exercise training (Hamadeh et al. 2005a). Implications for postmenopausal and amenorrhoeic athletes are as yet unclear. Further research is warranted to determine the applicability of these findings to women, with and without menses or on varying forms of hormonal contraception, and the extent to which possible alterations in BCAA metabolism influence muscle growth and repair.

Conclusions

There may well be menstrual cycle and/or female sex hormone effects on the metabolism of other nutrients or supplements of particular importance to women engaged in regular physical training, but research is limited. We focus on those with the most significant effects and summarise these in Table 6.2. We encourage future researchers to explore the specific effects and nutrient interactions modified by normal fluctuations and alterations in female sex hormones. As the majority of acute response and training studies delineating the impact of nutrients on exercise

Table 6.2 Summary of practical applications of nutrients with respect to female sex hormone alteration

Practical applications
Lower resting muscle glycogen in the follicular phase can be overcome by CHO loading but an increase in total energy intake may be required.
Pre-exercise feeding and/or CHO ingestion negate the oestrogen-induced reduction in gluconeogenesis during endurance exercise (>50 % VO_2max).
Female athletes need to pay extra attention to recovery nutrition in the luteal phase to offset the increase in protein catabolism.
Oestrogen and progesterone affect the hormonal and neural control of thirst, sodium regulation, and fluid retention, increasing the risk of hyponatraemia during the luteal phase of the menstrual cycle.
Hormone therapy in menopausal women lowers the threshold for osmotic AVP release, increased basal plasma volume expansion and decreased urine output, resulting in greater fluid retention.
Oestrogen enhances antioxidant capacity in females.
Supplementing with dietary sources of antioxidants may be prudent in those with amenorrhoea or in menopause, but may still not compensate for lack of oestrogen.
Fish oil (omega-3 fatty acid source) may aid in inflammatory disorders such as dysmenorrhoea and those associated with menopause.
Vitamin D and calcium play a role in fertility, possibly in dysmenorrhoea as well as bone health; however, they cannot fully compensate for lack of oestrogen.
Branched chain amino acid oxidation may be greater when oestrogen is low; this may have dietary implications for in those with amenorrhoea or in menopause, particularly when training regularly and/ or on low energy diets.

tolerance and impact have been conducted in males, recommendations for females are often based on male responses. We, as researchers that have undertaken intervention studies with females in varying phases of the menstrual cycle, realise the difficulties and time commitment necessary for this type of work and implore granting bodies to commit dedicated funds for more systematic study such that the knowledge base concerning women eventually equals that of men.

Acknowledgements The authors would like to thank Dr James D. Cotter for his insightful suggestions.

References

Akova B, Surmen-Gur E, Gur H, Dirican M, Sarandol E, Kucukoglu S. Exercise-induced oxidative stress and muscle performance in healthy women: role of vitamin E supplementation and endogenous oestradiol. Eur J Appl Physiol. 2001;84(1-2):141–7.

Almond CS, Shin AY, Fortescue EB, Mannix RC, Wypij D, Binstadt BA, et al. Hyponatremia among runners in the Boston Marathon. N Engl J Med. 2005;352(15):1550–6.

Ayres S, Baer J, Ravi Subbiah MT. Exercised-induced increase in lipid peroxidation parameters in amenorrheic female athletes. Fertil Steril. 1998;69(1):73–7. doi:10.1016/S0015-0282(97)00428-7. http://dx.doi.org.

Baer J, Taper L, Gwazdauskas F, Walberg J, Novascone M, Ritchey S, et al. Diet, hormonal, and metabolic factors affecting bone mineral density in adolescent amenorrheic and eumenorrheic female runners. J Sports Med Phys Fitness. 1992;32(1):51–8.

Baeza I, De Castro NM, Arranz L, Fdez-Tresguerres J, De la Fuente M. Ovariectomy causes immunosenescence and oxi-inflamm-ageing in peritoneal leukocytes of aged female mice similar to that in aged males. Biogerontology. 2011;12(3):227–38. doi:10.1007/s10522-010-9317-0. http://dx.doi.org.

Bailey S, Zacher C, Mittleman K. Effect of menstrual cycle phase on carbohydrate supplementation during prolonged exercise to fatigue. J Appl Physiol. 2000;88:690–7.

Berger NJA, Campbell IT, Wlkerson DP, Jones AM. Influence of acute plasma volume expansion on VO2 kineitics, VO2peak, and performance during high-intensity cycle exercise. J Appl Physiol. 2006;101:707–14.

Bisson DL, Dunster GD, O'Hare JP, Hampton D, Penney MD. Renal sodium retention does not occur during the luteal phase of the menstrual cycle in normal women. Br J Obstet Gynaecol. 1992;99:247–52.

Blakesmith SJ, Lyons-Wall PM, George C, Joannou GE, Petocz P, Samman S. Effects of supplementation with purified red clover (Trifolium pratense) isoflavones on plasma lipids and insulin resistance in healthy premenopausal women. Br J Nutr. 2003;89(4):467–74.

Broad E, Cox G. What is the optimal composition of an athlete's diet? Eur J Sport Sci. 2008;8(2):57–65.

Burke L. Re-examining high-fat diets for sports performance: did we call the 'nail in the coffin' too soon? Sports Med. 2015;45 Suppl 1:S33–49.

Burke L, Hawley J, Schabort E, St Clair Gibson A, Mujika I, Noakes T. Carbohydrate loading failed to improve 100-km cycling performance in a placebo-controlled trial. J Appl Physiol. 2000;88:1284–90.

Campbell S, Febbraio M. Effect of ovarian hormones on mitochondrial enzyme activity in fat oxidation pathway of skeletal muscle. Am J Physiol Endocrinol Metab. 2001;281:E803–8.

Campbell S, Febbraio M. Effect of ovarian hormones on GLUT4 expression and contraction-stimulated glucose uptake. Am J Physiol Endocrinol Metab. 2002;282:E1139–46.

Campbell S, Angus D, Febbraio M. Glucose kinetics and exercise performance during phases of the menstrual cycle: effect of glucose ingestion. Am J Physiol Endocrinol Metab. 2001;281: E817–25.

Campbell MJ, Woodside JV, Honour JW, Morton MS, Leathem AJ. Effect of red clover-derived isoflavone supplementation on insulin-like growth factor, lipid and antioxidant status in healthy female volunteers: a pilot study. Eur J Clin Nutr. 2004;58(1):173–9.

Casazza G, Jacobs K, Suh S-H, Miller B, Horning M, Brooks G. Menstrual cycle phase and oral contraceptive effects on triglyceride mobilisation during exercise. J Appl Physiol. 2004;97:302–9.

Cassidy A, Bingham S, Setchell KD. Biological effects of a diet of soy protein rich in isoflavones on the menstrual cycle of premenopausal women. Am J Clin Nutr. 1994;60(3):333–40.

Cederroth CR, Nef S. Soy, phytoestrogens and metabolism: a review. Mol Cell Endocrinol. 2009;304(1–2):30–42. doi:10.1016/j.mce.2009.02.027. http://dx.doi.org.

Cermak N, van Loon L. The use of carbohydrates during exercise as an ergogenic aid. Sports Med. 2013;43:1139–55.

Charkoudian N, Johnson JM. Modification of active cutaneous vasodilation by oral contraceptive hormones. J Appl Physiol. 1997;83(6):2012–8.

Charkoudian N, Johnson JM. Reflex control of cutaneous vasoconstrictor system is reset by exogenous female reproductive hormones. J Appl Physiol. 1999;87(1):381–5.

Charkoudian N, Stachenfeld NS. Reproductive hormone influences on thermoregulation in women, Comprehensive Physiology. Hoboken: Wiley; 2011.

Charkoudian N, Stephens DP, Pirkle KC, Kosiba WA, Johnson JM. Influence of female reproductive hormones on local thermal control of skin blood flow. J Appl Physiol. 1999;87(5):1719–23.

Chung S-C, Goldfarb AH, Jamurtas AZ, Hegde SS, Lee J. Effect of exercise during the follicular and luteal phases on indices of oxidative stress in healthy women. Med Sci Sports Exerc. 1999;31(3):409–13.

Cornelli U, Belcaro G, Cesarone MR, Finco A. Analysis of oxidative stress during the menstrual cycle. Reprod Biol Endocrinol. 2013;11:74. doi:10.1186/1477-7827-11-74. http://dx.doi.org.

Correia-Oliveira C, Bertuzzi R, Dal'Molin Kiss M, Lima-Silva A. Strategies of dietary carbohydrate manipulation and their effects of performance in cycling time trials. Sports Med. 2013;43:707–19.

D'Eon T, Sharoff C, Chipkin S, Grow D, Ruby B, Braun B. Regulation of exercise carbohydrate metabolism by estrogen and progesterone in women. Am J Physiol Endocrinol Metab. 2002;283:E1046–55.

Deutch B, Jørgensen EB, Hansen JC. Menstrual discomfort in Danish women reduced by dietary supplements of omega-3 PUFA and B 12 (fish oil or seal oil capsules). Nutr Res. 2000;20(5):621–31.

Devries M, Hamadeh M, Phillips S, Tarnopolsky M. Menstrual cycle phase and sex influence muscle glycogen utilization and glucose turnover during moderate-intensity endurance exercise. Am J Physiol Regul Integr Comp Physiol. 2006;291:R1120–8.

Drinkwater BL, Nilson K, Ott S, Chesnut CH. Bone mineral density after resumption of menses in amenorrheic athletes. JAMA. 1986;256(3):380–2.

Druyan A, Makranz C, Moran D, Yanovich R, Epstein Y, Heled Y. Heat tolerance in women: reconsidering the criteria. Aviat Space Environ Med. 2012;83(1):58–60. doi:10.3357/ASEM.3130.2012.

Eijsvogels TMH, Scholten RR, van Duijnhoven NTL, Thijssen DHJ, Hopman MTE. Sex difference in fluid balance responses during prolonged exercise. Scand J Med Sci Sports. 2013;23(2):198–206. doi:10.1111/j.1600-0838.2011.01371.x.

Foran SE, Flood JG, Lewandrowski KB. Measurement of mercury levels in concentrated over-the-counter fish oil preparations: is fish oil healthier than fish? Arch Pathol Lab Med. 2003;127(12):1603–5.

Fortney SM, Wenger CB, Bove JR, Nadel ER. Effect of hyperosmolality on control of blood flow and sweating. J Appl Physiol. 1984;57:1688–95.

Frey MAB, Riddle J, Charles JB, Bungo MW. Blood and urine responses to ingesting fluids of various salt and glucose-concentrations. J Clin Pharmacol. 1991;31(10):880–7.

Gagnon D, Kenny GP. Sex modulates whole-body sudomotor thermosensitivity during exercise. J Physiol. 2011;589(24):6205–17. doi:10.1113/jphysiol.2011.219220.

Gagnon D, Kenny GP. Sex differences in thermoeffector responses during exercise at fixed requirements for heat loss. J Appl Physiol. 2012;113(5):746–57. doi:10.1152/japplphysiol.00637.2012.

Gagnon D, Jay O, Lemire B, Kenny GP. Sex-related differences in evaporative heat loss: the importance of metabolic heat production. Eur J Appl Physiol. 2008;104(5):821–9. doi:10.1007/s00421-008-0837-0.

Greenleaf JE, Looft-Wilson R, Wisherd JL, McKenzie MA, Jensen CD, Whittam JH. Pre-Exercise hypervolemia and cycle ergometer endurance in men. Biol Sport. 1997;14:103–14.

Greenleaf JE, Jackson CG, Geelen G, Keil LC, Hinghofer-Szalkay H, Whittam JH. Plasma volume expansion with oral fluids in hypohydrated men at rest and during exercise. Aviat Space Environ Med. 1998a;69(9):837–44.

Greenleaf JE, Looft-Wilson R, Wisherd JL, Jackson CG, Fung PP, Ertl AC, et al. Hypervolemia in men from fluid ingestion at rest and during exercise. Aviat Space Environ Med. 1998b;69(4):374–86.

Hackney, AC. Effects of the menstrual cycle on resting muscle glycogen content. Horm Metab Res. 1990;22:647.

Hamadeh M, Devries M, Tarnopolsky M. Estrogen supplementation reduces whole body leucine and carbohydrate oxidation and increases lipid oxidation in men during endurance exercise. J Clin Endocrinol Metab. 2005;90(6):3592–9.

Hansen P, McCarthy T, Pasia E, Spina R, Gulve E. Effects of ovariectomy and exercise training on muscle GLUT-4 content and glucose metabolism in rats. J Appl Physiol. 1996;80(5):1605–11.

Hashimoto H, Ishijima T, Hayashida H, Suzuki K, Higuchi M. Menstrual cycle phase and carbohydrate ingestion alter immune response following endurance exercise and high intensity time trial performance test under hot conditions. J Int Soc Sports Nutr. 2014;11:39.

Hausswirth C, Le Meur Y. Physiological and nutritional aspects of post-exercise recovery: specific recommendations for female athletes. Sports Med. 2011;41(10):861–82. doi:10.2165/11593180-000000000-00000. http://dx.doi.org.

Hawley J, Palmer G, Noakes T. Effects of 3 days of carbohydrate supplementation on muscle glycogen content and utilisation during a 1-h cycling performance. Eur J Appl Physiol. 1997;75:407–12.

Hew-Butler T, Rosner MH, Fowkes-Godek S, Dugas JP, Hoffman MD, Lewis DP, et al. Statement of the third international exercise-associated hyponatremia consensus development conference, Carlsbad, California, 2015. Clin J Sport Med. 2015;25(4):303–20.

Hightower JM, Moore D. Mercury levels in high-end consumers of fish. Environ Health Perspect. 2003;111(4):604.

Hiroshoren N, Tzoran I, Makrienko I, Edoute Y, Plawner MM, Itskovitz-Eldor J, Jacob G. Menstrual cycle effects on the neurohumoral and autonomic nervous systems regulating the cardiovascular system. J Clin Endocrinol Metab. 2002;87(4):1569–75.

Houghton BL, Holowatz LA, Minson CT. Influence of progestin bioactivity on cutaneous vascular responses to passive heating. Med Sci Sports Exerc. 2005;37(1):45–51. discussion 2.

Houltham S, Rowlands D. A snapshot of nitrogen balance in endurance-trained women. Appl Physiol Nutr Metab. 2014;39:219–25.

Howatson G, van Someren K. The prevention and treatment of exercise-induced muscle damage. Sports Med. 2008;38(6):483–503.

Ishunina TA, Swaab DF. Vasopressin and oxytocin neurons of the human supraoptic and paraventricular nucleus; size changes in relation to age and sex. J Clin Endocrinol Metab. 1999;84(12):4637–44.

James A, Lorraine M, Cullen D, Goodman C, Dawson B, Palmer T, et al. Muscle glycogen supercompensation: absence of a gender-related difference. Eur J Appl Physiol. 2001;85:533–8.

Jeukendrup A. Nutrition for endurance sports: marathon, triathlon, and road cycling. J Sport Sci. 2011;29 Suppl 1:S91–9.

Joo MH, Maehata E, Adachi T, Ishida A, Murai F, Mesaki N. The relationship between exercise-induced oxidative stress and the menstrual cycle. Eur J Appl Physiol. 2004;93(1-2):82–6.

Jukic AM, Steiner AZ, Baird DD. Association between serum 25-hydroxyvitamin D and ovarian reserve in premenopausal women. Menopause. 2015;22(3):312–6. doi:10.1097/GME.0000000000000312. http://dx.doi.org.

Kang AK, Duncan JA, Cattran DC, Floras JS, Lai V, Scholey JW, Miller JA. Effect of oral contraceptives on the renin angiotensin system and renal function. Am J Physiol Regul Integr Comp Physiol. 2001;280:R807–13.

Kawahata A. Sex differences in sweating. In: Ito S, Ogata H, Yoshimura H, editors. Essential problems in climatic physiology. Kyoto, Japan: Nankodo Publ; 1960.

Keane K, Salicki R, Goodall S, Thomas K, Howatson G. Muscle damage response in female collegiate athletes after repeated sprint activity. J Strength Cond Res. 2015;29(10):2802–7.

Kehrer JP. Free radicals as mediators of tissue injury and disease. Crit Rev Toxicol. 1993;23(1):21–48. doi:10.3109/10408449309104073.

Klapcinska B, Sadowska-Krepa E, Manowska B, Pilis W, Sobczak A, Danch A. Effects of a low carbohydrate diet and graded exercise during the follicular and luteal phases on the blood antioxidant status in healthy women. Eur J Appl Physiol. 2002;87(4-5):373–80.

Kobayashi R, Shimomura Y, Murakami T, Nakai N, Fujitsuka N, Otsuka M, et al. Gender difference in regulation of branched-chain amino acid catabolism. Biochem J. 1997;327(Pt 2):449–53.

Kolka MA, Stephenson LA. Effect of luteal phase elevation in core temperature on forearm blood flow during exercise. J Appl Physiol. 1997a;82(4):1079–83.

Kolka MA, Stephenson LA. Resetting the thermoregulatory set-point by endogenous estradiol or progesterone in women. Ann N Y Acad Sci. 1997b;813:204–6.

Kriengsinyos W, Wykes L, Goonewardene L, Ball R, Pencharz P. Phase of menstrual cycle affects lysine requirement in healthy women. Am J Physiol Endocrinol Metab. 2004;287:E489–96.

Kuipers H, Saris W, Brouns F, Keizer H, ten Bosch C. Glycogen synthesis during exercise and rest with carbohydrate feeding in males and females. Int J Sports Med. 1989;10 Suppl 1:S63–7.

Kushi LH, Folsom AR, Prineas RJ, Mink PJ, Wu Y, Bostick RM. Dietary antioxidant vitamins and death from coronary heart disease in postmenopausal women. N Engl J Med. 1996;334(18): 1156–62. doi:10.1056/NEJM199605023341803.

Lamont L, Lemon P, Bruot B. Menstrual cycle and exercise effects on protein catabolism. Med Sci Sports Exerc. 1987;19(2):106–10.

Lariviere F, Moussalli R, Garrel D. Increased leucine flux and leucine oxidation during the luteal phase of the menstrual cycle in women. Am J Physiol Endocrinol Metab. 1994;267:E422–8.

Latour M, Shinoda M, Lavoie J-M. Metabolic effects of physical training in ovariectomized and hyperestrogenic rats. J Appl Physiol. 2001;90:235–41.

Lavoie J, Dionne N, Helie R, Brisson G. Menstrual cycle phase dissociation of blood glucose homeostasis during exercise. J Appl Physiol. 1987;62(3):1084–9.

Mack GW, Nadel ER. Body fluid balance during heat stress in humans. Comprehensive Physiology: Wiley; 2010.

Maskarinec G, Williams AE, Inouye JS, Stanczyk FZ, Franke AA. A randomized isoflavone intervention among premenopausal women. Cancer Epidemiol Biomarkers Prev. 2002;11(2): 195–201.

Massafra C, Buonocore G, Gioia D, Sargentini I. Changes in the erythrocyte antioxidant enzyme system during transdermal estradiol therapy for secondary amenorrhea. Gynecol Endocrinol. 1996;10(3):155–8.

Matute M, Kalkhoff R. Sex steroid influence on hepatic gluconeogenesis and glycogen formation. Endocrinology. 1973;92:762–8.

Maughan RJ, Leiper JB, Shirreffs SM. Factors influencing the restoration of fluid and electrolyte balance after exercise in the heat. Br J Sports Med. 1997;31(3):175–82.

Maughan RJ, Shirreffs SM, Leiper JB. Errors in the estimation of hydration status from changes in body mass. J Sports Sci. 2007;25(7):797–804. doi:10.1080/02640410600875143.

McCarty MF. Vascular nitric oxide, sex hormone replacement, and fish oil may help to prevent Alzheimer's disease by suppressing synthesis of acute-phase cytokines. Med Hypotheses. 1999;53(5):369–74.

McLay R, Thomson C, Williams S, Rehrer N. Carbohydrate loading and female endurance athletes: effects of menstrual-cycle phase. Int J Sport Nutr Exerc Metab. 2007;17(2):189–205.

Mee JA, Gibson OR, Doust J, Maxwell NS. A comparison of males and females' temporal patterning to short- and long-term heat acclimation. Scand J Med Sci Sports. 2015;25:250–8. doi:10.1111/sms.12417.

Mei J, Yeung SS, Kung AW. High dietary phytoestrogen intake is associated with higher bone mineral density in postmenopausal but not premenopausal women. J Clin Endocrinol Metab. 2001;86(11):5217–21.

Mestre-Alfaro A, Ferrer MD, Sureda A, Tauler P, Martinez E, Bibiloni MM, et al. Phytoestrogens enhance antioxidant enzymes after swimming exercise and modulate sex hormone plasma levels in female swimmers. Eur J Appl Physiol. 2011;111(9):2281–94. doi:10.1007/s00421-011-1862-y. http://dx.doi.org.

Michos C, Kiortsis DN, Evangelou A, Karkabounas S. Antioxidant protection during the menstrual cycle: the effects of estradiol on ascorbic-dehydroascorbic acid plasma levels and total antioxidant plasma status in eumenorrhoic women during the menstrual cycle. Acta Obstet Gynecol Scand. 2006;85(8):960–5.

Moran DS, Shapiro Y, Laor A, Izraeli S, Pandolf KB. Can gender differences during exercise-heat stress be assessed by the physiological strain index? Am J Physiol Regul Integr Comp Physiol. 1999;276(6):R1798–804.

Moreira AC, Silva AM, Santos MS, Sardão VA. Phytoestrogens as alternative hormone replacement therapy in menopause: What is real, what is unknown. J Steroid Biochem Mol Biol. 2014;143:61–71. doi:10.1016/j.jsbmb.2014.01.016. http://dx.doi.org.

Morrow C, Naumburg EH. Dysmenorrhea. Prim Care. 2009;36(1):19–32.

Nhan S, Anderson KE, Nagamani M, Grady JJ, Lu LJ. Effect of a soymilk supplement containing isoflavones on urinary F2 isoprostane levels in premenopausal women. Nutr Cancer. 2005;53(1):73–81.

Nicklas B, Hackney AC, Sharp R. The menstrual cycle and exercise: performance, muscle glycogen, and substrate responses. Int J Sports Med. 1989;10:264–9.

Obayashi M, Shimomura Y, Nakai N, Jeoung NH, Nagasaki M, Murakami T, et al. Estrogen controls branched-chain amino acid catabolism in female rats. J Nutr. 2004;134(10):2628–33.

Oian P, Tollan A, Fadnes HO, Noddeland H, Maltau JM. Transcapillary fluid dynamics during the menstrual cycle. Am J Obstet Gynecol. 1987;156(4):952–5.

O'Keeffe K, Keith R, Wilson G, Blessing D. Dietary carbohydrate intake and endurance exercise performance of trained female cyclists. Nutr Res. 1989;9:819–30.

Oosthuyse T, Bosch A. The effect of the menstrual cycle on exercise metabolism. Implications for exercise performance in eumenorrhoeic women. Sports Med. 2010;40(3):207–27.

Patisaul HB, Jefferson W. The pros and cons of phytoestrogens. Front Neuroendocrinol. 2010;31(4):400–19. doi:10.1016/j.yfrne.2010.03.003. doi:http://dx.doi.org.

Paul D, Mulroy S, Horner J, Jacobs K, Lamb D. Carbohydrate-loading during the follicular phase of the menstrual cycle: effects on muscle glycogen and exercise performance. Int J Sport Nutr Exerc Metab. 2001;11:430–41.

Peternelj T-T, Coombes JS. Antioxidant supplementation during exercise training. Sports Med. 2011;41(12):1043–69.

Pitkin RM, Reynolds WA, Williams GA, Hargis GK. Calcium-regulating hormones during the menstrual cycle. J Clin Endocrinol Metab. 1978;47(3):626–32.

Rahbar N, Asgharzadeh N, Ghorbani R. Effect of omega-3 fatty acids on intensity of primary dysmenorrhea. Int J Gynaecol Obstet. 2012;117(1):45–7.

Rauch L, Rodger I, Wilson G, Belonje J, Dennis S, Noakes T, et al. The effects of carbohydrate loading on muscle glycogen content and cycling performance. Int J Sport Nutr. 1995;5:25–36.

Rauch H, St Clair Gibson A, Lambert E, Noakes T. A signaling role for muscle glycogen in the regulation of pace during prolonged exercise. Br J Sports Med. 2005;39:34–8.

Rechichi C, Dawson B, Goodman C. Athletic performance and oral contraceptive. Int J Sport Physiol Perform. 2009;4:151–62.

Reznik Dolins K, Boozer C, Stoler F, Bartels M, DeMeersman R, Contento I. Effect of variable carbohydrate intake on exercise performance in female endurance cyclists. Int J Sport Nutr Exerc Metab. 2003;13:422–35.

Rosner MH, Bennett B, Hew-Butler T, Hoffman MD. Exercise-associated hyponatremia. In: Simon EE, editor. Hyponatremia: evaluation and treatment. New York, NY: Springer New York; 2013. p. 175–92.

Rowlands D, Wadsworth D. Effect of high-protein feeding on performance and nitrogen balance in female cyclists. Med Sci Sports Exerc. 2011;43(1):44–53.

Roy B, Luttmer K, Bosman M, Tarnopolsky M. The influence of post-exercise macronutrient intake on energy balance and protein metabolism in active females participating in endurance training. Int J Sport Nutr Exerc Metab. 2002;12:172–88.

Salazar FJ, Llinas MT. Role of nitric oxide in the control of sodium excretion. News Physiol Sci. 1996;11:62–7.

Sar M, Stumpf W. Simultaneous localization of [3 H] estradiol and neurophysin I or arginine vasopressin in hypothalamic neurons demonstrated by a combined technique of dry-mount autoradiography and immunohistochemistry. Neurosci Lett. 1980;17(1):179–84.

Sedlock D. The latest on carbohydrate loading: a practical approach. Curr Sports Med Rep. 2008;7(4):209–13.

Sherman W, Costill D, Fink W, Miller J. The effect of exercise-diet manipulation on muscle glycogen and its subsequent utilisation during performance. Int J Sports Med. 1981;2:114–8.

Shimomura Y, Obayashi M, Murakami T, Harris RA. Regulation of branched-chain amino acid catabolism: nutritional and hormonal regulation of activity and expression of the branched-chain alpha-keto acid dehydrogenase kinase. Curr Opin Clin Nutr Metab Care. 2001;4(5):419–23.

Simpson LO. The etiopathogenesis of premenstrual syndrome as a consequence of altered blood rheology: a new hypothesis. Med Hypotheses. 1988;25(4):189–95.

Sims ST, Rehrer NJ, Bell ML, Cotter JD. Preexercise sodium loading aids fluid balance and endurance for women exercising in the heat. J Appl Physiol. 2007a;103(2):534–41. doi:10.1152/japplphysiol.01203.2006.

Sims ST, van Vliet L, Cotter JD, Rehrer NJ. Sodium loading aids fluid balance and reduces physiological strain of trained men exercising in the heat. Med Sci Sports Exerc. 2007b;39(1):123–30. doi:10.1249/01.mss.0000241639.97972.4a.

Sjödin B, Westing YH, Apple FS. Biochemical mechanisms for oxygen free radical formation during exercise. Sports Med. 1990;10(4):236–54.

Stachenfeld NS. Hormonal changes during menopause and the impact on fluid regulation. Reprod Sci. 2014;21(5):555–61. doi:10.1177/1933719113518992.

Stachenfeld NS, Keefe DL. Estrogen effects on osmotic regulation of AVP and fluid balance. Am J Physiol Endocrinol Metab. 2002;283(4):E711–21.

Stachenfeld NS, Dipietro L, Palter SF, Nadel ER. Estrogen influences osmotic secretion of AVP and body water balance in postmenopausal women. Am J Physiol Regul Integr Comp Physiol. 1998;274(1):R187–95.

Stachenfeld NS, Silva C, Keefe DL, Kokoszka CA, Nadel ER. Effects of oral contraceptives on body fluid regulation. J Appl Physiol. 1999;87(3):1016–25.

Stachenfeld NS, Silva C, Keefe DL. Estrogen modifies the temperature effects of progesterone. J Appl Physiol. 2000;88(5):1643–9.

Stachenfeld NS, Keefe DL, Palter SF. Estrogen and progesterone effects on transcapillary fluid dynamics. Am J Physiol Regul Integr Comp Physiol. 2001a;281(4):R1319–29.

Stachenfeld NS, Splenser AE, Calzone WL, Taylor MP, Keefe DL. Selected Contribution: Sex differences in osmotic regulation of AVP and renal sodium handling. J Appl Physiol. 2001b;91(4):1893–901.

Stephens DP, Bennett LA, Aoki K, Kosiba WA, Charkoudian N, Johnson JM. Sympathetic non-noradrenergic cutaneous vasoconstriction in women is associated with reproductive hormone status. Am J Physiol Heart Circ Physiol. 2002;282(1):H264–72.

Stephenson LA, Kolka MA. Plasma volume during heat stress and exercise in women. Eur J Appl Physiol. 1988;57:373–81.

Stephenson LA, Kolka MA. Esophageal temperature threshold for sweating decreases before ovulation in premenopausal women. J Appl Physiol. 1999;86(1):22–8.

Stephenson LA, Kolka MA, Francesconi R, Gonzales RR. Circadian variations in plasma renin activity, catecholamines, and aldosterone during exercise in women. Eur J Appl Physiol. 1989;58:756–64.

Stumpf WE, Denny ME. Vitamin D (soltriol), light, and reproduction. Am J Obstet Gynecol. 1989;161(5):1375–84.

Stupka N, Tiidus PM. Effects of ovariectomy and estrogen on ischemia-reperfusion injury in hindlimbs of female rats. J Appl Physiol. 2001;91(4):1828–35.

Suh S-H, Casazza G, Horning M, Miller B, Brooks G. Luteal and follicular glucose fluxes during rest and exercise in 3-h postabsorptive women. J Appl Physiol. 2002;93:42–50.

Suh S-H, Casazza G, Horning M, Miller B, Brooks G. Effects of oral contraceptives on glucose flux and substrate oxidation rates during rest and exercise. J Appl Physiol. 2003;94:285–94.

Sun F-H, Wong S-S, Chen S-H, Poon T-C. Carbohydrate electrolyte solutions enhance endurance capacity in active females. Nutrients. 2015;7:3739–50.

Tarnopolsky M, Atkinson S, Phillips S, MacDougall J. Carbohydrate loading and metabolism during exercise in men and women. J Appl Physiol. 1995;75:2134–41.

Tarnopolsky M, Bosman M, MacDonald J, Vadeputte D, Martin J, Roy B. Post-exercise protein-carbohydrate and carbohydrate supplements increase muscle glycogen in men and women. J Appl Physiol. 1997;83(6):1877–83.

Tarnopolsky M, Zawada C, Richmond L, Carter S, Shearer J, Graham T, et al. Gender differences in carbohydrate loading are related to energy intake. J Appl Physiol. 2001;91:225–30.

Temesi J, Johnson N, Raymond J, Burdon C, O'Connor H. Carbohydrate ingestion during endurance exercise improves performance in adults. J Nutr. 2011;141:890–7.

Thys-Jacobs S. Micronutrients and the premenstrual syndrome: the case for calcium. J Am Coll Nutr. 2000;19(2):220–7.

Thys-Jacobs S, McMahon D, Bilezikian JP. Cyclical changes in calcium metabolism across the menstrual cycle in women with premenstrual dysphoric disorder. J Clin Endocrinol Metab. 2007;92(8):2952–9.

Tranquilli A, Mazzanti L, Cugini A, Cester N, Garzett G, Romanini C. Transdermal estradiol and medroxyprogesterone acetate in hormone replacement therapy are both antioxidants. Gynecol Endocrinol. 1995;9(2):137–41.

Van Pelt R, Gozansky W, Schwartz R, Kohrt W. Intravenous estrogens increase insulin clearance and action in postmenopausal women. Am J Physiol Endocrinol Metab. 2003;285:E311–7.

Verney EB. The antidiuretic hormone and the factors which determine its release. Proc R Soc Lond B Biol Sci. 1947;135(878):25–106.

Vina J, Borras C, Gambini J, Sastre J, Pallardo FV. Why females live longer than males: control of longevity by sex hormones. Sci Aging Knowledge Environ. 2005;2005(23), e17.

Walker J, Heigenhauser G, Hultman E, Spriet L. Dietary carbohydrate, muscle glycogen content, and endurance performance in well-trained women. J Appl Physiol. 2000;88:2151–8.

Wallis G, Yeo S, Blannin A, Jeukendrup A. Dose-response effects of ingested carbohydrate on exercise metabolism in women. Med Sci Sports Exerc. 2007;39(1):131–8.

Wismann J, Willoughby D. Gender differences in carbohydrate metabolism and carbohydrate loading. J Int Soc Sports Nutr. 2006;31(1):28–34.

Zderic T, Coggan A, Ruby B. Glucose kinetics and substrate oxidation during exercise in the follicular and luteal phases. J Appl Physiol. 2001;90:447–53.

Zittermann A, Geppert J, Baier S, Zehn N, Gouni-Berthold I, Berthold HK, et al. Short-term effects of high soy supplementation on sex hormones, bone markers, and lipid parameters in young female adults. Eur J Nutr. 2004;43(2):100–8.

Chapter 7
The Effect of Sex Hormones on Ligament Structure, Joint Stability and ACL Injury Risk

Sandra J. Shultz

Introduction

While more physically active males injure their anterior cruciate ligament (ACL) due to their greater exposure to high risk sport activity (Gianotti et al. 2009), high school and college age females are two to five times more likely to suffer a non-contact ACL injury compared to similarly trained males (Hootman et al. 2007; Prodromos et al. 2007). This increased risk in females occurs around 13–14 years of age (Csintalan et al. 2008; Gianotti et al. 2009; Shea et al. 2004), when females begin to markedly differ from males in hormone secretion and their physical characteristics such as body composition, joint laxity (Shultz et al. 2008; Svenningsen et al. 1989; Wilmore and Costill 1999), and hip and knee control during sport related activity (Ford et al. 2010; Schmitz et al. 2009). As such, hormones have often been implicated in the ACL injury risk equation, because they underlie most of the sex differences in physical characteristics that emerge after puberty, and because they have the potential to impact collagen metabolism, ligament remodeling, and the structural integrity of the ACL in a way that may increase the potential for ligament failure. Before examining these hormone effects, the chapter first highlights the inherent complexity of studying sex hormone profiles in physically active females. We then focus primarily on what we know about the impact of sex hormones on collagen metabolism, ligament remodeling, and structural integrity of the ACL, and how this may impact ACL injury risk. The impact of oral contraceptive hormones and the hormone relaxin is also discussed.

S.J. Shultz, Ph.D., A.T.C., F.N.A.T.A. (✉)
Department of Kinesiology, University of North Carolina at Greensboro,
1400 Spring Garden St, Greensboro, NC 27412, USA
e-mail: sjshultz@uncg.edu

Complexity of Studying Hormone Profiles in Physically Active Females

It is well accepted that hormone profiles in women change considerably over the course of the menstrual cycle. These changes are often described relative to a typical 28-day cycle where the follicular phase represents the first half of the cycle (days 1–14) and the luteal phase represents the latter half of the cycle (days 15–28), with ovulation occurring between days 10 and 14. The time of ovulation is then subsequently used to identify the time of peak estrogen concentrations, and 7 days later the time of peak progesterone and the secondary peak in estrogen concentrations in the mid luteal phase. These typical cycle events have often been used as a calendar framework for determining relative injury risk across the menstrual cycle (Hewett et al. 2007). When examining hormone effects of relevant risk factors (e.g., joint laxity), measurements are commonly collected at three time points; one sample each to depict when both hormone concentrations are low (a day during menses), when estrogen rises unopposed near ovulation (days 10–14) and when both estrogen and progesterone are elevated during the luteal phase (day 21). While a serum or urine sample is sometimes obtained to confirm that the hormone milieu of interest was actually captured, more often than not cycle characteristics are assumed based on calendar days alone.

Unfortunately, the sampling approaches described above are fraught with error given the large variability in hormone profiles among women. For example, Landgren et al. reported that while the mean follicular and luteal phase lengths in 68 women were 15 and 13 days respectively, the actual length of the follicular and luteal phases ranged from 9 to 23 days and 8 to 17 days, respectively (Landgren et al. 1980). Shultz et al. (2004) reported similar findings when measuring daily serum sex hormone concentrations in 22 women who reported normal and consistent menstrual cycles lasting 28–32 days (Table 7.1). These data not only demonstrated the large variations in the timing of cycle events (cycle length, timing of ovulation, timing of the subsequent

Table 7.1 Variability in sex hormone profile characteristics in eumenorrheic females

Cycle characteristic	Range in values
Cycle length	24–36 days
Day of positive ovulation test	Day 9 to Day 20
Day of first estradiol peak near ovulation	Day 8 to Day 25
Day of progesterone rise (<2 ng/mL)	Day 11 to Day 27
Day of progesterone peak	Day 15 to Day 27
Peak estradiol concentration	86–295 pg/mL
Peak progesterone concentration	3.6 to 26.8 ng mL
Peak testosterone concentration	37–115 ng/mL

Data from Shultz et al. (2004). Data are representative of a single investigative study and are not intended to imply "clinical reference range" values

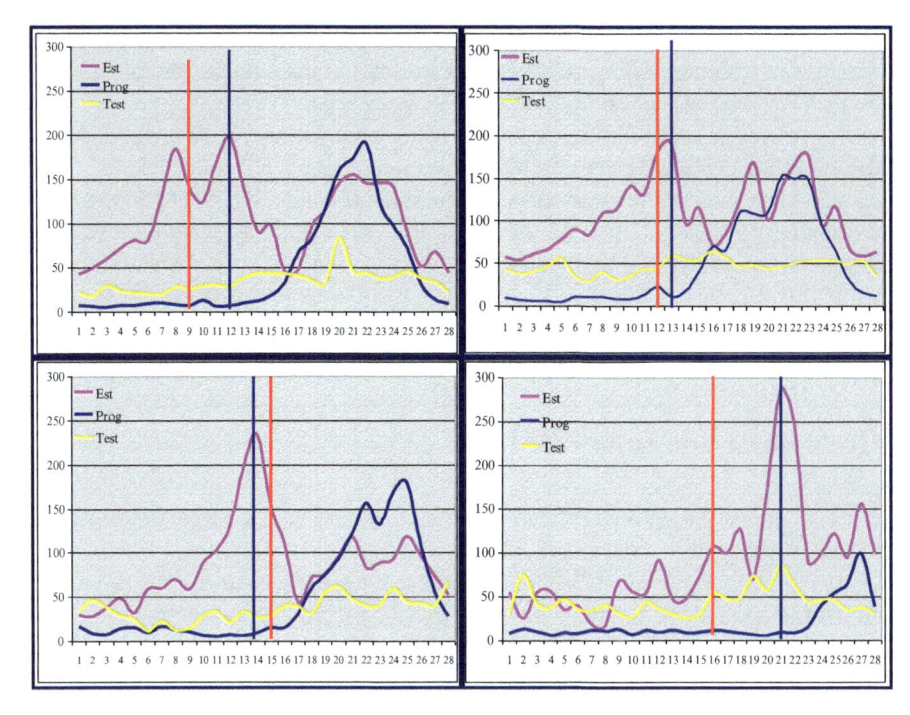

Fig. 7.1 Comparative timing of menstrual cycle events in 4 women who each had 28 day cycle lengths. *Red bar* indicates the day the ovulation test strip tested positive. Individual subject data (previously unpublished) derived from the study by Shultz et al. (2004)

rises and peaks in estrogen and progesterone) but also in the peak concentrations values obtained. Although testosterone concentrations are much lower in women than men, and as such their effects have received less attention than those of estrogen and progesterone, these concentrations also vary widely in women.

The variations observed in the timing of specific cycle events (e.g., ovulation, day of peak concentrations) are not simply a function of different cycle lengths. This is exemplified in data obtained from four different women (unpublished) who each had a 28 day cycle length (Fig. 7.1). The red line in each graph indicates the day that the ovulation test strip tested positive for the surge in luteinizing hormone. Of the four women, only one actually ovulated within the typical 10–14-day window. Further, the timing of peak estradiol levels (blue line) is not consistent relative to the day of ovulation, occurring within one day in two women, but occurring 3–5 days later in two other women. Capturing the progesterone peak at day 21 was more consistent, but was entirely missed in one female. Hence, if one uses calendar days alone, the hormone milieu of interest may be missed in the majority of women, yielding inaccurate findings.

It is also important to note that when measuring a particular risk factor or documenting an injury at a particular time in the cycle, the hormone milieu at the time of risk factor measurement or injury may not be the most relevant. Research indicates that the impact of changing hormones on ligament tissue may occur at some time delay (Shultz et al. 2004), suggesting that the hormone milieu in the days preceding the day of testing or injury may be more telling as to the impact of sex hormones on the variables of interest than the hormone concentrations obtained on the day of testing.

Together, this variability suggests that using a particular day or range of days of the menstrual cycle to depict a particular hormone event in all women is likely inaccurate. As we proceed through this chapter, is important to appreciate this variability among physically active females, and that our sampling techniques/research designs when examining hormone effects often do not adequately account for this variability. Because of this, there is much that is still unknown about cyclic hormone effects on ligament structure and function, and ACL injury risk.

Cycle Phase and Injury Risk

Because women are exposed to large variations in their hormone concentrations across the menstrual cycle, a number of studies have retrospectively examined whether ACL injury risk is disproportionately greater at certain times of the menstrual cycle (Adachi et al. 2008; Arendt et al. 2002; Beynnon et al. 2006; Myklebust et al. 1998, 2003; Slauterbeck et al. 2002; Wojtys et al. 1998, 2002). These retrospective studies generally report a greater number of injuries than expected during the follicular as compared to ovulatory phase (Table 7.2. However, among studies that identified the follicular phase as being the phase of greater risk, some reported a greater proportion of injuries early in the follicular phase during the perimenstrual days when hormone levels are nearing or at their nadirs (Myklebust et al. 1998, 2003; Slauterbeck et al. 2002) while others reported a greater proportion of injuries late in follicular phase near the time of ovulation when estrogen begins to rapidly rise (Adachi et al. 2008; Wojtys et al. 1998, 2002). While the hormone profile surrounding these two times points are quite different, they are alike in that both time points represent transitional periods of the menstrual cycle when hormone concentrations are rapidly changing. However, the actual hormone milieu or phase at the time of injury may be very difficult to accurately characterize in these retrospective studies.

In the majority of these studies, cycle phase was determine based on calendar counting methods based on subject self-recall of her menstrual cycle characteristics over previous months. Unfortunately, these methods have been found to be quite inaccurate (Small et al. 2007; Wojtys et al. 2002). Only three studies collected blood or urine samples to compliment calendar counting methods to better determine the hormone milieu at the time of injury. These samples were obtained within 2 h (Beynnon et al. 2006), 24 h (Wojtys et al. 2002) and 72 h (Slauterbeck et al. 2002) of the injury event. However, it is difficult to determine retrospectively from this single hormone sample what the hormone milieu may have been at the time of injury. As previously discussed, individuals vary considerably in the timing, magnitude and phasing of hormone concentrations within a cycle, and hormone concentrations can change substantially within hours near the time of menses and ovulation. The inaccuracy in ascertaining cycle phase from a single hormone sample was confirmed by

Table 7.2 ACL injury risk and menstrual cycle phase

Study	Normalized day of the cycle																											
	1	2	3	4	5	6	7	8	9	10	11	12	13	14	15	16	17	18	19	20	21	22	23	24	25	26	27	28
	Follicular phase														Luteal phase													
Myklebust et al. (1998) ($N=17$)[a]	29%*							12%							6%							53%*						
Myklebust et al. (2003) ($N=46$)[a]	50%*							26%							11%							13%						
Wojtys et al. (1998) ($N=28$)[a]	13%									29%*					58%													
Wojtys et al. (2002) ($N=51$)[a,b]	23%									43%*					34%													
Adachi et al. (2008) ($N=18$)[a]	11%									73%*					17%													
Arendt et al. (2002) ($N=83$)[a]	64%*														36%													
Beynnon et al. 2006 ($N=46$)[a,b]	74%*														26%													
Ruedl et al. 2009 ($N=93$)[a]	57%														43%													
Slauterbeck et al. 2002 ($N=37$)[a,b]	70%*														30%													

Menstrual cycle phase determine by [a]Calendar counting or [b]Hormone assessment
With permission, from S.J. Shultz, 2007

Tourville et al. (2016). Specifically, retrospective classification of menstrual cycle phase using self-reported menstrual cycle questionnaire data and a single hormone sample taken at a random date after a mock injury was not able to accurately classify the cycle phase that the women were in at the time of injury.

Even if research advances were able to accurately determine the hormone milieu at the time of injury, there is much that remains unknown about the mechanisms that underlie this potential relationship between menstrual cycle phase and ACL injury. First, research has yet to identify how the time of injury occurrence aligns with the hormone changes responsible for the increased risk, and therefore what hormone actions are most relevant to target in injury prevention efforts. Second, the specific mechanisms through which sex hormones are impacting soft tissues and the potential for ligament failure are largely unknown. While there is good evidence that sex hormones have the potential to exert substantial influence on collagen metabolism and the structural integrity of the ACL, understanding these mechanisms is complicated for several reasons. In addition to the known variability in the timing and magnitude of hormone concentrations changes between women as previously described (see previous section), there are also variations in cycle characteristics within a given female from month to month, including the occurrence of anovulatory cycles (Lenton et al. 1983; Shultz et al. 2011b). Because not all women go on to injure their ACL, understanding how this intraindividual and interindividual variability affects risk may be critically important. There is also evidence of a time and dose dependent effect by which soft tissues changes may occur in response to hormone concentration changes (Shultz et al. 2004; Yu et al. 2001), which complicates our ability to align the timing of injury occurrence to the hormone concentrations that may be responsible for that risk. Finally, it is unlikely that any effect is due to a single hormone, but rather represents a complex interaction among multiple hormones (Shultz et al. 2004; Yu et al. 2001; Dragoo et al. 2011a) and other relevant factors such as an individual's genotypic profile (Posthumus et al. 2009; Shultz et al. 2015) and exercise habits (Lee et al. 2004) that together may determine the extent to which a female is susceptible to injury. To address many of these challenges, prospective study designs that track a female's hormone profiles over several months would be required. Unfortunately, this approach is impractical given the relative infrequency in which these injuries occur.

Effect of Sex Hormones on Collagen Metabolism, Tissue Remodeling, and Ligament Structure

It is well accepted that steroidal hormone factors have the potential to exert substantial influence on soft tissue structures composed of collagen, including the ACL. Tissues exposed to estradiol are reported to increase both collagen synthesis (Dyer et al. 1980; Hassager et al. 1990; Ho and Weissberger 1992; Hosokawa et al. 1981) and absorption (Dyer et al. 1980; Fischer 1973), indicating increased metabolic activity. Structural changes in tissue have also been observed in response to estrogen exposure, noting decreases in total collagen and protein content, and fiber diameter and density

(Abubaker et al. 1996; Dubey et al. 1998; Hama et al. 1976). These tissue responses appear to be enhanced with exposure to both estrogen and progesterone (Abubaker et al. 1996; Dubey et al. 1998), but are diminished when the tissue is exposed to either progesterone or testosterone alone (Abubaker et al. 1996; Hama et al. 1976; Shikata et al. 1979). While these findings are based on a variety of connective tissues and research models, the general consensus from the literature is that collagen structure and metabolism are greatly influenced by sex hormones.

These investigations, along with the identification of sex hormone receptors on the human ACL (Dragoo et al. 2003; Hamlet et al. 1997; Liu et al. 1996), have led to considerable interest in how sex hormones might modify the structural integrity of the ACL (Hamlet et al. 1997; Liu et al. 1996; Yu et al. 1997). Investigations in this area include both animal and human models that have primarily examined the effects of estrogen (with or without progesterone) on collagen metabolism and the mechanical properties of the ACL.

Effect on Collagen Metabolism

The effect of estrogen on collagen metabolism of the ACL has primarily been examined in animal (Seneviratne et al. 2004; Liu et al. 1997) and human cell culture models (Yu et al. 1999, 2001).

Yu et al. (1999, 2001) examined human ACL tissue in cell culture to prospectively evaluate the effects of both physiologic and supraphysiologic levels of 17β-estradiol (range 2.9 pg/mL–2500 pg/mL) and progesterone on cell proliferation and collagen synthesis in vitro. These studies revealed two relevant findings. First they observed progressive decreases in fibroblast proliferation and Type 1 procollagen synthesis as estradiol levels progressively increased, which eventually leveled off at supraphysiologic levels. Increasing levels of progesterone attenuated this inhibitory effect, and when estradiol levels were controlled, increasing progesterone levels actually resulted in dose dependent increases in fibroblast proliferation and Type 1 procollagen synthesis. The second relevant finding is that these hormone effects were transient, with the most pronounced effects observed in the initial days after hormone exposure (days 1 and 3), which then began to attenuate within 7 days of exposure. These results suggest that large, transient changes in progesterone and estrogen concentrations across the menstrual cycle may influence ACL metabolism and collagen synthesis in an interactive, dose and time-dependent manner.

Results from animal model studies on the other hand reveal conflicting findings. Liu et al. (1997) prospectively examined female rabbit ACLs in cell culture after 2 weeks of exposure to control (0 pg/ml) physiologic (2.9, 25, and 250 pg/mL) and supraphysiologic (2500 and 25,000 pg/mL) concentrations of estradiol. A decrease in collagen synthesis and fibroblast proliferation was noted with increasing concentrations of estradiol, starting with physiological levels of 25 pg/mL, compared to a control group with no exposure to estradiol. Conversely, Seneviratne et al. (2004) prospectively examined sheep ACL fibroblasts in cell culture 4 and 6 days after being subjected to somewhat similar incremental doses of estradiol [2.2 (control), 5, 15, 25, 250, and 2500 pg/mL], and found no difference in fibroblast proliferation and collagen synthesis at any concentration level. Because of the limited and conflicting studies in this area, it is difficult to draw meaningful conclusions at this time. Differences in the study designs, including the length of estradiol exposure and the control group that was used, make it somewhat difficult to directly compare results between studies. Where Liu et al. (1997) used a control group that received no estradiol, and examine changes after 2 weeks of exposure, Seneviratne et al. (2004) compared their data to a control group receiving 2.2 pg/mL after 4 and 6 days following exposure. Yu et al. (1999) also compared their data to a control group that received no estradiol, and was the only study to look at transient changes that occurred within days of exposure.

Effect on Mechanical Properties

Estrogen effects on the ultimate mechanical properties of the ACL have been limited to animal models, including rabbit (Slauterbeck et al. 1999; Hattori et al. 2010; Komatsuda et al. 2006), sheep (Strickland et al. 2003), and monkey (Wentorf et al. 2006). Using a prospective, matched control design, Slauterbeck et al. (1999) examined the ultimate failure load on the ACL in ovariectomized rabbits with and without 30 days of exposure to estradiol concentrations consistent with pregnancy levels. While biomechanical testing revealed the estrogen-treated ACLs failed at a 10 % lower load compared to control ACLs, these results were limited to supraphysiological levels of estradiol exposure. More recently, Komatsuda et al. (Komatsuda et al. 2006) examine mechanical properties in ovariectomized rabbits receiving different physiological [no (control), low and medium concentrations] or supraphysiologic levels (high concentrations) of estradiol over 5 weeks. Those administered high concentrations (supraphysiologic) demonstrated a decrease in ultimate tensile stress and linear stiffness compared to those administered medium (high physiologic) concentrations who had the highest values of all groups (but not significantly more than control or low concentration groups).

Studies investigating the effects of estrogen on mechanical properties at more physiological levels have not consistently demonstrated an effect (Hattori et al. 2010; Strickland et al. 2003; Wentorf et al. 2006). In subsequent analyses of the work by Komatsuda et al. (2006) those administered medium concentrations of estradiol had less tissue elasticity than controls as measured by scanning acoustic microscopy (lower sound speed and attenuation) (Hattori et al. 2010). Strickland et al. (2003) examined the biomechanical properties of sheep knee ligaments 6 months following random assignment to sham-operated, ovariectomy, ovariectomy + estradiol implant, as well as low dose and high dose raloxifene (estrogen receptor agonist) groups. For this study, estradiol was administered at concentrations near 2 pg/ml, which was deemed similar to that experienced during the normal luteal phase of their estrus cycle. While the ultimate stress of the ram was greater than the ewes, they observed no difference in ligament strength (maximum force, stiffness, energy to failure) between groups. Similar findings were reported by Wentorf et al. (2006), who examined the mechanical properties of the ACLs and patellar tendons obtained from Cynomolgus macaque monkeys two years after they were divided into sham operated and ovariectomized groups. They found no difference in any of the mechanical or material properties tested, including failure load, stiffness, elongation at failure, ultimate stress or strain, or energy at failure. A strength of the latter study is that monkeys were examined, who closely mirror the estrogen levels and cyclic variations of the human menstrual cycle (Goodman et al. 1977).

While these studies suggest that mechanical properties of the ACL may not be substantially altered after prolonged exposure to different physiological concentrations of estrogen (6 months to 2 years) (Strickland et al. 2003; Wentorf et al. 2006), the tissue may be more affected by acute changes (5 weeks) (Hattori et al. 2010; Yu et al. 2001). Future studies should examine more acute, physiological changes in estradiol concentrations that women experience, and include sex hormones other than estrogen (either in combination or isolation), as estrogen alone may not be responsible for changes in ligament properties. Given the attenuating hormone effects on collagen metabolism over time described by Yu et al. (1999, 2001), and the cyclic variations that occur in sex hormones across the female menstrual cycle, examining both acute and chronic effects seems prudent. Finally, more studies using human and primate models are recommended. While data from various animal studies have improved our understanding of the effects of estradiol on mechanical properties of the ligament, their clinical relevance to the human ACL is uncertain since non-primates have estrous cycles rather than menstrual cycles, and therefore experience very different hormone profiles (Griffin et al. 2006).

Effect on Ligament Laxity

While direct biomechanical measurement of the mechanical properties of the ACL are not possible to obtain in vivo, indirect, noninvasive clinical measures of knee laxity may provide important insights into the structural integrity of the ACL, and the biological processes that may mediate this structural integrity.

Knee Laxity as a Risk Factor for ACL Injury

Anterior knee laxity (the magnitude of anterior displacement of the tibia on the femur when an anterior directed load is applied to the posterior tibia) is often used to characterize an individual's knee laxity, because the ACL acts as the primary restraint to this motion (Butler et al. 1980). It is well documented that females have greater anterior knee laxity compared males (Scerpella et al. 2005; Rozzi et al. 1999; Shultz et al. 2005; Beynnon et al. 2005; Uhorchak et al. 2003; Nguyen and Shultz 2007), and both prospective and retrospective studies have consistently identified an association between greater magnitudes of anterior knee laxity and greater risk of ACL injury. When examine prospectively in US military cadets, the risk of

ACL injury was 2.7 times greater when females had AKL values ≥1 SD above the mean (Uhorchak et al. 2003). When examined retrospectively, ACL-injured females had 19–26% (>0.6–0.8 SD) greater laxity in their un-injured knee compared to controls. In a recent prospective cohort study with a nested, matched case–control analysis that examined multiple ACL injury risk factors in high school and college female athletes, anteroposterior knee laxity was a significant predictor in the final multivariate model along with greater body mass index (BMI = weight in kilograms/height in meters^2) and having a parent with history of ACL injury. Specifically, females with knee laxity values 1sd (2.7) and 2 sd (5.4 mm) above the mean had a 70% and 140% greater risk of suffering an ACL injury (Beynnon 2016).

There are two likely mechanisms through which greater knee laxity is associated with a greater risk of ACL injury. One is a *biomechanical mechanism* where the ACL acts as a passive restraint to control tibial motion during weight bearing tasks. Studies have shown that greater knee laxity is associated with greater anterior tibial translation of the tibia on the femur during the transition of the knee from non-weight bearing to weight bearing (Shultz et al. 2006b), a stiffer (less absorptive) landing upon ground contact that leads to greater knee extensor loads (Shultz et al. 2010b, 2013) and greater knee valgus motion and moments during landing (i.e., a more inward collapse of the knee) (Shultz and Schmitz 2009), all of which have the potential to increase loading of the ACL during weight bearing activities.

The second potential mechanism is a *biological mechanism*, where a more lax ligament may represent a structurally weaker ligament that is more prone to failure or more likely to fail (as compared to a less lax ligament) a given critical load. A more lax ACL has been associated with less collagen fiber density (fibers per unit area) and lower mechanical properties (less strain/stress at failure) (Chandrashekar et al. 2006; Hashemi et al. 2008). Because ligament laxity is not solely a function of ligament and body size, these sex differences are thought to result primarily from metabolic/remodeling processes that regulate the material properties of the ligament (Comerford et al. 2005; Chandrashekar et al. 2006). This is supported by animal studies, where greater laxity was associated with ligament biomarkers indicative of greater collagen turnover (Comerford et al. 2005; Quasnichka et al. 2005), more immature cross links (Quasnichka et al. 2005), and lower failure loads (Comerford et al. 2005; Quasnichka et al. 2005; Wang et al. 2006). Given the potent effects of sex hormones on collagen metabolism previously described, the changing sex hormone concentrations that female's experience likely play a critical role in the biological processes that contribute to their greater magnitudes of knee laxity, thus their greater risk of ACL injury.

Sex Hormone Effects on Knee Laxity

While boys and girls have similar magnitudes of knee laxity prior to puberty, upon maturation females maintain higher levels of knee laxity while knee laxity in males decreases to a greater extent (Flynn et al. 2000; Shultz et al. 2008). This results in females having, on average, greater knee laxity than males throughout adulthood (Scerpella et al. 2005; Rozzi et al. 1999; Shultz et al. 2005; Beynnon et al. 2005; Uhorchak et al. 2003; Nguyen and Shultz 2007). However, it is important to note that the magnitude of knee laxity can vary widely in both sexes, and therefore not all women have greater knee laxity than males. Additionally, females are unique in that they experience substantial changes in knee laxity across their menstrual cycle. Studies have largely concluded that knee laxity is generally greater in the periovulatory days of the cycle and, to a lesser extent, in the mid luteal days of the cycle compared to the days of menses (Deie et al. 2002; Eiling et al. 2007; Heitz 1999; Park et al. 2009a; Shultz et al. 2004; Zazulak et al. 2006; Khowailed et al. 2015; Lee et al. 2014). When sex hormones and knee laxity changes are tracked and compared daily across one complete menstrual cycle, knee laxity was observed to change on average 3–4 days following changes in sex hormone concentrations (Shultz et al. 2004). When this time delay was accounted for, changes in estradiol, progesterone, testosterone and their interactions explained on average $63 \pm 7.7\%$ of the variance in knee laxity changes (compared to 5.4% and 26% when changes in estradiol alone or in combination with progesterone and testosterone were examined without accounting for this time delay) (Shultz et al. 2004). However, the magnitude of change in knee laxity was quite variable among the women studied (range 1.5–5.3 mm) and was found to be more pronounced in response to rising concentrations of estradiol and testosterone in women who had lower minimum estradiol and higher minimum progesterone concentrations at menses (a more androgenic environment) (Shultz et al. 2006a). This individual variability in hormone profiles and knee laxity responsiveness is important for clinicians and scientists to understand, as it may expose some women to a greater risk of injury compared to others. For example, studies have shown that those who experience greater acute increases in knee laxity are more likely to move toward higher risk biomechanics when knee laxity is increased, including greater anterior tibial translation during the transition from non-weight bearing to weight bearing (Shultz et al. 2011a), greater knee stiffness upon landing (Shultz et al. 2013), and greater dynamic knee valgus movement and forces during landing and cutting maneuvers (Park et al. 2009b; Shultz et al. 2012a).

To further understand the mechanisms by which sex hormone changes may lead to knee laxity changes, Shultz et al. (2012b) completed a secondary analysis of their data by assaying serum markers of collagen production (CICP; C-terminal propeptide of collagen type-I) and degradation (ICTP; carboxyterminal telopeptide of type I collagen) and insulin-like growth factor (IGF-I; a mediator of collagen production) (Malloy 2003). Their purpose was to determine if normal physiological changes in hormone concentrations across the menstrual cycle were sufficient to stimulate changes in collagen metabolism, and if these changes in collagen metabolism coincided with the changes in knee laxity observed. They also compared eumenorrheic females to females taking oral contraceptives (who were expected to maintain more stable hormone concentrations). Based on prior study findings (Hansen et al. 2008; Hansen et al. 2009; Wreje et al. 2000; Yu et al. 2001), Shultz et al. hypothesized that concentrations of CICP, ICTP and IGF-I would generally be lower (i.e., collagen production and synthesis depressed) during days of the cycle when estradiol levels were elevated, and that greater suppression of collagen synthesis (greater decreases in CICP, ICTP and IGF-I concentrations) would be associated with greater anterior knee laxity. Results revealed that serum levels of CICP and ICTP tended to be higher during the days of menses, then decreased during the periovulatory and luteal days compared to menses while IGF-I values stayed relatively stable (Shultz et al. 2012b). This decrease in CICP and ICTP was most pronounced in the initial days post ovulation when estrogen was rising unopposed, and this effect began to attenuate in the early luteal phase once progesterone began to rise. When these data were compared to women taking oral contraceptives, eumenorrheic women generally had lower CICP and ICTP concentrations, and tended to demonstrate more variability in these concentration changes across time compared to women on oral contraceptives. However, in both groups, decreasing CICP concentrations and increasing IGF-I concentrations predicted increasing anterior knee laxity across the cycle ($R^2 = 0.310$ and 0.400). While these results tend to support the findings from in vitro cell culture models that increasing estradiol concentrations have the potential to influence collagen synthesis and ligament integrity in a dose dependent and negative manner, this study represents a fairly rudimentary step in attempting to understand these mechanisms. When markers of Type I collagen synthesis and degradation are measured in the serum, they represent changes from a variety of collagen tissue and do not directly represent the local environment of the knee (Hansen et al. 2008, 2009). Additionally the temporal sequencing of these changes was not examined, which makes it difficult to ascertain the sequencing of these events with the times in the cycle when ACL injury risk may be elevated (Renstrom et al. 2008). Further research examining these mechanisms is warranted.

Summary

It is clear that sex hormones have the potential to have a profound effect on collagen metabolism in a way that may impact the structural integrity of the ACL, and thus the stability of the knee and risk of ligament injury. However, there is much we do not know about the mechanisms through which these hormone actions occur, the time dependency of these actions, or the hormone profiles that are most likely to contribute to an inferior collagen structure or a more lax ligament. It should also be noted that the majority of in vivo studies examining hormone effects on knee laxity and injury risk are limited to eumenorrheic females with "normal" cycles that are consistent month to month. Menstrual dysfunction in exercising females is common, and reported to be as high as 50% (DeSouza et al. 2010; Thein-Nissenbaum et al. 2014; Tourville et al. 2016; Vescovi 2011), and current sampling techniques cannot distinguish between ovulatory and anovulatory cycles. Given the high prevalence of menstrual function, it is equally important to examine relationships between sex hormones, collagen metabolism, ligament behavior, and ACL injury risk in oligomenorrheic and amenorrheic females. In fact, limited research suggests that the risk for severe musculoskeletal injury may be somewhat higher in high school female athletes who experience menstrual cycle disturbances (i.e., those with 9 or fewer cycles in previous year and those with primary amenorrhea) (Thein-Nissenbaum et al. 2012). Moreover, a large percentage of physically active females use oral contraceptives, which may also differentially exert their influence on ligament structures. The effect of oral contraceptive use will be covered in the next section.

Contraceptive Hormones

A large portion of physically active females use oral contraceptives (OC) for a variety of reasons. Research estimates that 8–14% of adolescents, and 27–42% of collegiate females (and as high as 70% in collegiate soccer athletes) use birth control hormones of some kind (Agel et al. 2006; Beals and Manore 2002; Miller et al. 1999; Paulus et al. 2000; Thein-Nissenbaum et al. 2014). Because contraceptive hormones stabilize and lower endogenous sex hormone levels, it is often theorized that these stabilizing effects would have a protective effect against ACL injury. To date, however, there is no strong evidence in the literature for or against a protective effect of oral contraceptives (Renstrom et al. 2008; Shultz et al. 2015). Of the previously epidemiological studies examining cycle phase and ACL injury risk, four included both oral contraceptive and non-oral contraceptive users. When conducting group sub-analyses, cycle specific injury trends were actually quite similar between the groups (Arendt et al. 2002; Ruedl et al. 2009; Slauterbeck et al. 2002; Wojtys et al. 2002). While there were fewer oral contraceptive users represented in these studies (suggesting they may be at lower risk), comparative risk between OC users and nonusers could not be determined without knowing the proportion of OC users vs. nonusers in the larger populations from which these subjects were obtained. Of the two studies that included a control group to account for proportional population statistics, there was no evidence that OC users were at lower risk for ACL injury (Agel et al. 2006; Ruedl et al. 2009). However, in a recent case–control study using national insurance claims data from 2002 to 2012 (Gray et al. 2016), the risk associated with OC use may change over time. In this study, ACL reconstructed females did not differ from controls in OC usage when all subjects were considered. However, when the population was stratified by age, ACL reconstructed females who were 15–19 years of age were 18% *less* likely to use OC in the 12 months preceding the injury date than matched controls, while those who were 25–34 years of age were 15% *more* likely to use OCPs than matched controls. While this may suggest that the duration of OCP use may modify its effect on ACL injury risk over time, this study was not limited to injuries associated with sport (i.e., it included recreational and accidental ACL injuries), and only represents those who underwent ACL reconstruction. Because athletes are more likely to use OCs and seek reconstructive surgery so that they can continue sport participation, this may have introduced a bias in the proportional use of OCPs in

ACL-reconstructed cases versus control subjects. Thus, there remains no clear evidence that the use of OCPs negatively or positively impacts ACL injury.

Although contraceptive hormones stabilize and lower endogenous hormone levels (Clark et al. 2001; Coney and DelConte 1999; Henzyl 2001; London et al. 1992), they are also biologically active and able to exert their influence on soft tissue structures. While it is often posited that contraceptive hormones provide a more stable, predictable hormone environment, this environment may differ widely depending on how the contraceptive hormone is administered. For example, dosing can be monophasic or triphasic, and therefore concentrations may or may not vary over the 21 pill days of the cycle. The concentration of exogenous estradiol (ethinyl estradiol) and progesterone (progestogen) can also differ, and can be as much as three to five times and one to two times higher, respectively, than normal, physiological endogenous levels (Burrows and Peters 2007). Also, while ethinyl estradiol is the only form of synthetic estrogen used in OCs, multiple progestogens are used (e.g., levonorgestrel, norethindrone, desogestrel, norgestimate, gestodene). Because the type, potency, and androgenicity of these progestogens may differ, the extent to which the progestogen counteracts the estrogenic effects may also differ (Burrows and Peters 2007).

These variations in oral contraceptive preparations may in part explain the inconsistent findings when comparing the effects of OCs on collagen metabolism, tissue structure and knee joint laxity. Wreje et al. compared serum markers of collagen synthesis and degradation prior to and following 2 months administration of an oral contraceptive that contained a progestogen with high androgenicity in healthy women. They reported lower concentrations of serum markers of collagen synthesis and degradation after OC administration as compared to pre-administration when measured during the luteal phase (Wreje et al. 2000). Hansen and colleagues compared local markers of tendon collagen synthesis and collagen fibril diameters during the luteal days of women on OCs (which contained high estradiol dosing and a progestogen with low androgenicity) compared to days of menses in eumenorrheic women (when hormones are at their nadirs). They observed reduced markers of collagen synthesis and smaller tendon fibril diameters in women using OCs (Hansen et al. 2008, 2009). However, in subsequent analyses, they found no detrimental effects on tendon biomechanical properties, tendon fibril characteristics or collagen cross-linking when comparing women who were long term users of OC versus non-OC users (Hansen et al. 2015). In other work comparing OCP vs. eumenorrheic females across multiple days of the cycle, women on various types of OCs were reported to have *higher* concentrations of markers of both collagen synthesis and degradation (CICP and ICTP), and these differences were most pronounced when eumenorrheic women were at peak estradiol concentrations in the post ovulatory/early luteal days of the cycle (Shultz et al. 2012b). In all three studies, IGF-I concentrations (a mediator of collagen production) were reported to be lower in women using oral contraceptives, particularly when comparisons were made in the luteal phase (Hansen et al. 2008, 2009; Shultz et al. 2012b; Wreje et al. 2000).

In studies comparing knee laxity in OC users and nonusers, one study observed no group differences in knee laxity (Pokorny et al. 2000) while another observed lower knee laxity in OC users (Martineau et al. 2004) when a single sample was measured on a random day during the cycle. When laxity changes were compared at different phases of the menstrual cycle, OC users were reported to have less anterior knee laxity than nonusers at all points, but this was most pronounced when knee laxity was increased in eumenorrheic women during ovulatory and luteal test days (Lee et al. 2014). When compared daily across the menstrual cycle, similar laxity values were observed for OC and eumenorrheic females across the majority of test days except for the early luteal phase (post estrogen peak, before the rise in progesterone levels) when eumenorrheic females were found to increased their laxity values (Shultz et al. 2012b). In both studies (Lee et al. 2014; Shultz et al. 2012b), laxity values were more stable over time in women using OCs versus eumenorrheic women.

It is difficult to build a clear consensus of the effects of OC use on collagen metabolism and knee laxity in the aforementioned studies because they vary so much in the timing of sample(s) acquisition as well as in the type of OC administered (e.g., dosage of ethinyl estradiol and progestogen delivered, consistency of hormone concentrations over the cycle, and the androgenicity of progestogen). Because the patterns of variability in these serum markers and knee laxity values are different across the cycle in OC users versus eumenorrheic females (Gorai et al. 1998; Shultz et al. 2012b), it is difficult to compare findings when samples were acquired at a single random time point or at different phases of the cycle. Further, correlational analyses in a small sample of OC users reported by Shultz et al. (2012b) suggests that the OCs that contained progestogens with greater androgenicity were more likely to be associated with decreases in IGF-I (marker of collagen production) and ICTP (marker of collagen degradation) concentrations than OCs that contained progestogens with lower androgenicity. Hence there remains insufficient evidence to determine if OCs (or certain types of OCs) have a negative or positive effect on collagen metabolism, tissue integrity, and injury risk.

In summary, there is no clear evidence of either a positive or negative effect of OC usage on ligament structural integrity or ACL injury risk potential. Clearly, more work is needed to fully understand the impact of chronic oral contraceptive use on these outcomes in physically active females. This includes the need to gain a better understanding of how the different hormone preparations (some more androgenic than others) differentially impact collagen metabolism and ligament integrity, as well as other relevant tissues such as muscle and tendon.

Relaxin

Although relaxin has been traditionally considered a pregnancy hormone responsible for relaxing pelvic ligaments in preparation for labor (Samuel et al. 2007), it is also detectable in the serum of nonpregnant females (Dragoo et al. 2011b; Johnson et al. 1993; Pehrsson et al. 2007; Stewart et al. 1990; Wolf et al. 2013b; Wreje et al. 1995). Relaxin is typically lower during the follicular phase, then rises by day 6 and peaks within 8–10 days following the LH surge at ovulation (Bryant et al. 1975; Johnson et al. 1993; Stewart et al. 1990; Wreje et al. 1995). However, actual levels can vary widely among females within this window, with some having undetectable levels and others having unusually high levels that are similar to pregnancy concentrations (Dragoo et al. 2011b; Stewart et al. 1990). Additionally, some women are reported to have episodic peaks during the follicular phase (Bryant et al. 1975) while others have abnormally high values throughout the cycle (Bryant et al. 1975; Stewart et al. 1990). These interindividual variations in relaxin levels are likely in part due to large, interindividual variability in the timing and magnitude of sex steroid concentrations (Shultz et al. 2004, 2011b), as relaxin secretion is thought to be largely regulated by estradiol (Dragoo et al. 2011b; Johnson et al. 1993; Wreje et al. 1995).

Relaxin and Collagen Metabolism

Relaxin is a member of the insulin superfamily of peptide hormones which initiate their actions by binding to receptors on the cell surface, utilizing cellular signaling pathways to further transmit messages, ultimately resulting in altered cellular function. Relaxin-2 is the predominant circulating form of relaxin in humans (Sherwood 2004). While it is difficult to study the effect of relaxin on collagen metabolism in human knee ligaments in situ, in vivo, and in vitro animal studies and human cell culture studies suggest that relaxin administered at physiological levels can have a profound effect on soft tissue remodeling (ligament fibrocartilage, articular cartilage, tendon, and dermal). Specifically, circulating relaxin increases expression of relaxin receptors on target tissues (Kang et al. 2014), leading to dose-dependent increases in the expression of matrix metalloproteinases (MMPs) *for* collagenases (MMPs 1 and 13), gelatinases (MMP 2 and 9), and stromelysins (MMP 3) that breakdown fibrillar collagens, fibrocartilage, and extracellular matrix proteins (Naqvi et al. 2005; Takano et al. 2009; Unemori and Amento 1990). Relaxin also decreases the expression of Type I, III, and IV collagen in a dose-dependent manner (Kang et al. 2014; Takano et al. 2009; Unemori and Amento 1990), and modestly reduces expression of tissue inhibitors (TIMPs) that regulate collagenase activity (Takano et al. 2009; Unemori and Amento 1990). These collagenolytic effects have also been shown in fibrotic and healing tissues where collagen synthesis and deposition (thus scar formation) were greatly reduced (Kang et al. 2014; Negishi et al. 2005). The net effect of this tissue remodeling is a less organized (Unemori et al. 1993) and less dense (both in fiber diameter and density) collagen structure (Naqvi et al. 2005; Unemori et al. 1993). Because these same tissue properties have been associated with a more lax (less stiff) and structurally weaker ligament in ACL animal models (Comerford et al. 2005; Dragoo et al. 2009; Fleming et al. 2011; Quasnichka et al. 2005; Hashem et al. 2006), these findings provide strong evidence of the potential for relaxin to alter ligament structure and function in ways that may contribute to greater ligament laxity and risk of ACL injury.

Because of the stability of collagen, the aforementioned changes are thought to be more chronic in nature (Dragoo et al. 2011a), thus are more likely to explain the higher baseline laxity values in females. However, there is also evidence that relaxin may contribute to acute elongation of the ligament by interrupting interfibrillar bonds, allowing the fibers to slip and reorient (Wood et al. 2003). This collagen sliding has been demonstrated in rat tail tendon where a fluorescent dye was used to label collagen fibers, and changes in fiber orientation were observed over 48 h while the tendon was under strain (Wood et al. 2003). Tendons treated with relaxin demonstrated significantly more creep than controls within 3 h of relaxin exposure (3 % vs. 1 % of tendon length), and this creep gradually increased over 48 h (10–12 % vs. 1 %). Hence, acute collagen fiber sliding provides a plausible explanation for the acute increases in knee laxity that are commonly observed in females during the luteal phase of the menstrual cycle (i.e., similar in timing to the rise in relaxin concentrations) (Shultz et al. 2004, 2010a; Deie et al. 2002; Heitz 1999). This collagen fiber sliding may also explain why greater relaxin concentrations were associated with decreased tendon stiffness ($r^2 = 0.31$), but not changes in cross-sectional area, when human tendon force-elongation characteristics were examined across three times points in the menstrual cycle (Pearson et al. 2011).

Relaxin and ACL Injury Epidemiology

Relaxin receptors have been identified on the human ACL (Dragoo et al. 2003; Faryniarz et al. 2006; Galey et al. 2003), and are therefore capable of directly impacting ACL laxity and structural integrity. Relaxin receptors on the human ACL are reported to be more prevalent in females vs. males (Dragoo et al. 2003; Faryniarz et al. 2006; Galey et al. 2003) and in younger vs. older women (Galey et al. 2003). Since collagen is the main load bearing structure of the ACL, the acute and chronic effects of relaxin on collagen organization and content previously described suggest that higher serum relaxin concentrations may lead to clinically relevant increases in laxity and weakness of the ACL (Dragoo et al. 2003). This is supported by a recent prospective study of Division I female athletes where relaxin levels were threefold higher and more variable in those who suffered an ACL injury compared to non-injured controls (6.0 ± 8.1 vs. 1.8 ± 3.4 pg/mL), and females with relaxin levels greater than 6.0 pg/mL were four times more likely to suffer an ACL injury (Dragoo et al. 2011a). While the authors theorized this increased risk was likely due to altered ligament laxity and strength (Dragoo et al. 2011a, 2012), they did not measure knee laxity in these women to determine if higher relaxin levels resulted in clinically observable differences in the mechanical behavior of the ligament. The likelihood of greater knee laxity in these individuals is supported by an animal model where guinea pig ACLs treated with relaxin at pregnancy levels were 13 % more lax and 36–49 % weaker (Dragoo et al. 2009). Other retrospective work indirectly corroborate these findings, as both serum relaxin and knee laxity values were significantly higher in females with a history of ACL injury compared to un-injured controls (Arnold et al. 2002).

Despite compelling evidence that relaxin may profoundly affect ligament properties, few studies have examined associations between relaxin and joint laxity in eumenorrheic females. While three studies reported no significant correlations between serum relaxin levels and general joint laxity (Wolf et al. 2013a, b, 2014), relaxin was sampled at a single time point, and was not timed with the mid-luteal phase when relaxin is known to be elevated. Thus, it is unlikely that peak relaxin levels were obtained in many of these women, which may very well explain the large proportion of females with undetectable levels (58–80 %). Only 1 study examined anterior knee laxity, obtaining weekly samples of serum relaxin and anterior knee laxity for 4 weeks in 57 collegiate nonpregnant females (8 of which were ACL injured) (Arnold et al. 2002). While both serum relaxin and anterior knee laxity were higher in ACL-injured vs. non-injured, no significant within day correlations were identified. However, a single sample was obtained each week, and the timing of each sample relative to known hormone events was not controlled (Arnold et al. 2002). Considering the relatively transient peak in relaxin (Johnson et al. 1993; Stewart et al. 1990; Wreje et al. 1995), it is unlikely that this study accurately captured peak relaxin in all females, thus the magnitude of change in relaxin among these women. It is also unknown whether the relaxin concentrations obtained on the day of laxity testing would sufficiently characterize the relationship between relaxin and either baseline or cyclic increases in laxity.

Prior studies have also not controlled for circulating sex hormone concentrations. Sex hormones have the potential to alter the effect of relaxin on collagen structure and metabolism (Dehghan et al. 2014a, b; Hashem et al. 2006; Naqvi et al. 2005) and circulating estradiol is thought to be the primary regulator of relaxin secretion (Johnson et al. 1993; Wreje et al. 1995). In ovariectomized rabbits, relaxin secretion increased when primed with estradiol, and total collagen content in knee articular and temporomandibular joint (TMJ) fibrocartilage decreased with administration of relaxin, estradiol, and relaxin+estradiol while it was maintained with relaxin+progesterone or relaxin+estradiol+progesterone (Hashem et al. 2006). In rabbit cell cultures, MMP-1 and MMP-2 expression were 1.7 fold higher when relaxin and relaxin+estradiol were administered at normal physiological levels, and this was substantially greater than when estradiol was administered alone (Naqvi et al. 2005). In ovarectomized rats, relaxin+estrogen and relaxin+progesterone resulted in a dose-dependent increase in relaxin protein and mRNA expression in medial collateral ligaments and patellar tendons (Dehghan et al. 2014a), while relaxin+testosterone downregulated this response and subsequently inhibited an increase in passive knee motion that was observed with relaxin administration alone (Dehghan et al. 2014a, b). Although relaxin and estrogen are strongly correlated within a day (Johnson et al. 1993; Wreje et al. 1995), and estrogen is thought to be the primary regulator of relaxin secretion (Johnson et al. 1993), estrogen does not appear to enhance or alter relaxin's effect on target tissue (thus may not be critical to control for when examining the effects of relaxin) (Dehghan et al. 2014a, b; Hashem et al. 2006; Naqvi et al. 2005). However, because progesterone and testosterone are reported to modify relaxin expression in target tissues, it may be important to control for these hormone levels when examining associations between relaxin, knee laxity and ACL injury risk. The potential for progesterone and testosterone to downregulate relaxin expression and subsequently inhibit an increase in passive knee motion (Dehghan et al. 2014a, b) may also explain in part the highly variable associations previously observed between sex hormone changes and knee laxity changes in eumenorrheic women (Shultz et al. 2004, 2006a).

Together, these findings strongly suggest that future in vivo studies examining the relationship between relaxin, knee laxity, and ACL injury risk in normal menstruating females should: (1) time the sampling of relaxin to known hormone events (i.e., rather than calendar days of the cycle), (2) ideally obtain serial measures around the time that relaxin is known to be at its nadir and peak levels in order to fully capture an individual's relaxin profile, and (3) account for circulating sex hormone concentrations to control for their moderating effects when characterizing these relationships.

Summary and Future Directions

Greater knee joint laxity has consistently been associated with a greater risk of ACL injury. Females have greater and more variable knee laxity than males both in terms of absolute magnitude and in the cyclic increases and decreases they experience across their menstrual cycle, and are at a greater risk for ACL rupture. While greater laxity in vivo has been shown to have detrimental biomechanical effects on knee stability during sport activity, cadaveric and animal studies suggest that this greater laxity is also associated with a less dense, less organized, and structurally weaker ligament. While this inferior ligament structure is thought to result from metabolic and remodeling processes that influence ligament structural integrity, the factors that differentially regulate these processes in females versus males remain poorly understood.

What is clear is that sex hormones and other hormones such as relaxin likely play a role in these processes given their potential to exert tremendous influences on the metabolism and structural and mechanical properties of soft tissue structures. However, the extent to which normal physiological variations in these hormones impact the structural and mechanical properties of the ACL in a way that renders it more susceptible to injury in vivo remain poorly understood. This is in part because of the large variability in hormone profiles in physically active women, and the potential time dependency of the tissues responsiveness to hormones, which make it difficult to understand these relationships without prospectively tracking hormone concentrations and variables or outcomes of interest over time. Understanding this variability and time dependency is critical if we are to better align the time of injury occurrence with acute changes in ACL structure and metabolism, and understand how the rate of increase or time duration of elevated hormone concentrations impact the responsiveness of the ligament (Shultz et al. 2015). Unfortunately, the study designs commonly used in this area of research fall well short of the complexity of these issues. The scientific community must become more vigilant in verifying the hormonal milieu at the time of and prior to the time of injury or outcome measurement of interest. This will likely require multiple samples taken over repeated days to accurately characterize a female's hormone environment.

Moreover, it is becoming increasingly evident that there is no one hormone that acts independently to exert these effects, but rather there is likely a complex interaction among multiple hormones and other relevant factors such as exercise status and one's genetic makeup. It is also critical that we expand our study designs to women taking contraceptive hormones and who experience menstrual dysfunction, given their high prevalence in physically active females. Despite these challenges, this remains an important area of study if we are to fully elucidate the underlying mechanisms for the increased risk of ACL injury in females, and develop the most effective intervention strategies to mitigate that risk.

Acknowledgements Selected text is reprinted or adapted, with permission, from S.J. Shultz, 2007, Hormonal influences on ligament biology. In *Understanding and preventing noncontact ACL injuries,* by American Orthopaedic Society for Sports Medicine, edited by T.E. Hewett, S.J. Shultz, and L.Y. Griffin (Champaign, IL: Human Kinetics), 219-238.

References

Abubaker AO, Hebda PC, Gunsolley JN. Effects of sex hormones on protein and collagen content of the temporomandibular joint disc of the rat. J Oral Maxillofac Surg. 1996;54:721–7.
Adachi N, Nawata K, Maeta M, Kurozawa Y. Relationship of the menstrual cycle phase to anterior cruciate ligament injuries in teenage female athletes. Arch Orthop Trauma Surg. 2008;128(5): 473–8.
Agel J, Bershadsky B, Arendt EA. Hormonal Therapy: ACL and Ankle Injury. Med Sci Sports Exerc. 2006;38(1):7–12.
Arendt EA, Bershadsky B, Agel J. Periodicity of noncontact anterior cruciate ligament injuries during the menstrual cycle. J Gend Specif Med. 2002;5(2):19–26.
Arnold C, VanBell C, Rogers V, Cooney T. The relationship between serum relaxin and knee joint laxity in female athletes. Orthopedics. 2002;25(6):669–73.
Beals KA, Manore ML. Disorders of the female athlete triad among collegiate athletes. Int J Sport Nutr Exerc Metab. 2002;12:281–92.
Beynnon BD, Bernstein I, Belisle A, Brattbakk B, Devanny P, Risinger R, Durant D. The effect of estradiol and progesterone on knee and ankle joint laxity. Am J Sports Med. 2005;33(9): 1298–304.
Beynnon BD, Johnson RJ, Braun S, Sargent M, Bernstein I, Skelly JM, Vacek PM. The relationship between menstrual cycle phase and anterior cruciate ligament injury: A case-control study of recreational alpine skiers. Am J Sports Med. 2006;34(5):757–64.
Beynnon BD, Vacek PM, Tourville TW, Sturnick DR, Gardner-Morse M, Holterman LA, Smith HC, Slauterbeck J, Hashemi J, Shultz SJ, Johnson RJ. Multivariate analysis of the risk factors for first-time non-contact ACL injury in high school college athletes; A prospective cohort study with a nested, matched case-control analysis. Am J Sports Med. 2016;44(6):1492–501.
Bryant GD, Panter ME, Stelmasiak T. Immunoreactive relaxin in human serum during the menstrual cycle. J Clin Endocrinol Metab. 1975;41(6):1065–9.
Burrows M, Peters CE. The influence of oral contraceptives on athletic performance in female athletes. Sports Med. 2007;37(7):557–74.
Butler DL, Noyes FR, Grood ES. Ligamentous restraints to anterior-posterior drawer in the human knee. J Bone Joint Surg. 1980;62-A(2):259–70.
Chandrashekar N, Mansour JM, Slauterbeck J, Hashemi J. Sex-based differences in the tensile properties of the human anterior cruciate ligament. J Biomech. 2006;39:2943–50.
Clark MK, Sowers M, Levy BT, Tenhundfeld P. Magnitude and variability of sequential estradiol and progesterone concentrations in women using depot medroxyprogesterone acetate for contraception. Fertil Steril. 2001;75(5):871–7.

Comerford EJ, Tarlton JF, Innes JF, Johnson KA, Amis AA, Bailey AJ. Metabolism and composition of the canine anterior cruciate ligament relate to differences in knee joint mechanics and predisposition to ligament rupture. J Orthop Res. 2005;23:61–6.

Coney P, DelConte A. The effects of ovarian activity of a monophasic oral contraceptive with 100 μg levonorgestrel and 20 μg ethinyl estradiol. Am J Obstet Gynecol. 1999;181(5):S53–8.

Csintalan RP, Inacio MC, Funahashi TT. Incidence rate of anterior cruciate ligament reconstructions. Perm J. 2008;12(3):17–21.

Dehghan F, Muniandy S, Yusof A, Salley N. Sex-steroid regulation of relaxin receptor isoforms (RXFP1 & RXFP2) expression in the patellar tendon and lateral collateral ligament of female WKY rats. Int J Med Sci. 2014a;11(2):180–91.

Dehghan F, Muniandy S, Yusof A, Salley N. Testosterone reduces knee passive range of motion and expression of relaxin receptor isoforms via 5α-Dihydrotestosterone and androgen receptor binding. Int J Mol Sci. 2014b;15:619–4634.

Deie M, Sakamaki Y, Sumen Y, Urabe Y, Ikuta Y. Anterior knee laxity in young women varies with their menstrual cycle. Int Orthop. 2002;26:154–6.

DeSouza MJ, Toombs RJ, Scheid JL, O'Donnell EO, West SL, Williams NI. High prevalence of subtle and severe menstrual disturbances in exercising women: confirmation using daily hormone measures. Hum Reprod. 2010;25(2):491–503.

Dragoo JL, Lee RS, Benhaim P, Finerman GAM, Hame SL. Relaxin receptors in the human female anterior cruciate ligament. Am J Sports Med. 2003;31(4):577–84.

Dragoo JL, Padrez K, Workman R, Lindsey DP. The effect of relaxin on the female anterior cruciate ligament: Analysis of mechanical properties in an animal model. Knee. 2009;16(1):69–72.

Dragoo JL, Castillo TN, Braun HJ, Ridley BA, Kennedy AC, Golish SR. Prospective correlation between serum relaxin concentration and anterior cruciate ligament tears among elite collegiate female athletes. Am J Sports Med. 2011a;39(10):2175–80.

Dragoo JL, Castillo TN, Korotkova TA, Kennedy AC, Kim HJ, Stewart DR. Trends in serum relaxin concentration among elite collegiate female athletes. Int J Womens Health. 2011b;3:19–24.

Dragoo JL, Braun HJ, Durham JL, Chen MR, Harris AH. Incidence and risk factors for injuries to the anterior cruciate ligament in National Collegiate Athletic Association football: data from the 2004–2005 through 2008–2009 National Collegiate Athletic Association Injury Surveillance System. Am J Sports Med. 2012;40(5):990–5. doi:10.1177/0363546512442336.

Dubey RK, Gillespie DG, Jackson EK, Keller PJ. 17B-Estradiol, its metabolites, and progesterone inhibit cardiac fibroblast growth. Hypertension. 1998;31(2):522–8.

Dyer R, Sodek J, Heersche JM. The effect of 17 B-Estradiol on collagen and noncollagenous protein synthesis in the uterus and some periodontal tissues. Endocrinology. 1980;107:1014–21.

Eiling W, Bryant AL, Petersen W, Murphy A, Hohmann E. Effects of menstrual cycle hormone fluctuations on musculoskeletal stiffness and knee joint laxity. Knee Surg Sports Traumatol Arthrosc. 2007;15(2):126–32.

Faryniarz DA, Bhargave M, Lajam C, Attia ET, Hannafin JA. Quantitation of estrogen receptors and relaxin binding in human anterior cruciate ligament fibroblasts. In Vitro Cell Dev Biol Anim. 2006;42:176–81.

Fischer GM. Comparison of collagen dynamics in different tissues under the influence of estradiol. Endocrinology. 1973;93:1216–8.

Fleming BC, Vajapeyam S, Connolly SA, Margarian EM, Murray MM. The use of magnetic resonance imaging to predict ACL graft structural properties. J Biomech. 2011;44:2843–6.

Flynn JM, Mackenzie W, Kolstad K, Sandifer E, Jawad AF, Galinat B. Objective evaluation of knee laxity in children. J Pediatr Orthop. 2000;20:259–63.

Ford KR, Shapiro R, Myer GD, VanDenBogert AJ, Hewett TE. Longitudinal sex differences during landing in knee abduction in young athletes. Med Sci Sports Exerc. 2010;42(10):1923–31.

Galey S, Konieczko EM, Arnold CA, Cooney TE. Immunohistological detection of relaxin binding in anterior cruciate ligaments. Orthopaedics. 2003;26(12):1201–4.

Gianotti SM, Marshall SW, HUme PA, Bunt L. Incidence of anterior cruciate ligament injury and other knee injuries: A national population-based study. J Sci Med Sport. 2009;12:622–7.

Goodman AL, Descalzi CD, Johnson DK, Hodgen GD. Composite pattern of circulating LH, FSH, estradiol, and progesterone during the menstrual cycle in cynomolgus monkeys. Proc Soc Exp Biol Med. 1977;155(4):479–81.

Gorai I, Taguchi Y, Chaki O, Kikuchi R, Nakayama M, Yang BC, Yokota S, Minaguchi H. Serum soluble interleukin-6 receptor and biochemical markers of bone metabolism show significant variations during the menstrual cycle. J Clin Endocrinol Metab. 1998;83(2):326–32.

Gray AM, Gugala Z, Baillargeon J. Effects of oral contraceptive use on anterior cruciate ligament injury epidemiology. Med Sci Sports Exerc. 2016;48(4):648–54.

Griffin LY, Albohm MJ, Arendt EA, Bahr E, Beynnon BD, DeMaio M, Dick RW, Engebretsen L, Garrett WE, Gilchrist J, Hannafin JA, Hewett TE, Huston LJ, Johnson RJ, Lephart SM, Ireland ML, Mandelbaum BR, Mann B, Marks PH, Marshall SW, Myklebust G, Noyes FR, Powers C, Shields C, Shultz SJ, Silvers H, Slauterbeck J, Taylor D, Teitz CC, Wojtys EM, Yu B. Update on ACL Prevention: Theoretical and Practical Guidelines. Am J Sports Med. 2006;34(9):1512–32.

Hama H, Yamamuro T, Takeda T. Experimental studies on connective tissue of the capsular ligament. Influences of aging and sex hormones. Acta Orthop Scand. 1976;47:473–9.

Hamlet WP, Liu SH, Panossian V, Finerman GA. Primary immunolocalization of androgen target cells in the human anterior cruciate ligament. J Orthop Res. 1997;15(5):657–63.

Hansen M, Koskinen SO, Petersen SG, Doessing S, Frystyk J, Flyvbjerg A, Westh E, Magnusson SP, Kjaer M, Langberg H. Ethinyl oestradiol administration in women suppresses synthesis of collagen in tendon in response to exercise. J Physiol. 2008;586(12):3005–16.

Hansen M, Miller BF, Holm L, Doessing S, Petersen SG, Skovgaard D, Frystyk J, Flyvbjerg A, Koskinen S, Pingel J, Kjaer M, Langberg H. Effect of administration of oral contraceptives in vivo on collagen synthesis in tendon and muscle connective tissue in young women. J Appl Physiol. 2009;106:1435–43.

Hansen M, Couppe C, Hansen CSE, Skovgaard D, Kovanen V, Larsen J, Aagaard P, Magnussson SP, Kjaer M. Impact of oral contraceptive use and menstrual phases on patellar tendon morphology, biomechanical composition, and biomechanical properties in female athletes. J Appl Physiol. 2015;114:998–1008.

Hashem G, Zhang Q, Hayami T, Chen J, Wang W, Kapila S. Relaxin and B-estradiol modulate targeted matrix degradation in specific synovial joint fibrocartilages: progesterone prevents matrix loss. Arthritis Res Ther. 2006;8(4):R98.

Hashemi J, Chandrashekar N, Mansouri H, Slauterbeck J, Hardy DM. The Human Anterior Cruciate Ligament: Sex Differences in Ultrastructure and Correlation with Biomechanical Properties. J Orthop Res. 2008;26:945–50.

Hassager C, Jensen LT, Podenphant J, Riis BJ, Christiansen C. Collage synthesis in postmenopausal women during therapy with anabolic steroid or female sex hormones. Metabolism. 1990;39:1167–9.

Hattori K, Sano H, Komatsuda T, Saijo Y, Sugita T, Itoi E. Effect of estrogen on tissue elasticity of the ligament proper in rabbit anterior cruciate ligament: measurements using scanning acoustic microscopy. J Orthop Sci. 2010;15(584-588).

Heitz NA. Hormonal changes throughout the menstrual cycle and increased anterior cruciate ligament laxity in females. J Athl Train. 1999;343(2):144–9.

Henzyl MR. Norgestimate: From the laboratory to three clinical indications. J Reprod Med. 2001;46(7):647–61.

Hewett TE, Zazulak BT, Myer GD. Effects of the menstrual cycle on anterior cruciate ligament injury risk. Am J Sports Med. 2007;35(4):659–68.

Ho KKY, Weissberger AJ. Impact of short-term estrogen administration on growth hormone secretion and action: Distinct route-dependent effects on connective and bone tissue metabolism. J Bone Miner Res. 1992;7:821–7.

Hootman JM, Dick R, Agel J. Epidemiology of collegiate injuries for 15 sports: summary and recommendations for injury prevention initiatives. J Athl Train. 2007;42(2):311–9.

Hosokawa M, Ishii M, Inoue K, Yao CS, Takeda T. Estrogen induces different responses in dermal and lung fibroblasts: Special reference to collagen. Connect Tissue Res. 1981;9:115–20.

Johnson MR, Carter G, Grint C, Lightman SL. Relationship between ovarian steroids, gonadotropins and relaxin during the menstrual cycle. Acta Endocrinol. 1993;129(2):121–5.

Kang Y, Choi Y, Yun C, Park J, Suk K, Kim H, Park M, Lee B, Lee H, Moon S. Down-regulation of collagen synthesis and matrix metalloproteinase expression in myofibroblasts from Dupuytren nodule using adenovirus-mediated relaxin gene therapy. J Orthop Res. 2014;32(4):515–23.

Khowailed IA, Petrofsky JS, Lohman E, Daher N, Mohamed O. 17B-Estradiol induced effects on anterior cruciate ligament laxness and neuromuscular activation patterns in female runners. J Women Health. 2015;24(8):670–80.

Komatsuda T, Sugita T, Sano H, Kusakabe T, Watanuki M, Yohsizumi Y, Murakami T, Hashimoto M, Kokubub S. Does estrogen alter the mechanical properties of the anterior cruciate ligament. Acta Orthop Scand. 2006;77(6):973–80.

Landgren BM, Unden AL, Deczfalusy E. Hormonal profile of the cycle in 68 normal menstruating women. Acta Endocrinol. 1980;94:89–98.

Lee C, Liu X, Smith CL, Zhang X, Hsu H, Wang D, Luo ZP. The combined regulation of estrogen and cyclic tension on fibroblast biosynthesis derived from anterior cruciate ligament. Matrix Biol. 2004;23:323–9.

Lee H, Petrofsky JS, Daher N, Berk L, Laymon M. Differences in anterior cruciate ligament elasticity and force for knee flexion in women: oral contraceptive users versus non-oral contraceptive users. Eur J Appl Physiol. 2014;114:285–94.

Lenton EA, Lawrence GF, Coleman RA, Cooke ID. Individual variation in gonadotropin and steroid concentrations and in the lengths of the follicular and luteal phases in women with regular menstrual cycles. Clin Reprod Fertil. 1983;2:143–50.

Liu SH, Al-Shaikh RA, Panossian V, Finerman GM. Primary immunolocalization of estrogen and progesterone target cells in the human anterior cruciate ligament. J Orthop Res. 1996;14:526–33.

Liu SH, Al-Shaikh RA, Panossian V, Finerman GA, Lane JM. Estrogen affects the cellular metabolism of the anterior cruciate ligament. Am J Sports Med. 1997;25(5):704–9.

London RS, Chapdelaine A, Upmalis D, Olson W, Smith J. Comparative contraceptive efficacy and mechanism of action of the norgestimate-containing triphasic oral contraceptive. Acta Obstet Gynecol Scand. 1992;71:9–14.

Malloy T, Wang Y, Murrell GAC. The roles of growth factors in tendon and ligament healing. Sports Med. 2003;33(5):381–94.

Martineau PA, Al-Jassir F, Lenczner E, Burman ML. Effect of the oral contraceptive pill on ligamentous laxity. Clin J Sports Med. 2004;14:281–6.

Miller KE, Sabo DF, Farrell MP, Barnes GM, Melnick MJ. Sports, sexual behavior, contraceptive use, and pregnancy among female and male high school students: testing cultural resource theory. Sociol Sport J. 1999;16:366–87.

Myklebust G, Maehlum S, Holm I, Bahr R. A prospective cohort study of anterior cruciate ligament injuries in elite Norwegian team handball. Scan J Med Sci Sports. 1998;8:149–53.

Myklebust G, Engebretsen L, Braekken IH, Skjolberg A, Olsen OE, Bahr R. Prevention of anterior cruciate ligament injuries in female team handball players: a prospective intervention study over three seasons. Clin J Sports Med. 2003;13(2):71–8.

Naqvi T, Duong TT, Hashem G, Shiga M, Zhang Q, Kapila S. MMP Induction by Relaxin Causes Cartilage Matrix Degradation in Target Synovial Joints: Receptor Profiles Correlate with Matrix Turnover. Arthritis Res Ther. 2005;7(1):R1–11.

Negishi S, Li Y, Usas A, Fu F, Huard J. The effect of relaxin treatment on skeletal muscle injuries. Am J Sports Med. 2005;33(12):1816–24.

Nguyen AD, Shultz SJ. Sex Differences in Lower Extremity Posture. J Orthop Sports Phys Ther. 2007;37(7):389–98.

Park SK, Stefanyshyn DJ, Loitz-Ramage B, Hart DA, Ronsky JL. Changing hormone levels during the menstrual cycle affect knee laxity and stiffness in healthy female subjects. Am J Sports Med. 2009a;37(3):588–98. doi:10.1177/0363546508326713.

Park SK, Stefanyshyn DJ, Ramage B, Hart DA, Ronsky JL. Alterations in knee joint laxity during the menstrual cycle in healthy women leads to increases in joint loads during selected athletic movements. Am J Sports Med. 2009b;37(6):1169–77.

Paulus D, Saint-Remy A, Jeanjean M. Oral contraception and cardiovascular risk factors among adolescents. Contraception. 2000;62:113–6.

Pearson SJ, Burgess KE, Onambele GL. Serum relaxin levels affect the in vivo properties of some but not all tendons in normally menstruating young women. Exp Physiol. 2011;96(7):681–8.

Pehrsson M, Westberg L, Landen M, Ekman A. Stable serum levels of relaxin throughout the menstrual cycle: A preliminary comparison of women with premenstrual dysphoria and controls. Arch Womens Ment Health. 2007;10:147–53.

Pokorny MJ, Smith TD, Calus SA, Dennison EA. Self-reported oral contraceptive use and peripheral joint laxity. J Orthop Sports Phys Ther. 2000;30(11):683–92.

Posthumus M, September AV, O'Cuinneagain D, van der Merwe W, Schwellnus MP, Collins M. The COL5A1 gene is associated with increased risk of anterior cruciate ligament ruptures in a female participants. Am J Sports Med. 2009;37:2234–40.

Prodromos CC, Han Y, Rogowski J, Joyce B, Shi K. A meta-analysis of the incidence of anterior cruciate ligament tears as a function of gender, sport, and a knee injury-reduction regimen. Arthroscopy. 2007;23(12):1320–5. e1326.

Quasnichka HL, Anderson-MacKenzie JM, Tarlton JF, Sims TJ, Billingham ME, Bailey AJ. Cruciate ligament laxity and femoral intercondylar notch narrowing in early-stage knee osteoarthritis. Arthritis Rheum. 2005;52(10):3100–9. doi:10.1002/art.21340.

Renstrom P, Ljungqvist A, Arendt E, Beynnon B, Fukubayashi T, Garrett W, Georgoulis T, Hewett TE, Johnson R, Krosshaug T, Mandelbaum B, Micheli L, Myklebust G, Roos E, Roos H, Schamasch P, Shultz S, Werner S, Wojtys E, Engebretsen L. Non-contact ACL injuries in female athletes: an International Olympic Committee current concepts statement. Br J Sports Med. 2008;42(6):394–412.

Rozzi SL, Lephart SM, Gear WS, Fu FH. Knee joint laxity and neuromuscular characteristics of male and female soccer and basketball players. Am J Sports Med. 1999;27(3):312–9.

Ruedl G, Ploner P, Linortner I, Schranz A, Fink C, Sommersacher R, Pocecco E, Nachbauer W, Burtscher M. Are oral contraceptive use and menstrual cycle phase related to anterior cruciate ligament injury risk in female recreational skiers? Knee Surg Sports Traumatol Arthrosc. 2009;17(9):1065–9.

Samuel CS, Lekgabe ED, Mookerjee I. The effects of relaxin on extracellular matrix remodeling in health and fibrotic disease. In: Agoulnik AI, editor. Relaxin and related peptides. Nottingham: Landes Bioscience and Springer Science+Business Media; 2007. p. 88–103.

Scerpella TA, Stayer TJ, Makhuli BZ. Ligamentous laxity and non-contact anterior cruciate ligament tears: a gender-based comparison. Orthopedics. 2005;28(7):656–60.

Schmitz RJ, Shultz SJ, Nguyen AD. Dynamic valgus alignment and functional strength in males and females during maturation. J Athl Train. 2009;44(1):26–32.

Seneviratne A, Attia E, Williams RJ, Rodeo SA, Hannafin JA. The Effect of estrogen on ovine anterior cruciate ligament fibroblasts. Am J Sports Med. 2004;32(7):1613–8.

Shea KG, Pfeiffer R, Wang JH, Curtin M, Apel PJ. Anterior cruciate ligament injury in pediatric and adolescent soccer players: an analysis of insurance data. J Pediatr Orthop. 2004;24(6):623–8.

Sherwood OD. Relaxin's physiological roles and other diverse actions. Endocr Rev. 2004;25(2):205–34.

Shikata J, Sanda H, Yamamuro T, Takeda T. Experimental studies of the elastic fiber of the capsular ligament: influence of aging and sex hormones on the hip joint capsule of rats. Connect Tissue Res. 1979;7:21–7.

Shultz SJ, Schmitz RJ. Effects of transverse and frontal plane knee laxity on hip and knee neuromechanics during drop landings. Am J Sports Med. 2009;37(9):1821–30.

Shultz SJ, Kirk SE, Johnson ML, Sander TC, Perrin DH. Relationship between sex hormones and anterior knee laxity across the menstrual cycle. Med Sci Sports Exerc. 2004;36(7):1165–74.

Shultz SJ, Kirk SE, Sander TC, Perrin DH. Sex differences in knee laxity change across the female menstrual cycle. J Sports Med Phys Fitness. 2005;45(4):594–603.
Shultz SJ, Gansneder BG, Sander TC, Kirk SE, Perrin DH. Absolute hormone levels predict the magnitude of change in knee laxity across the menstrual cycle. J Orthop Res. 2006a;24(2):124–31.
Shultz SJ, Shimokochi Y, Nguyen AD, Ambegaonkar JP, Schmitz RJ, Beynnon BD, Perrin DH. Nonweight-bearing anterior knee laxity is related to anterior tibial translation during transition from nonweight bearing to weight bearing. J Orthop Res. 2006b;24(3):516–23. doi:10.1002/jor.20040.
Shultz SJ, Nguyen A, Schmitz RJ. Differences in lower extremity anatomical and postural characteristics in males and females between maturation groups. J Orthop Sports Phys Ther. 2008;38(3):137–49.
Shultz SJ, Levine BJ, Nguyen AD, Kim HS, Montgomery MM, Perrin DH. A Comparison of cyclic variations in anterior knee laxity, genu recurvatum and general joint laxity across the menstrual cycle. J Orthop Res. 2010a;28:1411–7.
Shultz SJ, Schmitz RJ, Nguyen AD, Levine BJ. Joint laxity is related to lower extremity energetics during a drop jump landing. Med Sci Sports Exerc. 2010b;42(4):771–80. doi:10.1249/MSS.0b013e3181bbeaa6.
Shultz SJ, Schmitz RJ, Nguyen AD, Levine B, Kim H, Montgomery MM, Shimokochi Y, Beynnon BD, Perrin DH. Knee joint laxity and its cyclic variation influence tibiofemoral motion during weight acceptance. Med Sci Sports Exerc. 2011a;43(2):287–95. doi:10.1249/MSS.0b013e3181ed118d.
Shultz SJ, Wideman L, Montgomery MM, Levine BJ. Some sex hormone profiles are consistent over time in normal menstruating females: Implications for sports injury epidemiology. Br J Sports Med. 2011b;45:735–42. doi:10.1136/bjsm.2009.064931.
Shultz SJ, Schmitz RJ, Kong Y, Dudley WN, Beynnon BD, Nguyen AD, Kim H, Montgomery MM. Cyclic variations in multiplanar knee laxity influence landing biomechanics. Med Sci Sports Exerc. 2012a;44(5):900–9. doi:10.1249/MSS.0b013e31823bfb25.
Shultz SJ, Wideman L, Montgomery MM, Beasley KN, Nindl BC. Changes in serum collagen markers, IGF-I and knee joint laxity across the menstrual cycle. J Orthop Res. 2012b;30:1405–12. doi:10.1002/jor.22093.
Shultz SJ, Schmitz RJ, Cone JR, Copple TJ, Montgomery MM, Pye ML, Tritsch AJ. Multiplanar knee laxity increases during a 90-min intermittent exercise protocol. Med Sci Sports Exerc. 2013;45(8):1553–61. doi:10.1249/MSS.0b013e31828cb94e.
Shultz SJ, Schmitz RJ, Benjaminse A, Collins M, Ford K, Kulas AS. ACL Research Retreat VII: An update on anterior cruciate ligament injury risk factor identification, screening, and prevention. J Athl Train. 2015;50(10):1076–93. doi:10.4085/1062-6050-50.10.06.
Slauterbeck J, Clevenger C, Lundberg W, Burchfield DM. Estrogen level alters the failure load of the rabbit anterior cruciate ligament. J Orthop Res. 1999;17(405-408):405–8.
Slauterbeck JR, Fuzie SF, Smith MP, Clark RJ, Xu KT, Starch DW, Hardy DM. The menstrual cycle, sex hormones, and anterior cruciate ligament injury. J Athl Train. 2002;37(3):275–80.
Small CM, Manatunga AK, Marcus M. Validity of Self-Reported Menstrual Cycle Length. Ann Epidemiol. 2007;17:163–70.
Stewart DR, Celniker AC, Taylor CA, Cragun JR, Overstreet JW, Lasley BL. Relaxin in the peri-implantation period. J Clin Endocrinol Metab. 1990;70(6):1771–3.
Strickland SM, Belknap TW, Turner SA, Wright TM, Hannafin JA. Lack of hormonal influences on mechanical properties of sheep knee ligaments. Am J Sports Med. 2003;31(2):210–5.
Svenningsen S, Terjesen T, Auflem M, Berg V. Hip motion related to sex and age. Acta Orthop Scand. 1989;60(1):97–100.
Takano M, Yamaguchi M, Nakajima R, Fujita S, Kojima T, Kasai K. Effects of relaxin on collagen type I released by stretched human periodontal ligament cells. Orthod Craniofac Res. 2009;12:282–8.
Thein-Nissenbaum JM, Rauh MJ, Carr KE, Loud KJ, McGuine TA. Menstrual irregularity and musculoskeletal injury in female high school athletes. J Athl Train. 2012;47(1):74–82.

Thein-Nissenbaum JM, Carr KE, Hetzel S, Dennison E. Disordered eating, menstrual irregularity, and musculoskeletal injury in high school athletes: a comparison of oral contraceptive pill users and nonusers. Sports Health. 2014;6(4):313–20. doi:10.1177/1941738113498852.

Tourville T, Shultz SJ, Vacek P, Knudsen E, Bernstein I, Tourville K, Hardy DM, Slauterbeck J, Johnson R, Beynnon BD. Evaluation of an algorithm to predict menstrual cycle phase at the time of injury. J Athl Train. 2016;51(1):47–56.

Uhorchak JM, Scoville CR, Williams GN, Arciero RA, St Pierre P, Taylor DC. Risk factors associated with noncontact injury of the anterior cruciate ligament: a prospective four-year evaluation of 859 West Point cadets. Am J Sports Med. 2003;31(6):831–42.

Unemori EN, Amento EP. Relaxin modulates synthesis and secretion of procollagenase and collagen by human dermal fibroblasts. J Biol Chem. 1990;265(18):10681–5.

Unemori EN, Beck S, Lee WP, Xu Y, Siegel M, Keller G, Liggitt HD, Bauer EA, Amento EP. Human relaxin decreases collagen accumulation in vivo in two rodent models of fibrosis. J Invest Dermatol. 1993;101:280–5.

Vescovi JD. The menstrual cycle and anterior cruciate ligament injury risk: Implications of menstrual cycle variability. Sports Med. 2011;41(2):91–101.

Wang VM, Banack TM, Tsai CW, Flatow EL, Jepsen KJ. Variability in tendon and knee joint biomechanics among inbred mouse strains. J Orthop Res. 2006;24:1200–7.

Wentorf FA, Sudoh K, Moses C, Arendt EA, Carlson C. The Effects of estrogen on material and mechanical properties of the intra- and extra-articular knee structures. Am J Sports Med. 2006; 34(12):1948–52.

Wilmore JH, Costill DL. Physiology of sport and exercise. 2nd ed. Champaign: Human Kinetics; 1999.

Wojtys EM, Huston LJ, Lindenfeld TN, Hewett TE, Greenfield ML. Association between the menstrual cycle and anterior cruciate ligament injuries in female athletes. Am J Sports Med. 1998;26(5):614–9.

Wojtys EM, Huston LJ, Boynton MD, Spindler KP, Lindenfeld TN. The effect of the menstrual cycle on anterior cruciate ligament injuries in women as determined by hormone levels. Am J Sports Med. 2002;30(2):182–8.

Wolf JM, Cameron KL, Clifton KB, Owens BD. Serum relaxin levels in young athletic men are comparable with those in women. Orthopaedics. 2013a;36(2):128–31.

Wolf JM, Williams AE, Delaronde S, Leger R, Clifton KB, King KB. Relationship of serum relaxin to generalized and trapezial-metacarpal joint laxity. J Hand Surg Am. 2013b;38A:721–8.

Wolf JM, Scher DL, Etchill WE, Scott F, Williams AE, Delaronde S, King KB. Relationship of relaxin hormone and thumb carpometacarpal joint arthritis. Clin Orthop Relat Res. 2014;472(4): 1130–7.

Wood ML, Luthin WN, Lester GE, Dahners LE. Tendon creep is potentiated by NKISK and relaxin which produce collagen fiber sliding. Iowa Orthop J. 2003;23:75–9.

Wreje U, Kristiansson P, Aberg H, Bystrom B, Schoultz B. Serum levels of relaxin during the menstrual cycle and oral contraceptive use. Gynecol Obstet Invest. 1995;39:197–200.

Wreje U, Brynhildsen J, Aberg H, Bystrom B, Hammar M, VonSchoultz B. Collagen metabolism markers as a reflection of bone and soft tissue turnover during the menstrual cycle and oral contraceptive use. Contraception. 2000;61:265–70.

Yu WD, Hatch JD, Panossian V, Finerman GA, Liu SH (1997) Effects of estrogen on cellular growth and collagen synthesis of the human anterior cruciate ligament: an explanation for female athletic injury. In: 43rd Annual Meeting of the Orthopaedic Research Society, San Francisco, CA, February 9–13. Rider Dickerson, Inc, p 397

Yu WD, Liu SH, Hatch JD, Panossian V, Finerman GA. Effect of estrogen on cellular metabolism of the human anterior cruciate ligament. Clin Orthop Relat Res. 1999;366:229–38.

Yu WD, Panossian V, Hatch JD, Liu SH, Finerman GA. Combined effects of estrogen and progesterone on the anterior cruciate ligament. Clin Orthop Relat Res. 2001;383:268–81.

Zazulak BT, Paterno M, Myer GD, Romani WA, Hewett TE. The effects of the menstrual cycle on anterior knee laxity. Sports Med. 2006;36(10):847–62.

Chapter 8
Sex Hormones and Physical Activity in Women: An Evolutionary Framework

Ann E. Caldwell and Paul L. Hooper

Over recent decades, researchers, athletes, and coaches have been interested in understanding the bidirectional relationships between sex hormones and exercise in women. This interest comes from evidence suggesting that sex hormones are related to exercise both among highly active women and athletes as well as among sedentary women. In a laboratory-controlled study, for example, sedentary women in menses who were not using hormonal contraceptives had steeper increases in perceived exertion and pain during moderate intensity exercise (Caldwell Hooper et al. 2011). One potential explanation of this result is that estrogen has analgesic effects, and the absence of endogenous estrogen during the menstrual phase makes first-time moderate exercise relatively more aversive than during cycle phases with higher levels of estrogen. This is important because subjective experience (perception) of exercise has been shown to influence intentions to exercise and behavior (Kwan and Bryan 2010). That is, a more negative subjective experience may influence women's motivation to exercise again, and could affect the likelihood that sedentary women successfully take up exercise. This study shows that understanding the relationships between sex hormones and exercise can not only improve performance in highly trained athletes, but can also inform interventions aimed at increasing activity among sedentary women. Identifying female-specific approaches and barriers to making exercise more accessible and less aversive for women can make meaningful contributions to public health. To that end, the goal of this chapter is to present a framework from evolutionary biology, including life history theory, which can illuminate *why* sex hormones and exercise are related. This perspective

---

A.E. Caldwell, Ph.D. (✉)
Anschutz Health and Wellness Center, University of Colorado Denver, School of Medicine, Aurora, CO, USA
e-mail: ann.caldwell@ucdenver.edu

P.L. Hooper, Ph.D.
Department of Anthropology, Emory University, Atlanta, GA, USA

© Springer International Publishing Switzerland 2017
A.C. Hackney (ed.), *Sex Hormones, Exercise and Women*,
DOI 10.1007/978-3-319-44558-8_8

can lead to theoretically driven predictions about the bidirectional relationships between sex hormones and exercise among women that may not be considered from more strictly physiological approaches.

Life History Theory: An Evolutionary Framework for Understanding Sex Hormones and Exercise in Women

In general, an evolutionary approach aims to explain how behavior, and the underlying mechanisms that lead to behavior, have been shaped by natural selection. Natural selection operates through differential reproductive success—or fitness, in the evolutionary sense—as the genes of individuals who successfully survive and reproduce are passed on to subsequent generations at a relatively higher rate than the genes of those who reproduce less or not at all. The environmental forces that determine which traits or behaviors result in greater reproductive success are called selection pressures. Selection pressures differ considerably depending on an organism's natural environment, their ecological or social niche (their way of "making a living"), as well as age, sex, and physical condition.

Selection continues to act on traits, behaviors, and their underlying psychological and physiological mechanisms so long as they exhibit heritable variation that is associated with differential reproductive success. For traits or behaviors with one optimal solution within a species regardless of environment or individual condition, that trait or behavior will tend to become universal over time. However, when there is more than one optimal solution and/or the optimum depends on individual or environmental circumstances, variation will remain. A flexible system that responds to the individual and/or environmental circumstances with behaviors that increase the probability of reproductive success can evolve. Thus, while universality of a trait or behavior is often used as evidence that it has been shaped by evolutionary forces, this is not a necessary condition for evolved traits or behaviors. In the case of exercise and physical activity—the costs and benefits of which vary widely between individuals and environments—a flexible, condition-dependent system is more likely to have evolved.

Given the numerous mental and physical health benefits associated with exercise and the deleterious health outcomes related to physical inactivity in modern environments (Booth et al. 2012; Warburton et al. 2006; Kohl et al. 2012; Lee et al. 2012; Hillman et al. 2008), it is intuitively appealing that exercise might simply be a universally adaptive behavior in humans. Moreover, there is evidence that humans have anatomical (Bramble and Leiberman 2004) and neurological (Raichlen et al. 2012) adaptations for endurance activity. There is another side to the story, however, suggesting that physical *inactivity* and energy *conservation* are also adaptive in humans (Caldwell 2016).

Human patterns of activity have changed drastically over a relatively short amount of evolutionary time. Over the past 10,000 years—and especially in the last two centuries—humans have created novel environments that require very little physical energy expenditure in order to fulfill basic biological needs. Cumulative technological innovations have increased the efficiency of resource extraction, storage, and transportation. Why did humans create this environment that enables inactivity, in spite of adaptations that make endurance physical activity rewarding and relatively efficient?

From an evolutionary perspective, humans, like all other organisms, have evolved to strategically allocate time and energy in ways that increase the likelihood of reproductive success. This is the central premise of life history theory, the body of evolutionary thought that aims to understand how natural selection has shaped the division of time and energy between growth, reproduction, and maintenance across the lifespan (Stearns 1992; Charnov 1993; Hill and Kaplan 1999). Selection pressures arise from the interaction of an individual's condition within a given environment to determine optimal duration and rates of growth, age of reproductive maturation, pace of reproduction, rate and timing of reproductive decline, and senescence (Kaplan et al. 2010). Life history theory also fundamentally considers that there are inherent trade-offs between allocations to different (potentially) fitness-enhancing activities across the lifespan, because energy and time put toward one activity cannot be invested elsewhere. Because exercise explicitly requires energy expenditure, exercise necessarily trades off against growth, reproduction, and maintenance in important ways.

This drive to optimize energy allocation affects exercise and physical activity because allocation strategies have been shaped throughout human evolution to flexibly respond to factors—such as sex, age, environment, and individual condition—that influence the evolutionary fitness costs and benefits of physical activity. In humans and other mammals in particular, the energetic demands of reproduction are much higher for females than males, in terms of investment in sex cells (eggs vs sperm), gestation, and breastfeeding. As a result, the energetic trade-offs and opportunity costs of investing energy in physical fitness and activity/exercise tend to be higher for women of reproductive age than men.

Within the framework of life history theory, hormones are considered to be a physiological mechanism by which energy is allocated between competing short- and long-term demands of growth, reproduction, and maintenance (Worthman and Barrett-Connor 2002; Zera and Harshman 2001; Lancaster and Kaplan 2009). Energy expenditure in the form of physical activity or exercise similarly trades-off against these competing energetic demands, and is partially regulated through hormones (Caldwell 2016). Therefore, when considering the role of sex hormones and exercise, it is important to keep in mind that the primary function of sex hormones is their role in reproduction, and that traits and behaviors have been shaped over evolutionary time to increase the probability of reproductive success. A thorough understanding of how this system is predicted to operate can help illuminate *how and why* sex hormones and exercise are related.

One example of an exercise phenomenon which has been illumated by evolutionary principles is the decrease in physical activity across adolescence that is well documented in Western populations (Cumming et al. 2008; Thompson et al. 2003). Although epidemiological researchers tend to interpret this pattern of decrease as a by-product of the psychosocial stress of puberty, life history theory predicts that activity declines at this stage because pubertal adolescents increase the energy invested in growth and reproductive maturation, which trades off against exercise and non-obligatory forms of activity (e.g., active play, running games, riding bikes). Evidence supporting this interpretation comes from a study of activity levels of indigenous Tsimane' adolescents (Caldwell 2016). The Tsimane' are a small-scale society that lives in the Amazonian lowlands of Bolivia. They have a subsistence economy based on foraging and horticulture, with high levels of obligatory physical activity. Even in this setting, which shares many features with the conditions of our remote evolutionary past, decreases in objectively measured physical activity are seen in adolescence. These differences are predicted by Tanner stage of reproductive maturation, suggesting that reproductive maturation trades off against energy expenditure in the form of physical activity. Sex hormones are predicted to mediate these decreases, with higher levels of sex hormones predicting greater decreases in physical activity.

More generally, life history theory is an ideal theoretical framework for understanding exercise and sex hormones in women because they both influence and are influenced by life history parameters such as reproductive maturation, reproduction, and physical condition. This framework suggests that human physiology and psychology have been shaped by natural selection to maintain physical fitness and *selectively* engage in physical activity and exercise when the adaptive benefits outweigh the metabolic and opportunity costs (Caldwell 2016). When the benefits do not outweigh the costs, humans, like other animals, have evolved to conserve energy through behavioral and physiological shifts in energy allocation.

Another important consideration in employing evolutionary theory in this area is that over the vast majority of human history, optimal energy allocation strategies have been constrained by finite resource availability and resource scarcity (Shetty 1999; Vickers et al. 2003). Innate drives to conserve energy have only recently been coupled with massive abundances of calorically dense, easy-to-acquire foods. When environments change rapidly, or are vastly different from the environment in which selection was acting to shape a trait or behavior, a discordance or mismatch can occur (Eaton et al. 1988; Lieberman 2013; Eaton et al. 2002; Kaplan 1996). In these mismatched environments, previously adaptive behaviors or mechanisms may no longer increase reproductive success, and can even be detrimental to reproduction or survival. Energy-conserving behaviors and metabolic adaptations that increased the likelihood of survival and reproduction in environments with fewer and less predictable resources now lead to health disorders like obesity and cardiovascular disease, which can hinder reproduction in women (Metwally et al. 2007). One must thus consider the mechanisms and behaviors that would have been adaptive in the environments during the majority of human history, when selection was acting to shape them, rather than just those that are expected to be currently adaptive. Evolutionary theory can thus be informative for understanding the relationships between exercise and sex hormones that appear on the surface to be maladaptive, but are instead mismatched to current environments. In current environments, exercise and physical fitness significantly decrease the risks of chronic disease mortality and physical activity has been shown to induce epigenetic changes that decrease cancer risk (Bryan et al. 2013). Current environments therefore create the potential for selection to begin to favor higher levels of activity and exercise, because those who are more active and physically fit are more likely to live longer and be healthy enough to provide better support for offspring and grand-offspring relative to less active and physically fit individuals. This is particularly true in environments in which parental and grandparental investment significantly improves survival and reproduction of younger generations.

Reproductive Ecology, Sex Hormones and Exercise in Women

Given that selection operates through differential reproductive success, the effects of physical activity on reproductive function are central to an evolutionary framework. An evolutionary approach can also draw on important work in human reproductive ecology, a subfield of evolutionary anthropology that aims to understand the ways the human reproductive system responds to environmental cues (Jasienska 2013; Ellison 2001). Importantly, this body of research establishes that women's reproductive systems have evolved to be remarkably sensitive to energetic cues in the environment in order to shift effort adaptively.

Human females incur much higher energetic costs to reproduce compared to males. This imbalance begins at the level of the gamete, but energetic costs increase through pubertal maturation, gestation and breastfeeding. Child-birth also involves significant, potentially mortal, risks for females. The energetic trade-offs between reproduction and exercise or physical activity alone are substantial enough to help explain why exercise and sex hormones are related in women. Both activities can be hugely metabolically taxing. The metabolic costs of pregnancy during the third trimester are estimated to be around 465 kcal/day above prepregnancy levels, while breastfeeding can increase metabolic load by 625–700 kcal/day (Butte and King 2005). Research in reproductive ecology also shows that women's reproductive systems have physiological mechanisms that decrease the likelihood of conception in response to cues of short-term energetic stress, particularly through reductions in ovarian steroid hormone levels in response to low energy availability, negative energy balance, and high and low levels of energy flux (Ellison 2003). This makes conception less probable during unfavorable conditions when women are less capable of meeting the energetic demands of pregnancy and lactation.

Women's biological capacity to reproduce, or fecundity, is greatly influenced by sex hormones. Ovarian function varies along a continuum of fecundity, which can be assessed by sex hormones. Low levels of estradiol during the follicular phase or progesterone during the luteal phase have been shown to reflect decreased fecundity (Lipson and Ellison 1996). Menstrual cycle irregularities measured by a short luteal phase (<10 days), or by oligomenorrhea (cycle length >35 days) also signal potential disturbances in reproductive function and fecundity.

There is evidence that transient shifts in energy availability influence female fecundity in both Western and non-Western human samples, as well as in chimpanzees (Emery Thompson and Wrangham 2008). Low ovarian steroid levels have been observed among women in Western populations who have low energy availability (i.e., are losing weight, are restraining their intake below appetite, or have less stored fat, lower lipid profiles, or high energy expenditure through exercise or workload, reviewed in Ellison 2008; Vitzthum 2009). The combination of high energy expenditure and low energy intake has a particularly pronounced negative effect on fecundity (Ellison 2001). It is worth noting that even when food is not limited, increased energy expenditure has been shown to decrease sex hormones (e.g., (Jasienska and Ellison 2004; Jasienska et al. 2006; Williams et al. 2015).

Seminal research examining reproductive function and energy availability (dietary intake minus expenditure) has demonstrated that very low energy availability (less than 30 kcal/kg lean body mass per day) disrupts LH pulsatility, which is critical for reproductive function (Loucks and Thuma 2003; Loucks et al. 1994; Loucks et al. 1998). Building on this research, a recent study attempted to tease apart the effects of energy expenditure and negative energy balance on menstrual cycle irregularities in a randomized control trial of sedentary women in the US (Williams et al. 2015). In one condition, participants increased exercise, but had compensatory increases in energy intake to attain a neutral energy balance. In the other conditions, participants exercised *and* reduced caloric intake resulting in deficits of 15 %, 30 %, or 60 % across three conditions. Over three months, around 13 % of the women in the exercise-only condition experienced menstrual cycle irregularities (short luteal phase, <10 days, or inadequate urinary progesterone during the luteal phase, <5.0 μg/ml). In contrast, nearly all of those in the most extreme energy deficient condition (88 %) exhibited irregularities. In addition to demonstrating the dose–response nature of energetics on fecundity, this study demonstrated the individual differences in the responsive of the reproductive systems to energetic stress. While some women's reproductive systems were highly sensitive, showing menstrual irregularities even when energy expenditure was compensated by increased consumption, others were much more robust, and did not show signs of menstrual irregularities despite increased exercise *and* substantial caloric deficits.

What are the factors that underlie these individual differences? It can be difficult to know where to begin testing moderators of energetics and reproductive function/ fecundity. Does it have something to do with socioeconomic status, or ethnicity, or education, or other stressors? A life history framework predicts that reproductive responsiveness to energetic stress is influenced by prenatal and developmental environments, and factors that determine energetic trade-offs: age, parity, overall health and immune system, and previous experiences with physical activity and physical fitness. This framework would further predict that women whose reproductive system is particularly sensitive to energetic stress face higher costs of performing exercise than those whose system is more robust. Women facing higher costs are less likely to engage in exercise that is not related to tangible evolutionary fitness benefits (i.e., mating, parental investment). One can also test if there are psychological mediators between these relationships, such as whether women who have particularly responsive reproductive systems are less likely to feel motivated to or enjoy exercise when facing steep competing demands for reproductive function.

Relationships between energy expenditure and intake have been nicely illustrated in a natural experiment among the Tamang in Nepal. The Tamang practice small-scale agriculture and pastoralism, and they have seasonal variation in physical workloads—from moderately heavy in winter to very heavy during the monsoon season. Overall, Tamang women exhibit weight loss and decreased ovulation in the heavy-work monsoon season (38 % ovulating during the monsoon versus 71 % in the winter). Notably, however, this effect differed by age, with younger women (those aged 17–23) exhibiting negligible seasonal changes in ovarian function and no weight loss during the heavy work season compared to older menstruating women (Panter-Brick et al. 1993). Vitzthum (2009) hypothesized that acclimation to heavy work-loads and high energy consumption levels allow some Tamang women to buffer against ovarian suppression in the face of high energetic output. It could be that younger, non-lactating, and/or nulliparous women have a larger energy budget to put toward increasing the likelihood of becoming pregnant, and are therefore less affected by acute shifts in energy expenditure. Since the data are cross-sectional within one year, differences between age groups could also be driven by epigenetic factors that influenced the energetic phenotype of a cohort of women. Others have hypothesized that critical periods during development, where mothers provision offspring through the placenta or lactation, allow for the transfer of information about the mother's cumulative and current energetic status (Kuzawa and Quinn 2009). From this perspective, the information transferred to offspring is thought to provide cues of the energetic stress in the probable environment in which offspring will be born. Developing fetuses and babies can then adaptively shape their energetic phenotype to be more or less conservative. Maternal cues of energetic stress are thought to result in offspring with more conservatively calibrated energetic strategies that would be adaptive in environments with unpredictable food availability. This type of information transfer may lead to differences in the responsiveness of women's reproductive systems in the face of low energy availability. A more conservative energetic phenotype may be more sensitive to energetic stress, to decrease the likelihood of conception when it is unclear whether or not the energetic demands of the pregnancy will be able to be met.

A study by Jasienska and colleagues demonstrated that energetic stress during fetal development may affect the sensitivity of women's reproductive systems to increases in activity or workload. Among a sample of rural Polish women ($N=145$) who had moderate levels of physical activity, size at birth (measured by ponderal index, PI: kg/m^3 from medical records) moderated the relationship between physical activity and ovarian suppression measured by mid-follicular salivary estradiol. Those in relatively better energetic condition (higher PI) at birth did not demonstrate lower estradiol. In contrast, women who experienced a constrained fetal environment, reflected by low or moderate PI at birth, showed a heightened sensitivity of estradiol to increased physical activity. These results support the predictive adaptive response theory (Ellison and Jasienska 2007; Ellison 1990; Gluckman et al. 2005; Kuzawa et al. 2007; Kuzawa 2005; Lipson 2001), which hypothesizes that when a fetus develops in an environment with cues of constrained energetic resources, adaptive shifts in metabolism or energy allocation occur that favor energy conservation throughout life. Individuals' developmental environments may thus affect the extent to which their sex hormones and reproductive systems preemptively downregulate hormone production and fecundity in response to increases in physical activity or workload. In other words, developmental environments can moderate the relationships between sex hormones and exercise, leading to individual differences that vary in predictable ways.

Evolutionary research has established that energy balance influences female reproduction through a variety of pathways. Women who are energetically stressed tend to have shorter gestation periods and infants with lower birth weight (Ellison 2003; Kline et al. 1989). Energetics also modulate the length of time that breastfeeding women do not ovulate, termed lactational amenorrhea. As noted earlier, lactation is extremely energetically costly for women and typically leads to ovarian suppression (via endocrine mechanisms). The duration of lactational amenorrhea varies between and within populations, and is thought to be affected by energetic demands and fat stores available for producing breast milk and weaning practices (Kaplan et al. 2015). Women who have heavy daily workloads often breastfeed less frequently and begin to supplement children's diet with alternative food sources earlier, decreasing maternal levels of prolactin and reducing the drive for milk production (Panter-Brick and Pollard 1999). Decreased frequency of breastfeeding and/or food supplementation likely mediates the effect of energy expenditure on ovulatory suppression. Since reproduction involves such high metabolic investment from women, a reproductive system that adaptively responds to shifts in energy availability and expenditure may delay reproduction if it is unclear whether the energetic demands of pregnancy and/or lactation can be met (Ellison 2001; Vitzthum 2009; Jasienska 2003). Women's reproductive system appears to be particularly sensitive among those who had constrained fetal environments, and in response to transient shifts in energy availability. Consistent exercise (i.e., training), particularly if performed throughout life and paired with a healthy diet (so not in very low energy availability) is unlikely to have a detrimental effect on women's fecundity. In addition, some have suggested that one reason higher physical activity is associated with a lower risk of breast cancer is the reduction of ovarian steroids that is associated with physical activity and exercise (Jasienska et al. 2006; Key and Pike 1988; Kaaks and Lukanova 2002). In environments with contraception (where women experience many more menstrual cycles than historically), low levels of physical activity and exercise, and an abundance of calorically dense and highly palatable foods, estradiol levels may high enough to be detrimental to women's health.

Conclusions

An evolutionary perspective offers subtle but meaningful shifts in the interpretation of the existing literature on sex hormones and exercise. Moreover, it leads to theory-driven hypotheses regarding factors—such as individual condition and cues of resource scarcity—that can predictably influence individual differences in the relationships between sex hormones and exercise. Variation across individuals and contexts may contribute to the apparent inconsistency of past findings. Future research that aims to understand sex differences in sedentary and exercise behavior, and the psychology that underlies each, can draw on what is known about sex hormones, reproductive function and activity in the evolutionary life sciences.

There are five key messages that are derived from applying an evolutionary framework to understand the relationship between sex hormones and exercise.

- Natural selection favors physiological and behavioral adaptations that increase the probability of survival and reproductive success.
- Energy and time are finite resources, and the system that regulates energy allocation operates primarily through hormones, including sex hormones.
- Energy expended in exercise or physical activity trades-off against energy allocated to other activities, such as growth, reproduction, and maintenance.
- Reproduction is hugely energetically costly for women, and the female reproductive system has evolved to reduce fecundity in response to cues of transient increases in energy expenditure and reductions in energy intake. This responsiveness can lead to decreases in fecundity that lower the probability of reproductive success.
- Because an evolved propensity to decrease fecundity in response to increases in energy expenditure is potentially detrimental to reproductive success, this may create subconscious barriers to performing non-obligatory forms of physical activity and exercise in women.

By drawing on tools and insights from evolutionary biology, anthropology, and psychology, an evolutionary approach allows for an integrated approach to the mechanism, function, history, and ecology of sex hormones and exercise in women within a single framework.

References

Booth FW, Roberts CK, Laye MJ. Lack of exercise is a major cause of chronic diseases. Compr Physiol. 2012;2(2):1143–211. Available from: http://www.scopus.com/inward/record.url?eid=2-s2.0-84862234497&partnerID=40&md5=523f30209f96d6c968ce62a5e0cf518d.

Bramble DM, Leiberman D. Endurance running and the evolution of Homo. Nature. 2004;432: 345–52.

Bryan AD, Magnan RE, Caldwell Hooper AE, Harlaar N, Hutchison KE. Physical activity and differential methylation of breast cancer genes assayed from saliva: a preliminary investigation. Ann Behav Med. 2013;45(1):89–98.

Butte NF, King JC. Energy requirements during pregnancy and lactation. Public Health Nutr. 2005; 8(7a):1010–27. Available from: http://www.journals.cambridge.org/abstract_S136898000500131X.

Caldwell AE. Human physical fitness and activity: an evolutionary and life history perspective. Springer International: AG Switzerland; 2016.

Caldwell Hooper AE, Bryan AD, Eaton M. Menstrual cycle effects on perceived exertion and pain during exercise among sedentary women. J Womens Health (Larchmt). 2011;20(3):439–46. Available from: http://www.scopus.com/inward/record.url?eid=2-s2.0-79952741601&partnerID=tZOtx3y1.

Charnov E. Life history invariants: some explorations of symmetry in evolutionary ecology. Oxford: Oxford University Press; 1993.

Cumming SP, Standage M, Gillison F, Malina RM. Sex differences in exercise behavior during adolescence: is biological maturation a confounding factor. J Adolesc Health. 2008;42(5):480–5.

Eaton SB, Konner M, Shostak M. Stone agers in the fast lane: chronic degenerative diseases in evolutionary perspective. Am J Med. 1988;84(4):739–49.

Eaton SB, Strassman BI, Nesse RM, Neel JV, Ewald PW, Williams GC, et al. Evolutionary health promotion. Prev Med (Baltim). 2002;34(2):109–18.

Ellison PT. Human ovarian function and reproductive ecology. Am Anthropol. 1990;92:933–52.

Ellison PT. On fertile ground. Cambridge: Harvard Press; 2001.

Ellison PT. Energetics and reproductive effort. Am J Hum Biol. 2003;15:342–51.

Ellison PT. Energetics, reproductive ecology, and human evolution. Paleo Anthropol. 2008;2008:172–200.

Ellison PT, Jasienska G. Constraint, pathology, and adaptation: how can we tell them apart? Am J Hum Biol. 2007;19:622–30.

Emery Thompson M, Wrangham RW. Diet and reproductive function in wild female chimpanzees (Pan troglodytes schweinfurthii) at Kibale National Park. Uganda Am J Phys Anthropol. 2008;135(2):171–81.

Gluckman PD, Hanson MA, Spencer HG. Predictive adaptive responses and human evolution. Trends Ecol Evol. 2005;20:527–33.

Hill K, Kaplan H. Life history traits in humans: theory and empirical studies. Annu Rev Anthropol. 1999;28:397–430.

Hillman CH, Erickson KI, Kramer AF. Be smart, exercise your heart: exercise effects on brain and cognition. Nat Rev Neurosci. 2008;9(1):58–65.

Jasienska G. Energy metabolism and the evolution of reproductive suppression in the human female. Acta Bioitheoretica. 2003;51:1–18.

Jasienska G. The fragile wisdom: an evolutionary view on women's biology and health. Cambridge: Harvard University Press; 2013.

Jasienska G, Ellison PT. Energetic factors and seasonal changes in ovarian function in women from rural Poland. Am J Hum Biol. 2004;16:563–80.

Jasienska G, Ziomkiewicz A, Thune I, Lipson S, Ellison P. Habitual physical activity and estradiol levels in women of reproductive age. Eur J Cancer Prev. 2006;15:439–45.

Kaaks R, Lukanova A. Effects of weight control and physical activity in cancer prevention: role of endogenous hormone metabolism. Ann N Y Acad Sci. 2002;963:268–81. Available from: http://www.ncbi.nlm.nih.gov/entrez/query.fcgi?cmd=Retrieve&db=PubMed&dopt=Citation&list_uids=12095952.

Kaplan H. A theory of fertility and parental investment in traditional and modern human societies. Yearbook Phys Anthropol. 1996;39:91–135.

Kaplan H, Gurven M, Winking J, Hooper PL, Stieglitz J. Learning, menopause, and the human adaptive complex. Ann N Y Acad Sci. 2010;1204:30–42.

Kaplan HS, Bock J, Hooper PL. Fertility theory: Embodied-capital theory of human life history evolution. In: International Encyclopedia of Social and Behavioral Sciences, 2nd edition. James D. Wright, Elsevier, Amsterdam 2015:(9)28–34.

Key TJA, Pike MC. The role of oestrogens and progestagens in the epidemiology and prevention of breast cancer. Eur J Cancer Clin Oncol. 1988;24(1):29–43.

Kline J, Stein Z, Susser M. Conception to birth: epidemiology of prenatal development. New York: Oxford University Press; 1989.

Kohl HW, Craig CL, Lambert EV, Inoue S, Alkandari JR, Leetongin G, et al. The pandemic of physical inactivity: global action for public health. Lancet. 2012;380(9838):294–305.

Kuzawa CW. Fetal origins of developmental plasticity: are fetal cues reliable predictors of future nutritional environments? Am J Hum Biol. 2005;17:5–21.

Kuzawa CW, Quinn E. Developmental origins of adult function and health: evolutionary hypotheses. Annu Rev Anthropol. 2009;38(1):131–47.

Kwan BM, Bryan AD. Affective response to exercise as a component of exercise motivation: attitudes, norms, self-efficacy, and temporal stability of intentions. Psychol Sport Exerc. 2010;11(1):71–9.

Lancaster JB, Kaplan HS. The endocrinology of the human adaptive complex. In: Ellison PT, Gray PB, editors. Endocrinology of social relationships. Cambridge, MA: Harvard University Press; 2009. p. 95–119.

Lee IM, Shiroma EJ, Lobelo F, Puska P, Blair SN, Katzmarzyk PT, et al. Effect of physical inactivity on major non-communicable diseases worldwide: an analysis of burden of disease and life expectancy. Lancet. 2012;380(9838):219–29. Available from: http://dx.doi.org/10.1016/S0140-6736(12)61031-9.

Lieberman DE. The story of the human body: evolution, health, and disease. New York: Pantheon Books; 2013.

Lipson SF. Metabolism, maturation, and ovarian function. In: Ellison PT, editor. Reproductive ecology and human evolution. New York: Aldine de gruyter; 2001.

Lipson SF, Ellison PT. Comparison of salivary steroid profiles in naturally occurring conception and non-conception cycles. Hum Reprod. 1996;11:2090–6.

Loucks AB, Thuma JR. Luteinizing hormone pulsatility is disrupted at a threshold of energy availability in regularly menstruating women. J Clin Endocrinol Metab. 2003;88(1):297–311.

Loucks AB, Heath EM, Law T, Verdun M, Watts JR. Dietary restriction reduces luteinizing hormone (LH) pulse frequency during waking hours and increases LH pulse amplitude during sleep in young menstruating women. J Clin Endocrinol Metab. 1994;78(4):910–5.

Loucks AB, Verdun M, Heath EM. Low energy availability, not stress of exercise, alters LH pulsatility in exercising women. J Appl Physiol. 1998;84(1):37–46.

Metwally M, Li TC, Ledger WL. The impact of obesity on female reproductive function. Obes Rev. 2007;8(6):515–23.

Panter-Brick C, Pollard TM. Work and hormonal variation in subsistence and industrial contexts. In: Panter-Brick C, Worthman CM, editors. Hormones, health and behavior. Cambridge: University Press; 1999.

Panter-Brick C, Lotstein DS, Ellison PT. Seasonality of reproductive function and weight loss in rural Nepali women. Hum Reprod. 1993;8(5):684–90.

Raichlen DA, Foster AD, Gerdeman GL, Seillier A, Giuffrida A. Wired to run: exercise-induced endocannabinoid signaling in humans and cursorial mammals with implications for the 'runner's high'. J Exp Biol. 2012;215(8):1331–6.

Sherar LB, Esliger DW, Baxter-Jones ADG, Tremblay MS. Age and gender differences in youth physical activity: does physical maturity matter? Med Sci Sport Exerc. 2007;39(5):830–5.

Shetty PS. Adaptation to low energy intakes: the responses and limits to low intakes in infants, children and adults. Eur J Clin Nutr. 1999;53:S14–33.

Stearns SC. The evolution of life histories. Oxford: Oxford University Press; 1992.

Thompson AM, Baxter-Jones AD, Mirwald RL, Bailey DA. Comparison of physical activity in male and female children: does maturation matter? Med Sci Sport Exerc. 2003;35(10):1684–90.

Vickers MH, Breier BH, McCarthy D, Gluckman PD. Sedentary behavior during postnatal life is determined by the prenatal environment and exacerbated by postnatal hypercaloric nutrition. Am J Physiol Regul Integr Comp Physiol. 2003;285:R271–3.

Vitzthum VJ. The ecology and evolutionary endocrinology of reproduction in the human female. Am J Phys Anthropol. 2009;52:95–136.

Warburton DER, Nicol CW, Bredin SSD. Prescribing exercise as preventive therapy. CMAJ. 2006;174(7):961–74.

Williams NI, Leidy HJ, Hill BR, Lieberman JL, Legro RS, De Souza MJ. Magnitude of daily energy deficit predicts frequency but not severity of menstrual disturbances associated with exercise and caloric restriction. Am J Physiol Endocrinol Metab. 2015;308(1):E29–39. http://www.ncbi.nlm.nih.gov/pubmed/25352438.

Worthman CM, Barrett-Connor E. Endocrine pathways in differential well-being across the life course. In: Kuh Hardy RD, editor. A life course approach to women's health. Oxford: Oxford University Press; 2002. p. 197–232.

Zera AJ, Harshman LG. The physiology of life history trade-offs in animals. Annu Rev Ecol Syst. 2001;32:95–126.

Kuzawa CW, Gluckman PD, Hanson MA, Beedle AS. Evolution, developmental plasticity, and metabolic disease. In: Stearns SC, Koella JC, editors. Evolution in health and disease. 2nd ed. Oxford: Oxford University Press; 2007.

Chapter 9
Sex Hormones and Environmental Factors Affecting Exercise

Megan M. Wenner and Nina S. Stachenfeld

Introduction

Reproductive hormones and environmental conditions can influence physiological systems such as fluid regulation and thermoregulation, which in turn can impact exercise. There are numerous challenges with performing physiological studies on women due to the changing hormonal profiles that occur across the menstrual cycle, in addition to the various types of exogenous hormonal contraceptives used by women. Over the last 20 years, our laboratory has performed a number of research studies to examine sex and sex hormone effects on fluid regulation and temperature regulation in humans. In addition, our laboratory has developed a novel way to control reproductive hormone exposure in young women and to isolate the effects of individual sex hormones on physiological systems (discussed herein).

This chapter begins by addressing challenges in testing young, regularly menstruating, healthy women, who are not pregnant, have no chronic or acute disease, and are not medicated, much like the women (and men) recruited for physiological studies. Our purpose in beginning the chapter in this way is to emphasize that investigators need to take the same care in considering hormone milieu in both women and men as they do with any variable that can impact their findings.

M.M. Wenner, Ph.D.
Department of Kinesiology and Applied Physiology, University of Delaware, Newark, DE, USA

N.S. Stachenfeld, Ph.D. (✉)
Department of Obstetrics, Gynecology and Reproductive Sciences, The John B. Pierce Laboratory and Yale School of Medicine, New Haven, CT, USA
e-mail: nstach@jbpierce.org

Controlling Hormonal Effects During Human Physiological Studies

The primary roles of estrogens and progestogens are to create an environment hospitable for conception and the developing fetus. Research has also told us that gonadal hormones have important influences on organs and systems outside of reproduction. Moreover, physiological systems function differently within women, and sometimes these sex differences are due to their different hormonal milieu. A major research challenge, therefore, is to control female reproductive steroid hormone exposure to examine a physiological system of interest.

Estradiol is the predominant biologically active estrogen in young, healthy women so can exert a strong influence in physiological studies. While a number of estrogens are present in young, healthy women, 17 β-estradiol (referred to as just estradiol) is the most abundant and has the greatest activity on estrogen receptors. Both estradiol and estrone vary widely across the menstrual cycle in young women (Fig. 9.1; also, see Chap. 1). The most common method to minimize the hormone effects that confound research findings is to study women in the same phase of the menstrual cycle, usually in the early follicular phase (between days 1 and 7 following the onset of menses) when both estrogen and progesterone levels in the plasma are at their lowest levels (Fig. 9.1). This is a convenient method, but considering that women exist in this part of their cycle for only about 25% of their reproductive lives, it may not be the most clinically or physiologically relevant. Another aspect to consider is that focusing on plasma hormone levels to define hormonal impact does not take into account the potency of their associated receptors. Finally, even though estradiol and progesterone exposures are low relative to other phases of the cycle, these hormones are still considerably higher compared with those in men so their impact when drawing conclusions on sex differences, or when collapsing men and women into one experimental group, should not be ignored. Indeed, collapsing men and women into one group should be avoided when possible.

Hormonal contraceptives (usually combinations of different types of estrogens and progestins [see Chap. 1]) are also used to study hormonal effects in physiological studies. It has even become common to include women who are taking hormonal contraceptives within studies, and grouping them with men, or with other women who are not taking these hormones. A large proportion of European and US women take hormonal contraceptives, indicating high clinical applicability of findings. Hormonal contraceptives increase blood levels above endogenous estrogens and progesterone and provide a steady-state environment with which to compare with women not taking hormones. However, the hormones found in these contraceptives are simply not the same as endogenous hormones. Progestins in hormonal contraceptives differ in some of their basic hormonal actions compared with endogenous progesterone, including effects on peripheral circulation (Wenner et al. 2011a) and aldosterone function (Boschitsch et al. 2010) and differ in important ways with regard to synthesis, actions and androgenic properties (Speroff et al. 1999) and temperature regulation (Stachenfeld et al. 2000). Moreover, the types of progestogens or progestins in hormonal contraceptives are different from one contraceptive formula to another (Hapgood et al. 2014), but are often not distinguished

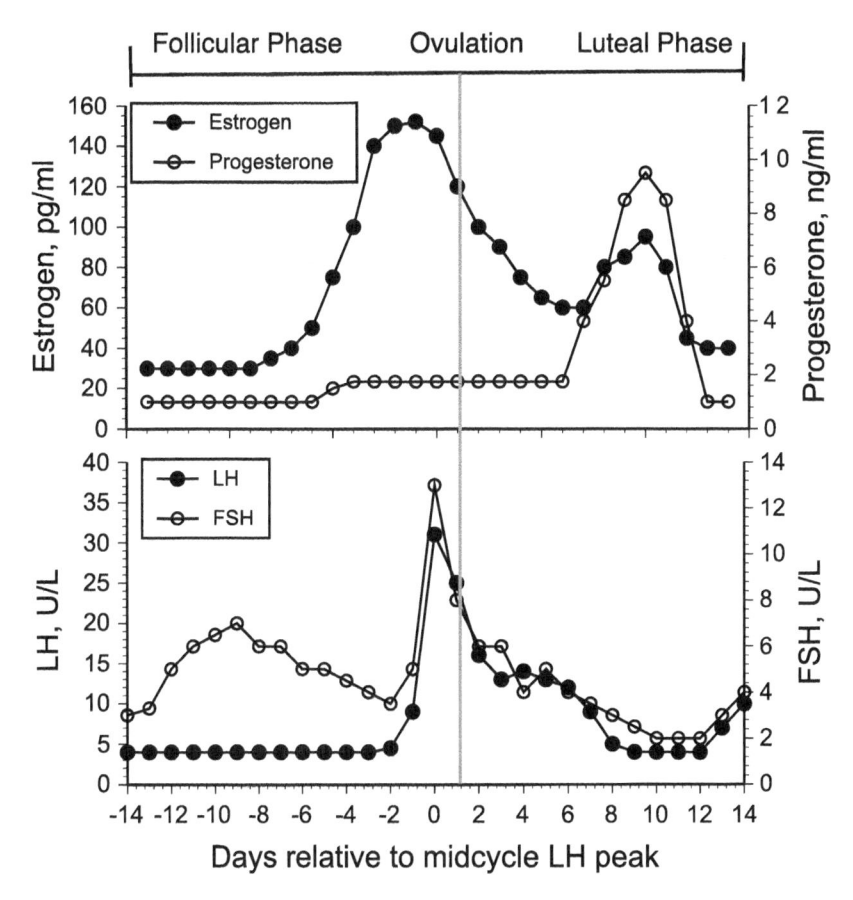

Fig. 9.1 Changes in 17β-estradiol (*top*) and progesterone (*bottom*) across the menstrual cycle. (Stachenfeld NS, Taylor HS. Sex hormone effects on body fluid and sodium regulation in women with and without exercise-associated hyponatremia. *J Appl Physiol.* 2008;107(3):864–72. Copyright 2008 The American Physiological Society. *Used with permission*)

within studies. For example, levonorgestrel, the most widely used progestin, has greater progestational, androgenic, and antiestrogen effects relative to norethindrone acetate or desogestrel, both of which minimize progestational and androgenic effects. Finally, drospirenone is derived from 17α-spirolactone and thus is an analog of spironolactone, a weak androgen *antagonist*. Thus while hormonal contraceptives can be a useful tool to control hormone exposure in women for physiological studies, care should be taken when choosing the contraceptive focusing on the hypothesis to be tested, all women should take the same contraceptive and women who are taking contraception should not be grouped with women who are not for any physiological studies.

Investigators also use the "placebo" week of the hormone contraceptive cycle, using weeks with their subjects on contraceptives as "high" hormone and weeks while taking placebo pills as "low" hormone phases (Charkoudian and Johnson 1999a). However, the placebo phase of the hormonal contraceptive pill cycle is not strictly a "low" hormonal phase. Immediately after stopping the hormonal contraceptives, blood or tissue levels of the exogenous estrogens or progestins or their metabolites can be elevated. At the very least, by the end of the 7-day placebo period, endogenous estrogens are variable across women (Creinin et al. 2002; Schlaff et al. 2004) and there are no consistent data on the impact of progestin metabolites still present in tissue during the placebo week in the contraception cycle. Thus, the placebo week during regular hormonal contraception is not a controlled period of low hormone exposure in women. A more controlled method is testing the women prior to and during beginning hormonal contraception administration. If the women are already taking contraception, they should go off the pills for at least a full menstrual cycle before beginning studies.

The most controlled method to examine hormonal effects on physiological systems in young women is temporary suppression of the menstrual cycle with a GnRH agonist (leuprolide acetate) or antagonist (ganirelix and cetrorelix acetate). This method requires subjects to use a small needle for subcutaneous injections of the drugs. It is more invasive than measuring changes in endogenous hormones over the course of the menstrual cycle, and less clinically relevant than examining changes over the course of the menstrual cycle or responses to hormonal contraceptives. Therefore, it is a method to be used when the questions posed are very specific to the hormone being tested. This method is ideal to examine causal inferences about hormonal effects on the system targeted for study and extends study to women with irregular menstrual cycles and to women with reproductive dysfunction. Briefly, leuprolide has greater GnRH receptor binding and decreased degradation than endogenous GnRH, so it is a potent inhibitor of gonadotropin secretion. Continuous leuprolide administration downregulates the hypothalamic–pituitary–ovarian axis, causing internalization and uncoupling of the GnRH receptors in the pituitary. Leuprolide administration leads to initial FSH stimulation and related steroidogenesis, followed by low or undetectable estrogen and progesterone concentrations within 7–14 days (Heritage et al. 1980) (Fig. 9.2). Additionally, Ganirelix and cetrorelix are synthetic decapeptides that compete with GnRH for receptor binding so function as competitive receptor antagonists, inducing rapid, reversible suppression of gonadotropin secretion and suppress estrogens and progesterone production 36–48 h of administration (Oberye et al. 1999a, b) (Fig. 9.2). When hormones are suppressed, estrogens, progestogens or androgens (or combinations) can be administered in a controlled fashion to test the hypothesis of interest.

These interventional methods are ideal to examine causal inferences about hormonal effects on any system targeted for study, including body fluid regulation (Stachenfeld and Keefe 2002; Stachenfeld et al. 2001a; Stachenfeld and Taylor 2005) cardiovascular function (Wenner et al. 2011a, b, 2013; Wenner and Stachenfeld 2012), and metabolism (Day et al. 2005; D'Eon et al. 2002). Both leuprolide or ganirelix acetate lead to suppression of estrogens and progesterone to postmenopausal levels, so women can experience vasomotor symptoms ("hot flashes"), breast tenderness, headaches, and transient mood changes, or some temporary mild water retention. Because ganirelix is taken for a shorter period, these symptoms are generally less severe.

Including women in physiological research is not only required by NIH, but is essential for women's health. The changing hormonal milieu in women across the menstrual cycle and as women age creates challenges for designing controlled

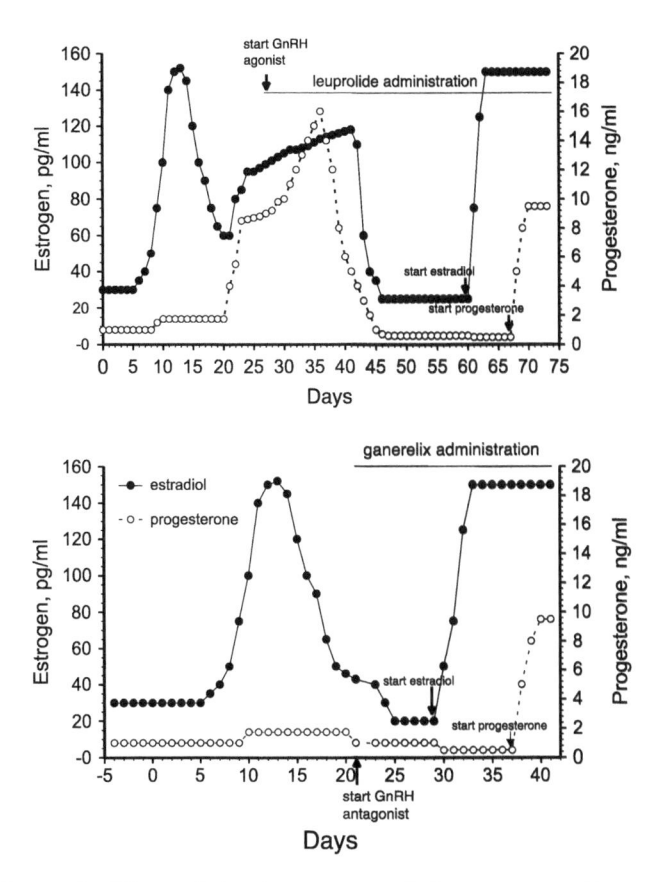

Fig. 9.2 Changes in 17β-estradiol and progesterone during treatment with a gonadotropin-releasing hormone (GnRH) agonist (leuprolide acetate) beginning on day 25 of a normal menstrual cycle, followed by treatment with two 17β-estradiol patches (0.1 mg) and oral progesterone (200 mg/day) (*left*). Changes in 17β-estradiol and progesterone during treatment with a GnRH antagonist (ganirelix acetate) beginning on day 25 of a normal menstrual cycle, followed by treatment with two 17β-estradiol patches (0.1 mg) and oral progesterone (200 mg/day) (*right*)

studies, can also provide an interesting environment to compare both sex hormone and sex differences. Investigators should consider hormone milieu in both women and men as they do with any variable that can impact their findings.

Water Regulation

Water is the largest component of the human body, representing from 60 % to 70 % of body weight. In a healthy, 60 kg woman, about 34 L of her body is composed of water. Athletes who generally have high lean muscle mass have a greater percentage of body water compared to sedentary individuals. Approximately 65 % of the body's water is contained in the cells (intracellular water), and approximately 5 % of the remaining extracellular water is in the blood stream (blood/plasma volume). Fluid within cells and outside of the vascular compartment cannot be immediately accessed during exercise, so only plasma volume is available for sweating and thermoregulation during exercise. Thus, it is this very small percentage of water (about 3.5 L in a normal woman) in the plasma that is used by the body's fluid regulatory and cardiovascular systems to control temperature, as well as stimulate thirst and modulate cardiac output and blood pressure.

Mechanisms that control fluid balance are complex and are influenced by reproductive hormones (Fig. 9.3). Both estradiol and progesterone can influence the complex and integrated neural and hormonal systems that have evolved to control thirst, fluid intake, sodium appetite, and renal fluid and sodium regulation (Fig. 9.3). In addition, sophisticated regulatory mechanisms have evolved to maintain body fluid volume and composition during challenges, including exercise, increases in water intake or deprivation. These regulatory mechanisms use receptors within the vasculature, brain, and gut that are sensitive to mechanical and chemical changes in water and electrolyte content, and whose effector systems act to modify rates of fluid intake and fluid output. For example, dehydration (hyperosmotic hypovolemia) leads to the sensory and behavioral responses of thirst and fluid intake and the phys-

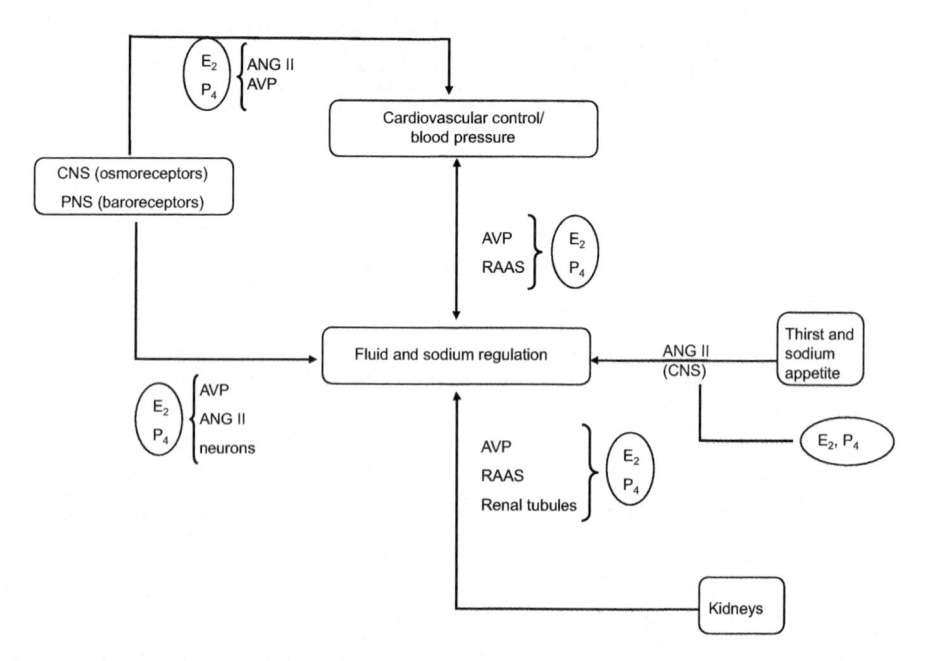

Fig. 9.3 Schematic to illustrate the complex control of fluid and sodium balance and the multiple ways in which estradiol (E2) and progesterone (P4) may influence these processes. AVP indicates arginine vasopressin; ANG II, angiotensin II; CNS, central nervous system; PNS, peripheral nervous system; RAAS, renin-angiotensin-aldosterone system (Stachenfeld NS. Sex hormone effects on body fluid regulation. *Exerc Sport Sci Rev.* 2008;36(3):152–9. Used *with permission*)

iological responses of sodium and water retention by the kidney (Fig. 9.3). During long-term exercise, a small percentage of athletes (1–13 %) retain water leading to a fall in plasma sodium concentration, or hyponatremia. Hyponatremia is the result of excess ingestion of hypotonic fluids (fluids with lower sodium concentration than is in the blood) combined with fluid retention (hypervolemic hyponatremia). Hyponatremia can also occur when excessive sodium is lost in sweating (hypovolemic hyponatremia).

Arginine vasopressin (AVP) is the primary hormone in the body involved in the retention of free water. Arginine vasopressin is synthesized in cell bodies of nuclei located in the anterior hypothalamus (AH), and axons from the AH project into the posterior pituitary where AVP is stored and released in response to central osmoreceptor stimulation. Osmotic regulation of AVP and thirst are linear, and a steeper slope indicates a greater sensitivity of the central osmoreceptors controlling thirst sensation and AVP synthesis and release from the AH and posterior pituitary (Fig. 9.4). A leftward shift in the intercept for this curve indicates an earlier threshold for the onset of thirst and AVP release, while a rightward shift in the intercept for this curve indicates a later threshold for the onset of thirst and AVP release. Likewise, changes in the steepness of this curve detect sensitivity. Arginine vasopressin and thirst are also sensitive to changes in intravascular fluid as sensed by peripheral baroreceptors, so are sensitive to changes in plasma volume during exercise, drinking or dehydration (Fig. 9.3).

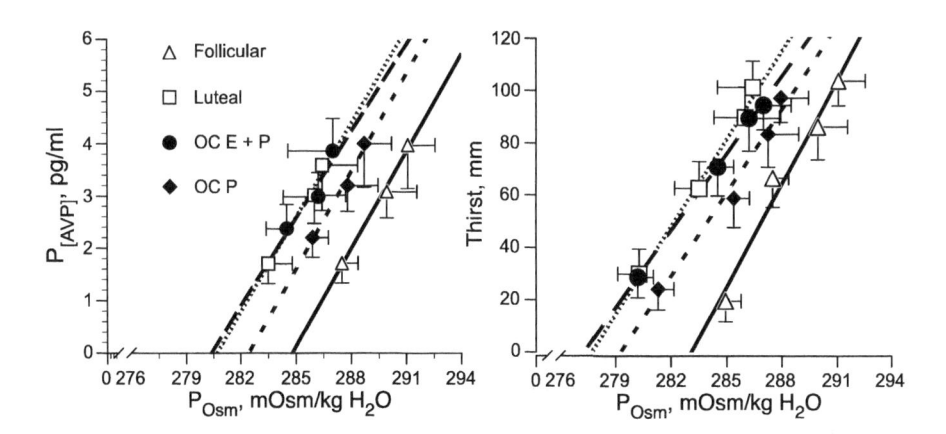

Osmotic regulation of arginine vasopressin and thirst during dehydration.

Fig. 9.4 Plasma arginine vasopressin (AVP) concentration and thirst sensation as a function of plasma osmolality (P_{Osm}) during 120 min of hypertonic (3.0 % NaCl) saline infusion the early follicular and mid luteal phases of the menstrual cycle, and during combined (ethinyl estradiol + progestin, OC E+P) and progestin-only (OC P) hormonal contraceptive administration. Note the high progesterone/progestin conditions (luteal phase, OC E+P, OC P) shifted the $P_{[AVP]}$-P_{Osm} curves to the left relative to the follicular phase (From Stachenfeld NS, Silva CS, Keefe DL, Kokoszka CA, Nadel ER. Effects of oral contraceptives on body fluid regulation. *J Appl Physiol.* 1999;87:1016–25. Copyright 1999 The American Physiological Society. Used with permission)

Sex Hormone Effects on Fluid Regulation

Both hypertonic saline infusion (3 % NaCl) and dehydration are used to increase plasma osmolality (P_{Osm}) under different sex hormone conditions to determine the effects of these hormones on the sensitivity and threshold on the linear relationship of $P_{[AVP]}$- P_{Osm} and thirst- P_{Osm} (Stachenfeld et al. 1998, 1999; Calzone et al. 2001). With these methods, the impact of estrogens and progesterone on osmotic control of AVP and thirst are examined by observing changes in the slope (sensitivity) and intercept (threshold) of the $P_{[AVP]}-P_{Osm}$ and thirst-P_{Osm} relationships (Stachenfeld et al. 1998, 1999; Calzone et al. 2001). The plasma hypertonicity associated with a 3 % NaCl infusion induces powerful and linear thirst responses and increases in $P_{[AVP]}$ and thirst. Moreover, hypertonic saline infusion increases P_{Osm} by as much as ~20 mOsmol/kg H_2O during a 2-h infusion so is a power AVP stimulus (Calzone et al. 2001). However, hypertonic saline infusion is not at all a dehydrated state, despite the large increases in P_{Osm}, thirst and $P_{[AVP]}$ because a large intravascular fluid expansion (~10–20 %) develops as water is drawn from cells in response to the increased osmotic pressure in the surrounding intracellular fluid in addition to the fluid infused (Stachenfeld and Keefe 2002; Calzone et al. 2001; Stachenfeld et al. 2001b). Under these conditions, the osmotic stimulus overwhelms the inhibitory input by the plasma volume expansion with regard to thirst and $P_{[AVP]}$ (Fig. 9.4) as well as renal fluid retention (Stachenfeld and Keefe 2002; Calzone et al. 2001; Stachenfeld et al. 2001b).

Estrogen receptors are present in the hypothalamic nuclei that produce AVP (Heritage et al. 1980; Sar and Stumpf 1980) and there are sex differences in the AVP neuron activity and size in these nuclei (Ishunina et al. 2000). Resting $P_{[AVP]}$ is greater in men than in women (in the early follicular phase) (Stachenfeld et al. 2001b; Claybaugh et al. 2000), although men have greater AVP sensitivity and blood pressure responses to hypertonic saline infusion (Stachenfeld et al. 2001b). With regard to sex hormone effects *within* women, the osmotic threshold for AVP release and thirst stimulation during both hypertonic saline infusion and exercise-induced dehydration is lower when using hormonal contraceptives containing estradiol compared to either the follicular phase or to hormonal contraceptives that contained only progestins. These findings are similar to those in postmenopausal women when compared to women taking estradiol (Stachenfeld et al. 1998) and support a role for estrogens in the osmotic regulation of AVP. Interestingly, free water clearance was unaffected during hypertonic saline infusion, dehydration, or rehydration in our younger subjects. This unchanged water and sodium balance in the face of estrogen-related shifts in osmotic AVP, thirst and drinking suggested *a shift in body water regulation to a lower plasma osmolality operating point* during estradiol exposure in young women. This shift in water regulation is in contrast to our earlier findings in postmenopausal women in whom estradiol administration increased osmotic production of AVP, but also resulted in greater water retention (Stachenfeld et al. 1998).

Exercise Effects on Fluid Balance

Environmental conditions (i.e., heat and humidity) and exercise type and intensity impact fluid and electrolyte loss that occurs with activity. During exercise, there is an increase in cardiac output as exercise intensity increases in order to meet the metabolic demands of the exercising skeletal muscle. The increase in cardiac output is due to increases in heart rate and stroke volume. However, in a hot environment, a large portion of cardiac output (up to 60%) is shifted from the core to the periphery (Rowell 1974), primarily to the skin for thermoregulation via sweating and cooling the body through evaporation.

Plasma volume expansion not only improves cardiovascular responses to exercise, but also increases internal water available for sweating thereby improving thermoregulation during exercise (Nadel et al. 1980; Fortney et al. 1983). These thermoregulatory improvements are due to the increase in cardiac output, as there is a greater ability for cutaneous vasodilation and heat dissipation in the periphery. In contrast, plasma or blood volume contraction (such as with hypovolemia or dehydration) limits the ability to effectively increase skin blood flow to dissipate heat (Fortney et al. 1983), as evident by a reduction in skin vascular conductance for a given core temperature (Tripathi et al. 1990). With exercise in the heat during hypovolemic or dehydrated states, without fluid and electrolytes replacement, sweating to dissipate heat is compromised, which can lead to heat illness (Sawka et al. 1992, 2007; Armstrong et al. 2007; Byrne et al. 2006).

Research laboratory studies have been conducted to examine thermoregulatory mechanisms, as highlighted in a number of review articles (Shibasaki et al. 2006; Gagnon and Kenny 2012a, b; Charkoudian and Stachenfeld 2014; Charkoudian 2015). In order to compare thermoregulatory function, cutaneous vasodilation or sweating is plotted as a function of core temperature. Both the threshold (core temperature at which either skin blood flow or sweating begins to increase) and/or the sensitivity (slope) are analyzed to determine effectiveness of heat dissipation (Fig. 9.5). The leftward shift in the threshold or set point for sweating indicates an earlier onset of sweating, or that sweating began at a lower core temperature. This commonly occurs with exercise training in the heat (acclimatization), and is an important adaptation because earlier sweating onset results in more effective core temperature maintenance (Roberts et al. 1977). While this is an important thermoregulatory advantage, this adaptation also requires greater attention to fluid and electrolyte intake, an important caveat for long training bouts. Thus, with adequate hydration and plasma volume, body water is available for sweating, there is less cardiovascular strain, and exercise performance is maintained. In contrast, with dehydration and the correlate reduction in plasma volume and cardiac output, there is typically a delayed core temperature set point for cutaneous vasodilation (Nadel et al. 1980) seen as a rightward shift in the threshold for vasodilation in the skin (Fig. 9.5) or sweating threshold. Further, for a given core temperature, both skin vasodilation and sweating rate are lower in dehydrated persons (Nadel et al. 1980; Sawka et al. 1992; Sawka and Wenger 1988). Thus, dehydration, or plasma volume

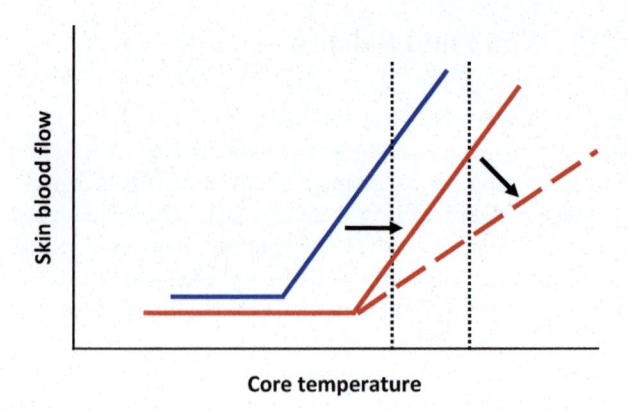

Fig. 9.5 Schematic example of graphs used in analysis of thermoregulatory effector mechanisms (primarily sweating and cutaneous vasodilation), showing the relevant effector as a function of core body temperature. As core temperature increases, a point is reached (the threshold) at which the heat dissipation mechanism begins to increase. The slope of the relationship after this threshold is referred to as the sensitivity of the response. A "rightward" shift in threshold and/or a decrease in sensitivity will decrease the amount of heat dissipation for a given core temperature, resulting in less efficient heat loss. *Vertical lines* show the change in the amount of a given effector response (at a given core temperature) caused by a shift in threshold or sensitivity. (From Charkoudian N, Stachenfeld N. Reproductive hormone influences on thermoregulation in women. *Compr Physiol*. 2014;4(2):793–804. Copyright 2014 The American Physiological Society. *Used with permission*)

contraction, results in less effective thermoregulation (i.e., high core temperature), increased cardiovascular strain, fatigue, limits exercise performance, and increases the risk for heat illness (Sawka et al. 1992, 2007; Armstrong et al. 2007; Byrne et al. 2006; Sawka and Wenger 1988).

Sex Differences in Thermoregulation

Sex differences in thermoregulation can influence fluid and electrolyte losses during exercise (Gagnon and Kenny 2012a, b; Charkoudian and Stachenfeld 2014; Charkoudian 2015). Most sex differences in thermoregulation are attributed to differences in body size, body composition, and fitness level (Gagnon and Kenny 2012a, b). Because of their smaller body size and lower lean mass, the amount of heat generated during exercise is typically lower in women compared to men. Women also generally have lower sweating rates compared to men due to their lower body size, although this is difficult to detect at lower exercise intensities (Gagnon and Kenny 2012b). Although sweating rates may differ between men and women, core temperature and cutaneous vasodilation during exercise in the heat are generally similar between the sexes. Thus, sex differences in thermoregulation are minimal, and likely not to influence exercise capacity for most young healthy people. However, because women lose less fluid and electrolytes from sweat during intense exercise in the heat, overconsumption of fluids can contribute to the higher incidence and more severe outcome of exercise associated hyponatremia in women compared to men (Almond et al. 2005).

There are important caveats to these statements regarding sex differences, however. The environment in which humans exercise also affects sex differences in thermoregulation (Shapiro et al. 1980). Heat production is mainly weight dependent, so women produce less heat during exercise due to their smaller body weight compared to men. In contrast, evaporation or cooling is mostly related to body surface area (BSA, i.e., *skin surface*) dependent, and thus, the sex with the higher BSA has the advantage (men). However, their greater body size and muscle mass induce greater heat production, so it is variable as to whether or not there are sex differences in dry heat. In contrast, in hot wet environments, evaporation is suppressed, so the greater BSA in men does not convey as great an advantage for sweating, while heat production remains the same. Because body weight is generally lower in women, core temperature increases less relative to men, so under hot wet conditions, women may fair better (Shapiro et al. 1980). In addition, of course, the slower sweating rates in women in the hot wet environment may convey an advantage to women who maintain better hydration.

Sex Hormone Effects Within Women During Exercise

As described above, sex hormones (specifically estrogens and progesterone) can impact fluid and electrolyte regulation. These hormones can also alter thermoregulatory mechanisms. Early studies conducted in women during the menstrual cycle demonstrated that sex hormones shift the core temperature threshold for sweating (Stephenson and Kolka 1999). During the luteal phase, there is a rightward shift in core temperature for the onset of sweating, such that for a given core temperature, sweating rates are lower in the luteal compared to follicular phase (Stephenson and Kolka 1999; Kolka and Stephenson 1989). The threshold for the onset of sweating during exercise in the preovulatory phase of the menstrual cycle, when estrogen is elevated independent of progesterone (Stephenson and Kolka 1999), is shifted leftward compared to the follicular phase, suggesting that estrogen lowers the threshold for the onset of sweating. Taken together with other studies, estrogen is likely associated with greater sweating rates for a given core temperature (Stachenfeld et al. 2000; Brooks-Asplund et al. 2000). Similar findings of a shift in core temperature due to changes in estrogen and progesterone exposure have also been reported in women using oral contraceptive pills (Rogers and Baker 1997; Charkoudian and Johnson 1999b). The sensitivity or slope of the sweating response does not appear to be influenced by changes in reproductive hormones. These data indicate that estrogen and progesterone have opposing effects on thermoregulatory mechanisms, and can alter the core temperature threshold for sweating to occur during exercise in the heat.

In order to directly determine whether estrogen opposes the progesterone-induced increase in core temperature threshold for sweating, women were tested during four different hormone conditions: the early follicular phase of menstrual cycle, the mid luteal phase of menstrual cycle, after 4 weeks of combined estradiol and progestin (OC-E+P) oral contraceptive pills, and after 4 weeks of progestin-only contraceptive pills (OC-P) (Stachenfeld et al. 2000). In this manner, changes in the onset of sweating during the menstrual cycle were assessed, and progestin effects on thermoregulation during exercise in the heat in the same women were isolated. Women were tested at rest, in response to passive heat stress, and during exercise (60 % of VO_{2peak} for 40 min) under each hormonal condition. Consistent with previous studies (Kolka and Stephenson 1989), core temperature was higher during the mid luteal compared to the early follicular phase of the menstrual cycle (Fig. 9.6). This change in resting core temperature is primarily due to the increase in progesterone, and consistent with increases in core temperature with progestin during OC-P compared to OC-E+P, follicular, and luteal phases (Stachenfeld et al. 2000). However, the addition of estrogen to progestin only pills *prevented* the rightward shift in core temperature. Furthermore, the onset of sweating occurred at a lower core temperature with the addition of estrogen to progestin pills (Fig. 9.6). As a result, for a given

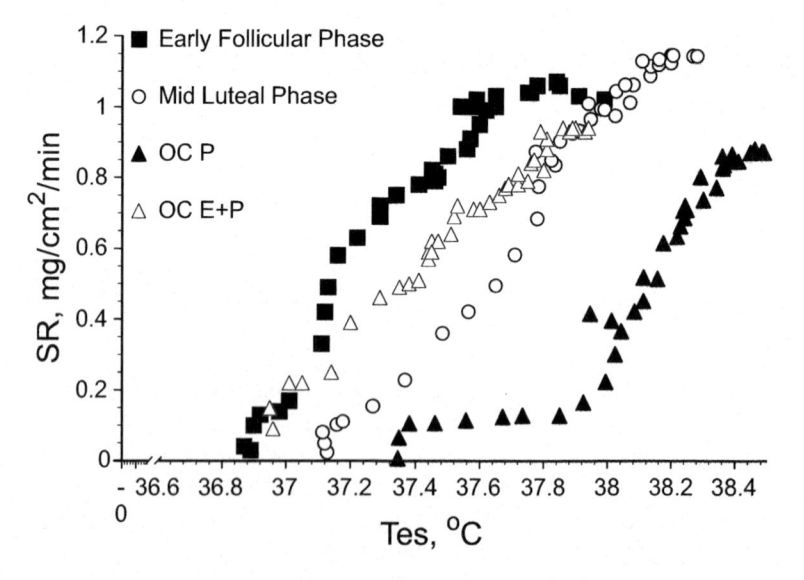

Fig. 9.6 Sweating rate (SR) as a function of core (esophageal) temperature during 40 min of exercise in the heat in young, healthy women during the early follicular and mid luteal phases of the menstrual cycle, and during combined (ethinyl estradiol + progestin, OC E+P) and progestin-only (OC P) hormonal contraceptive administration. Note the progestin alone condition (OC P) shifted the SR-°C curves to the right relative to the other conditions, and consistent with earlier data, mid luteal phase SR-°C curves were also shifted to the left relative to the early follicular phase (Kolka and Stephenson 1989; Stephenson et al. 1989) (Data are based on Stachenfeld NS, Silva C, Keefe DL. Estrogen modifies the temperature effects of progesterone. *J Appl Physiol.* 2000;88:1643–9. Copyright 2000. The American Physiological Society. Used with permission)

core temperature, sweating rates were greater in the presence of estrogen compared to the progestin only pills. This greater sweating rate with the addition of estrogen was also associated with a small plasma volume expansion that occurred with estrogen administration (Stachenfeld 2004). Conversely, the lower sweating rates during OC-P were associated with a significant plasma volume contraction (~3 %) that occurred with OC-P (Stachenfeld 2004). Throughout exercise, sweating sensitivity as represented by slopes of the relationship between sweat rate and core temperature were unaffected by hormone condition.

In summary, estrogens and progesterone/progestins have opposing effects on core temperature and the threshold for sweating onset, whereas the slope or sensitivity does not appear to be effected by fluctuations in sex hormones. Estrogen lowers the core temperature threshold for sweating promoting heat dissipation, whereas progesterone/progestins have the opposite effect. Although core temperature is higher and sweating onset is later in these circumstances, phase of the menstrual cycle or hormonal contraceptive use do not predict heat illness during exercise in women. Lastly, although sex hormones influence thermoregulation and sweating responses to exercise, it does not appear that these changes significantly impact exercise performance.

Training and Fitness Effects on Fluid and Electrolyte Requirements

Aerobic fitness may also influence fluid and electrolyte requirements during exercise. Exercise training can impact the sensitivity (or slope) and threshold of the relationships between core temperature, peripheral vasodilation, and sweating. For example, Roberts et al. demonstrated that 10 days of aerobic exercise training reduced the internal threshold for sweating and peripheral vasodilation in men and women, permitting greater heat dissipation (Roberts et al. 1977). Moreover, the sweating and blood flow are augmented if the exercise training is performed in the heat (acclimatization). While the responses to exercise training and acclimatization are similar between the sexes, women have lower sweating rates and a higher internal threshold for both sweating and peripheral vasodilation compared to men for a given core temperature (Hertig and Sargent 1963; Wyndham et al. 1965). Although these classic studies demonstrated important sex differences in sweating responses, they did not take into account the fluctuations in reproductive hormones that occur across the menstrual cycle.

As discussed earlier in this chapter, estrogen and progesterone also alter thermoregulatory sweating responses during exercise, so thermoregulation will change across the menstrual cycle. In order to determine fitness effects in women while minimizing the influence of hormonal fluctuations, Araki et al. (Araki et al. 1981) measured sweating responses to exercise in a hot environment in trained and untrained women during the same time period of phase menstrual cycle (within 7 days after menstruation, or when both estrogens and progesterone are low). The trained women demonstrated an earlier sweating onset compared to the untrained women. Furthermore, the untrained women underwent 60 days of exercise training and demonstrated improved thermoregulatory sweating responses. Therefore, exercise training can improve sweating responses in women so that they can more efficiently dissipate heat during exercise. The differences in sweating responses between trained and untrained women have been reproduced in subsequent studies (Kuwahara et al. 2005a, b), which also tested trained and untrained women during different phases of the menstrual cycle. In untrained women, sweating rate and skin blood flow responses to exercise in a thermoneutral environment were lower during the mid luteal compared to the mid follicular phase of the menstrual cycle (Kuwahara et al. 2005a). Furthermore, the internal temperature threshold at which sweating occurred was greater during the mid luteal phase of the menstrual cycle in untrained women (Kuwahara et al. 2005a). Interestingly, these menstrual cycle differences in sweating were not observed in trained women. Therefore, it seems possible that exercise training attenuates the impact of sex hormones on thermoregulation (Kuwahara et al. 2005a, b).

The greater sweating responses in trained women also indicate greater body fluid losses, so women need to be cognizant that as they improve their fitness or acclimatize to heat that their fluid and electrolyte requirements may change. Another important consideration is the lower tonicity of the sweat that can occur with training. The lower concentration of sodium in sweating is an important training adaptation because this lower electrolyte loss will balance the greater sweating rates achieved with training. It is also important to note that even though sweat sodium concentration is reduced with training, it remains highly variable across individuals, varying as much as 10–70 mEq/L (Sawka et al. 2007). Sims et al. (2007) showed that consumption of a high sodium beverage prior to exercise in the heat increased performance during the mid luteal phase of the menstrual cycle. Therefore, women should not only pay attention to fluid intake but also sodium intake, especially during exercise in the heat.

Temperature Regulation and Fluid Balance: Special Populations

Aging and Menopause

The menopausal transition is a period where significant physiological changes occur due to dramatic fluctuations in reproductive hormones, and can occur at different ages among women (Harlow et al. 2012). After menopause, estradiol and progesterone levels are significantly reduced compared to premenopausal women. This loss of estradiol can have significant implications on numerous physiological systems, such as bone, cardiovascular, and thermoregulatory (see Chap. 16). During the menopausal transition, women often experience symptoms such as vaginal dryness, hot flashes, and night sweats. Thus, fluctuations in reproductive hormones during this time period can also have important implications for thermoregulation and fluid balance.

Aging is associated with impairments in thermoregulation and thirst sensation during exercise in both sexes (Kenney and Anderson 1988; Stachenfeld et al. 1997). In perimenopausal (Tankersley et al. 1992) and postmenopausal (Brooks et al. 1997) women, estrogen therapy reduces core temperature at rest and during exercise. Furthermore, the core temperature threshold for sweating onset occurs lower with estrogen therapy in older women (Tankersley et al. 1992; Brooks et al. 1997). These improvements in thermoregulation may be one mechanism whereby estrogen therapy reduces the frequency and intensity of hot flashes. However, these thermoregulatory effects on core temperature and sweating were not apparent in postmenopausal women taking combined estrogen and progesterone hormone therapy (Brooks et al. 1997), suggesting that the effects of progesterone predominate over that of estrogen, similarly to what is observed in young women.

Although the mechanisms controlling skin blood flow and sweating during postmenopausal vasomotor symptoms (VMS) has not been established, a series of elegant studies has demonstrated that these physiological responses are controlled by similar autonomic mechanisms that contribute to peripheral changes in the thermoregulatory response during peripheral and core temperature heat challenges (Hubing et al. 2010; Low et al. 2008). Interestingly, while these mechanisms include a nitric oxide component, they are independent of prostaglandins (Hubing et al. 2010). These studies have also demonstrated a sympathetic cholinergic neural mechanism for skin blood flow increases during VMS (Low et al. 2011). Importantly, it appears that exercise training may improve subjective ratings of frequency and intensity of VMS events in postmenopausal women (Luoto et al. 2012).

With regard to fluid balance, the typical expansion in plasma volume that occurs with exercise training is impaired in postmenopausal women (Stachenfeld et al. 1998). However, estrogen administration induces basal transient fluid retention and plasma volume expansion, increases $P_{[AVP]}$, and reduces the osmotic set-point for AVP release in postmenopausal women (Stachenfeld et al. 1998). These changes are associated with water and sodium retention, which are likely due to a reduction in urine output because thirst and drinking patterns are not altered with estrogen administration. Lastly, although progesterone effects on fluid balance have been examined in young women, to our knowledge there are no data in postmenopausal women. Progestins and progesterone are commonly prescribed as part of hormone therapy regimens, so it is important to determine these effects on sodium and water balance.

Polycystic Ovary Syndrome

Polycystic ovary syndrome (PCOS) is the most common reproductive endocrinopathy (Barontini et al. 2001), affecting between 5 and 10% women of reproductive age (Tsilchorozidou et al. 2004), and is the most common cause of menstrual irregularity in young women. Approximately 75% of women with PCOS have the more severe reproductive and metabolic PCOS phenotype that is dominated by features of hyperandrogenism. This androgen excess (AE)-PCOS phenotype is typically associated with insulin resistance (IR), compensatory hyperinsulinemia, obesity, subcutaneous and visceral adiposity, dyslipidemia, enlarged adipocytes, hypoadiponectinemia, and oligoovulation or anovulation. AE-PCOS is also associated with obesity and metabolic syndrome (Rojas et al. 2014; Ehrmann et al. 2006; Legro et al. 2001). A sedentary lifestyle is a primary environmental risk factor for PCOS (Diamanti-Kandarakis et al. 2012; Diamanti-Kandarakis and Dunaif 2012). Physical activity independent of weight loss improves insulin sensitivity (Harrison et al. 2011; Hutchison et al. 2011) and improves reproductive function in PCOS (Harrison et al. 2011). Therefore, exercise is routinely prescribed for women with PCOS (Moran et al. 2006), although there are few data on exercise effects on women with PCOS. Obese women with PCOS appear to regulate temperature adequately during exercise in the heat, maintaining similar core temperature to obese women without PCOS, although with higher sweating rates even at mild exercise intensity, relative to control obese subjects (Stachenfeld et al. 2010). Women with PCOS sweat at a lower core temperature and more profusely relative to women without PCOS and this greater water loss was independent of obesity (Stachenfeld et al. 2010). These data suggest that women with PCOS should pay special attention to hydration during longer exercise periods. Finally, similar to lean women, estradiol administration lowered the sweating threshold in the control obese women, but had no effect on women with PCOS, who were insensitive to estradiol administration, with or without testosterone suppression (Stachenfeld et al. 2010). Despite the importance of physical activity in treating PCOS, there are no exercise guidelines for women with PCOS based on clinical or physiological data.

Conclusions

Including women in physiological research is essential for women's health, but creates challenges for designing controlled studies. Researchers cannot simply pool men and women into one group when they are included in physiological studies and cannot simply test women in one phase of the menstrual cycle. Regardless of methodology, the same attention to detail used to control the rest of the environment of our physiological studies should be paid to the hormonal environment when including women, female animals, cells or cell lines in research studies.

The primary female reproductive hormones—estrogens and progesterone—have physiological effects on fluid and electrolyte regulation and thermoregulation. These effects are most profound in lowering the set point for the regulation of thirst and the fluid/sodium regulation hormones, but do not typically induce fluid or sodium retention. Moreover, these hormones play an important role in reducing the core temperature sweating. Regardless of these physiological effects, there is not yet strong evidence that estrogens and progesterone/progestins impact performance significantly in younger or older women, or that they significantly increase the risk of heat illness.

Acknowledgments We gratefully acknowledge the intellectual contributions of Drs. Ethan Nadel PhD (posthumous), Gary Mack PhD, and Wendy Calzone, MS.; the technical assistance of Cheryl Leone, MA. and Andrew Grabarek BS.; the clinical support of Drs. Hugh Taylor and Celso Silva and Lubna Pal; and the cooperation of the volunteer subjects. These studies were supported, in part, by National Heart Lung Blood Institute R01 HL62240 and R01 HL71159, as well as the U.S. Army Medical and Research and Materiel Command under contract DAMD17-96-C-6093.

References

Almond CSD, Shin AY, Fortescue EB, Mannix RC, Wypij D, Binstadt BA, et al. Hyponatremia among runners in the Boston marathon. N Engl J Med. 2005;352:1550–6.
Araki T, Matsushita K, Umeno K, Tsujino A, Toda Y. Effect of physical training on exercise-induced sweating in women. J Appl Physiol. 1981;51(6):1526–32.
Armstrong L, Casa D, Millard-Stafford M, Moran D, Pyne S, Roberts W. American college of sports medicine position stand. Exertional heat illness during competition. Med Sci Sports Exerc. 2007;39:556–72.
Barontini M, Garcia-Rudaz MC, Veldhuis JD. Mechanisms of hypothalamic-pituitary-gonadal disruption in polycystic ovarian syndrome. Arch Med Res. 2001;32:544–52.
Boschitsch E, Mayerhofer S, Magometschnigg D. Hypertension in women: the role of progesterone and aldosterone. Climacteric. 2010;13(4):307–13.
Brooks EM, Morgan AL, Pierzga JM, Wladkowski SL, Gorman JT, Derr JA, et al. Chronic hormone replacement therapy alters thermoregulatory and vasomotor function in postmenopausal women. J Appl Physiol. 1997;83(2):477–84.
Brooks-Asplund EM, Cannon JG, Kenney WL. Influence of hormone replacement therapy and aspirin on temperature regulation in postmenopausal women. Am J Physiol. 2000;279:R839–48.
Byrne C, Lee JK, Chew SA, Lim CL, Tan EY. Continuous thermoregulatory responses to mass-participation distance running in heat. Med Sci Sports Exerc. 2006;38(5):803–10.
Calzone WL, Silva C, Keefe DL, Stachenfeld NS. Progesterone does not alter osmotic regulation of AVP. Am J Physiol Regul Integr Comp Physiol. 2001;281:R2011–20.
Charkoudian N, Johnson J. Altered reflex control of cutaneous circulation by female sex steroids is independent of prostaglandins. Am J Physiol. 1999a;276:H1634–40.
Charkoudian N, Johnson JM. Reflex control of cutaneous vasoconstrictor system is reset by exogenous female reproductive hormones. J Appl Physiol. 1999b;87:381–5.
Charkoudian N, Stachenfeld N. Reproductive hormone influences on thermoregulation in women. Compr Physiol. 2014;4(2):793–804.
Charkoudian N, Stachenfeld N. Sex hormone effects on autonomic mechanisms of thermoregulation in humans. Auton Neurosci. 2015;196:75–80.
Claybaugh JR, Sato AK, Crosswhite LK, Hassell LH. Effects of time of day, gender, and menstrual cycle phase on the human response to oral water load. Am J Physiol. 2000;279:R966–73.
Creinin MD, Lippman JS, Eder SE, Godwin AM, Olson W. The effect of extending the pill-free interval on follicular activity: triphasic norgestimate/35 μg ethinyl estradiol versus monophasic levonorgestrel/20 μg ethinyl estradiol. Contraception. 2002;66:147–52.
D'Eon TM, Sharoff C, Chipkin SR, Grow D, Ruby BC, Braun B. Regulation of exercise carbohydrate metabolism by estrogen and progesterone in women. A J Physiol Endocrinol Metab. 2002;283(5):E1046–55.
Day DS, Gozansky WS, Van Pelt RE, Schwartz RS, Kohrt WM. Sex hormone suppression reduces resting energy expenditure and β-adrenergic support of resting energy expenditure. J Clin Endocrinol Metab. 2005;90(6):3312–7.
Diamanti-Kandarakis E, Dunaif A. Insulin resistance and the polycystic ovary syndrome revisited: an update on mechanisms and implications. Endocr Rev. 2012;33(6):981–1030.

Diamanti-Kandarakis E, Christakou C, Marinakis E. Phenotypes and environmental factors: their influence in PCOS. Curr Pharm Des. 2012;18(3):270–82.

Ehrmann DA, Liljenquist DR, Kasza K, Azziz R, Legro RS, Ghazzi MN. Prevalence and predictors of the metabolic syndrome in women with polycystic ovary syndrome. J Clin Endocrinol Metab. 2006;91(1):48–53.

Fortney SM, Wenger CB, Bove JR, Nadel ER. Effects of plasma volume on forearm venous and cardiac stroke volumes during exercise. J Appl Physiol. 1983;55:884–90.

Gagnon D, Kenny GP. Does sex have an independent effect on thermoeffector responses during exercise in the heat? J Physiol. 2012a;590(Pt 23):5963–73.

Gagnon D, Kenny GP. Sex differences in thermoeffector responses during exercise at fixed requirements for heat loss. J Appl Physiol. 2012b;113(5):746–57.

Hapgood JP, Africander D, Louw R, Ray RM, Rohwer JM. Potency of progestogens used in hormonal therapy: toward understanding differential actions. J Steroid Biochem Mol Biol. 2014;142:39–47.

Harlow SD, Gass M, Hall JE, Lobo R, Maki P, Rebar RW, et al. Executive summary of the stages of reproductive aging workshop + 10: addressing the unfinished agenda of staging reproductive aging. J Clin Endocrinol Metab. 2012;97(4):1159–68.

Harrison CL, Lombard CB, Moran LJ, Teede HJ. Exercise therapy in polycystic ovary syndrome: a systematic review. Hum Reprod Update. 2011;17(2):171–83.

Heritage AS, Stumpf WE, Sar M, Grant LD. Brainstem catecholamine neurons are target sites for sex steroid hormones. Science. 1980;207:1377–9.

Hertig BA, Sargent 2nd F. Acclimatization of women during work in hot environments. Fed Proc. 1963;22:810–3.

Hubing KA, Wingo JE, Brothers RM, Del Coso J, Low DA, Crandall CG. Nitric oxide synthase inhibition attenuates cutaneous vasodilation during postmenopausal hot flash episodes. Menopause. 2010;17(5):978–82.

Hutchison SK, Stepto NK, Harrison CL, Moran LJ, Strauss BJ, Teede HJ. Effects of exercise on insulin resistance and body composition in overweight and obese women with and without polycystic ovary syndrome. J Clin Endocrinol Metab. 2011;96(1):E48–56.

Ishunina TA, Kruijver FPM, Balesar R, Swaab DF. Differential expression of estrogen receptor ∞ and ß immunoreactivity in the human supraoptic nucleus in relation to sex and aging. J Clin Endocrinol Metab. 2000;85:3283–91.

Kenney WL, Anderson RK. Responses of older and younger women to exercise in dry and humid heat without fluid replacement. Med Sci Sports Exerc. 1988;20(2):155–60.

Kolka M, Stephenson L. Control of sweating during the human menstrual cycle. Eur J Appl Physiol. 1989;58:890–5.

Kuwahara T, Inoue Y, Abe M, Sato Y, Kondo N. Effects of menstrual cycle and physical training on heat loss responses during dynamic exercise at moderate intensity in a temperate environment. Am J Physiol Regul Integr Comp Physiol. 2005a;288(5):R1347–53.

Kuwahara T, Inoue Y, Taniguchi M, Ogura Y, Ueda H, Kondo N. Effects of physical training on heat loss responses of young women to passive heating in relation to menstrual cycle. Eur J Appl Physiol. 2005b;94(4):376–85.

Legro RS, Kunselman AR, Dunaif A. Prevalence and predictors of dyslipidemia in women with polycystic ovary syndrome. Am J Med. 2001;111(8):607–13.

Low D, Davis S, Keller D, Shibasaki M, Crandall C. Cutaneous and hemodynamic responses during symptomatic postmenopausal women. Menopause. 2008;15:290–5.

Low DA, Hubing KA, Del Coso J, Crandall CG. Mechanisms of cutaneous vasodilation during the postmenopausal hot flash. Menopause. 2011;18(4):359–65.

Luoto R, Moilanen J, Heinonen R, Mikkola T, Raitanen J, Tomas E, et al. Effect of aerobic training on hot flushes and quality of life—a randomized controlled trial. Ann Med. 2012;44(6):616–26.

Moran LJ, Brinkworth G, Noakes M, Norman RJ. Effects of lifestyle modification in polycystic ovarian syndrome. Reprod Biomed Online. 2006;12(5):569–78.

Nadel ER, Fortney SM, Wenger CB. Effect of hydration state on circulatory and thermal regulations. J Appl Physiol. 1980;49:715–21.

Oberye JJL, Mannaerts BMJL, Huisman JAM, Timmer CJ. Pharmacokinetic and Pharmacodynamic characteristics of ganirelix (Antagon/Orgalutran). Part II. Dose-proportionality and gonadotropin suppression after multiple doses of ganirelix in healthy female volunteers. Fertil Steril. 1999a;72(6):1006–12.

Oberye JJL, Mannaerts BMJL, Huisman JAM, Timmer CJ. Pharmacokinetic and Pharmacodynamic characteristics of ganirelix (Antagon/Orgalutran). Part I. Absolute bioavailability of 0.25 mg of ganirelix after a single subcutaneous injection in healthy female volunteers. Fertil Steril. 1999b;72(6):1001–5.

Roberts MF, Wenger CB, Stolwijk JA, Nadel ER. Skin blood flow and sweating changes following exercise training and heat acclimation. J Appl Physiol. 1977;43:133–7.

Rogers SM, Baker MA. Thermoregulation during exercise in women who are taking oral contraceptives. Eur J Appl Physiol. 1997;75:34–8.

Rojas J, Chavez-Castillo M, Bermudez V. The role of metformin in metabolic disturbances during pregnancy: polycystic ovary syndrome and gestational diabetes mellitus. Int J Reprod Med. 2014;2014:797681.

Rowell LB. Human cardiovascular adjustments to exercise and thermal stress. Physiol Rev. 1974;54(1):75–159.

Sar M, Stumpf WE. Simultaneous localization of [3H]estradiol and neurophysin I or arginine vasopressin in hypothalamic neurons demonstrated by a combined technique of dry-mount autoradiography and immunohistochemistry. Neurosci Lett. 1980;17:179–84.

Sawka MN, Wenger CB. Physiological responses to acute exercise heat stress. In: Pandolf KB, Sawka MN, Gonzalez RR, editors. Human performance physiology and environmental medicine at terrestrial extremes. Indianapolis, IN: Benchmark; 1988. p. 97–151.

Sawka MN, Young AJ, Latzka WA, Neufer PD, Quigley MD, Pandolf KB. Human tolerance to heat strain during exercise: influence of hydration. J Appl Physiol. 1992;73:368–75.

Sawka MN, Burke LM, Eichner ER, Maughan RJ, Montain SJ, Stachenfeld NS. American College of Sports Medicine position stand. Exercise and fluid replacement. Med Sci Sports Exerc. 2007;39(2):377–90.

Schlaff WD, Lynch AM, Hughes HD, Cedars MI, Smith DL. Manipulation of the pill-free interval in oral conceptive pill users: the effect on follicular suppression. Am J Obstet Gynecol. 2004 ;190:943–51.

Shapiro Y, Pandolf KB, Avellini BA, Pimental NA, Goldman RF. Physiological responses of men and women to humid and dry heat. J Appl Physiol. 1980;49(1):1–8.

Shibasaki M, Davis SL, Cui J, Low DA, Keller DM, Durand S, et al. Neurally mediated vasoconstriction is capable of decreasing skin blood flow during orthostasis in the heat-stressed human. J Physiol. 2006;575(Pt 3):953–9.

Sims ST, Rehrer NJ, Bell ML, Cotter JD. Preexercise sodium loading aids fluid balance and endurance for women exercising in the heat. J Appl Physiol. 2007;103(2):534–41.

Speroff L, Glass RH, Kase NG. Steroid contraception clinical gynecological endocrinology and infertility. 4th ed. Baltimore: Williams & Wilkins; 1999. p. 873–9.

Stachenfeld NS. Sex hormone effects on body fluid regulation. Exerc Sport Sci Rev. 2008;36(3) :152–9.

Stachenfeld NS, Keefe DL. Estrogen effects on osmotic regulation of AVP and fluid balance. Am J Physiol. 2002;283:E711–21.

Stachenfeld NS, Taylor HS. Effects of estrogen and progesterone administration on extracellular fluid. J Appl Physiol. 2004;96:1011–8.

Stachenfeld NS, Taylor HS. Progesterone increases plasma and extracellular fluid volumes independent of estradiol. J Appl Physiol. 2005;98:1991–7.

Stachenfeld NS, Taylor HS. Sex hormone effects on body fluid and sodium regulation in women with and without exercise-associated hyponatremia. J Appl Physiol. 2008;107(3):864–72.

Stachenfeld NS, Mack GW, DiPietro L, Nadel ER. Mechanism for attenuated thirst in aging: role of central volume receptors. Am J Physiol. 1997;272:R148–57.

Stachenfeld NS, DiPietro L, Palter SF, Nadel ER. Estrogen influences osmotic secretion of AVP and body water balance in postmenopausal women. Am J Physiol. 1998;274:R187–95.

Stachenfeld NS, Silva CS, Keefe DL, Kokoszka CA, Nadel ER. Effects of oral contraceptives on body fluid regulation. J Appl Physiol. 1999;87:1016–25.

Stachenfeld NS, Silva C, Keefe DL. Estrogen modifies the temperature effects of progesterone. J Appl Physiol. 2000;88:1643–9.

Stachenfeld NS, Keefe DL, Palter SF. Effects of estrogen and progesterone on transcapillary fluid dynamics. Am J Physiol. 2001a;281:R1319–29.

Stachenfeld NS, Splenser AE, Calzone WL, Taylor MP, Keefe DL. Sex differences in osmotic regulation of AVP and renal sodium handling. J Appl Physiol. 2001b;91:1893–901.

Stachenfeld NS, Yeckel CW, Taylor HS. Greater exercise sweating in obese women with polycystic ovary syndrome compared with obese controls. Med Sci Sports Exerc. 2010;42(9):1660–8.

Stephenson LA, Kolka MA. Esophageal temperature threshold for sweating decreases before ovulation in premenopausal women. J Appl Physiol. 1999;86(1):22–8.

Stephenson LA, Kolka MA, Francesconi R, Gonzalez RR. Circadian variations in plasma renin activity, catecholamines and aldosterone during exercise in women. Eur J Appl Physiol. 1989;58:756–64.

Tankersley CG, Nicholas WC, Deaver DR, Mikita D, Kenney WL. Estrogen replacement therapy in middle-aged women: thermoregulatory responses to exercise in the heat. J Appl Physiol. 1992;73(4):1238–45.

Tripathi A, Mack GW, Nadel ER. Cutaneous vascular reflexes during exercise in the heat. Med Sci Sports Exerc. 1990;22:796–803.

Tsilchorozidou T, Overton C, Conway GS. The pathophysiology of polycystic ovary syndrome. Clin Endocrinol. 2004;60:1–17.

Wenner MM, Stachenfeld NS. Blood pressure and water regulation: understanding sex hormone effects within and between men and women. J Physiol. 2012;590(Pt 23):5949–61.

Wenner MM, Taylor HS, Stachenfeld NS. Progesterone enhances adrenergic control of skin blood flow in women with high but not low orthostatic tolerance. J Physiol. 2011a;589.4(4):975–86.

Wenner MM, Taylor HS, Stachenfeld N. Endothelin B receptor contribution to peripheral microvascular function in women with polycystic ovary syndrome. J Physiol. 2011b;589(19):4671–9.

Wenner MM, Haddadin AS, Taylor HS, Stachenfeld NS. Mechanisms contributing to low orthostatic tolerance in women: the influence of oestradiol. J Physiol. 2013;591(9):2345–55.

Wyndham CH, Morrison JF, Williams CG. Heat reactions of male and female Caucasians. J Appl Physiol. 1965;20(3):357–64.

Chapter 10
Exercise, Depression-Anxiety Disorders and Sex Hormones

Shannon K. Crowley

Introduction

The risk for many mental illnesses has a strong sex bias. In general, women have a higher prevalence of most affective disorders, whereas men have higher rates of substance use disorders (Kendler and Gardner 2014; Kessler et al. 1993). Depression, predicted to be the second leading cause of global disability burden by 2020, is twice as common in women compared to men and women are roughly twice as likely to suffer from anxiety disorders, such as panic disorder and trauma-related disorders [e.g., posttraumatic stress disorder (PTSD)] (Young and Pfaff 2014). The prevalence of depressive and anxiety disorders appears to be even higher during certain periods of a woman's life including, puberty, the reproductive years, and the menopause transition (Soares and Zitek 2008). While the exact mechanisms underlying sex differences in depression and anxiety rates across the female life span are currently unknown, chronic stress, early life adversity, and negative cognitive styles are more common in women than in men (Dunn et al. 2012; Matud 2004), and may contribute to the higher reports of depression and anxiety in women versus men. It has also been hypothesized that reproductive-related hormones may play a role in the development and maintenance of mood and anxiety disorders. The mechanisms underlying the influence of reproductive steroid hormones on affective regulation are still being understood. Chronic stress has been associated with the precipitation and exacerbation of depressive and anxiety disorders (Kendler et al. 2004; Brilman and Ormel 2001; Mundy et al. 2015; Eiland and McEwen 2012). Additionally, evidence suggests a reciprocal relationship exists between reproductive steroid hormones and stress-related systems (Handa et al. 1994). Therefore, one plausible pathway by which reproductive hormones may be associated with affective disorders is via an interaction with stress regulation.

S.K. Crowley, Ph.D. (✉)
Department of Exercise Science, North Carolina Wesleyan College, 3400 N Wesleyan Blvd, Rocky Mount, NC 27804, USA
e-mail: scrowley@ncwc.edu

Depression and anxiety are commonly associated with low levels of physical activity (Daumit et al. 2005; Goodwin 2003; Teychenne et al. 2015; Dugan et al. 2015), and even among individuals with mental illness, women with mood and anxiety disorders have increased odds of being physically inactive (Goodwin 2003). Mental health symptomatology may impede the initiation and motivation to engage in physical activity in affected individuals (Leventhal 2012). To date, however, there has been limited study of the relationship between reproductive-related mood and anxiety disorders and participation in physical activity.

Literature reviews maintain that exercise compares favorably to antidepressant medications as a first-line and/or adjuvant treatment for mild to moderate depression in adults (Mead et al. 2009; Lawlor and Hopker 2001; Byrne and Byrne 1993; Brown et al. 2013), and studies suggest that participation in physical activity may be protective against the development of mood and anxiety disorders (Kritz-Silverstein et al. 2001; Jacka et al. 2011; Rothon et al. 2010). The protective and treatment effects of physical exercise for depression and anxiety might be mediated through the positive impact of exercise on fundamental psychological processes of affective dysregulation (e.g., emotion regulation, mood), stress-processing systems, and/or comorbid conditions (e.g., sleep problems). This chapter aims to provide an overview of women's mood disorders, the role of sex hormones in the development and maintenance of women's reproductive-related mood disorders, and the associations among physical activity and women's reproductive-related mood disorders.

Women's Reproductive-Related Mood Disorders

Reproductive-related mood disorders in women consist of psychiatric disorders whose etiology and pathophysiology appears to be linked to reproductive-related processes. It is important to note that the current classification of "depression" occurring in the context of reproductive events may be somewhat delusive, as anxiety-like features are often predominant presenting symptoms in women with reproductive-related depressions (Yonkers 1997; Falah-Hassani et al. 2016). Moreover, studies indicate that women have a greater propensity to develop comorbid anxiety and depression than men (Angst and Vollrath 1991; Breslau et al. 1995; Howell et al. 2001; Yonkers 1997). There is evidence that symptoms associated with reproductive-related mood disorders may be associated with psychosocial events (e.g., early life adversity, chronic stress, social support) (Crowley et al. 2015a; Gordon et al. 2015, 2016; Kendler and Gardner 2014; Girdler et al. 2003), and/or hormone-mediated events (Gordon et al. 2016; Crowley et al. 2016; Schmidt et al. 2004; Schmidt and Rubinow 2009). Indeed, research suggests that some women may be differentially sensitive to changes in gonadal steroid hormones, including estrogen and progesterone (PROG) (Schiller et al. 2015; Soares and Zitek 2008), increasing vulnerability to the development of reproductive-related mood disorders during periods of gonadal steroid hormone flux. The increased prevalence of depression in women during periods of reproductive hormone change suggests a potential role of gonadal steroid hormones, perhaps via their interactions with behavior-modulating physiological systems, in the development and maintenance of women's mood and anxiety disorders.

Menstrually Related Mood Disorders (MRMDs)

Menstrually related mood disorders (MRMDs), including premenstrual syndrome (PMS) and premenstrual dysphoric disorder (PMDD), are characterized by the cyclic recurrence of emotional and physical symptoms during the luteal phase of the menstrual cycle that remit with the onset of menses. Epidemiological evidence suggests that, during their reproductive years, 15–20 % of women exhibit clinically relevant PMS, and 5–10 % of women meet diagnostic criteria for PMDD (Halbreich et al. 2003; Cohen et al. 2002). Women with MRMDs, PMDD in particular, report significant impairment which correlates strongly with affective symptoms (such as mood lability, irritability, anxiety/tension, and depressed mood) (Bloch et al. 1997; Ekholm and Backstrom 1994). However, somatic symptoms (e.g., breast tenderness, bloating, fatigue, joint pain) are also prevalent, affecting ~80 % of women with MRMDs (McHichi alami et al. 2002).

PMDD, the most severe form of an MRMD, results in luteal phase impairment equivalent to that of major depression, panic disorder, and post-traumatic stress disorder (PTSD) (Freeman and Sondheimer 2003; Halbreich et al. 2003). The DSM-V diagnosis of PMDD is based upon a premenstrual pattern of at least five physical, affective, and/or behavioral symptoms that are associated with significant distress or interference in role or social functioning, with the requirement that at least one of the key affective symptoms must be: (1) marked affective lability (mood swings, tearfulness, sensitivity to rejection); (2) marked irritability or anger; (3) marked depressed mood; or (4) marked anxiety or tension (American Psychiatric Association 2013). However, the DSM-V PMDD diagnostic criteria have been considered by some to be too restrictive, perhaps resulting in under-identification of women with PMDD (Freeman and Sondheimer 2003; O'Brien et al. 2011). Less severe than PMDD, PMS encompasses the cyclic recurrence of premenstrual symptoms with minimal impairment or distress (the presence of a mood symptom is not required for the PMS diagnosis) (Freeman 2003; Kessel 2000).

Hormonal regulation of the ovarian cycle in premenopausal women is characterized by a complex interaction of luteinizing hormone (LH), follicle-stimulating hormone (FSH), estrogen, and PROG (see Chap. 1). Menstruation marks the first day of the follicular phase, characterized by low and steady levels of PROG and estradiol (Farage et al. 2009). The ovulatory phase begins with a surge in LH and FSH, peak estrogen levels, and increasing PROG levels (Farage et al. 2009). Ending the cycle, the luteal phase is characterized by decreasing LH and FSH levels and peak PROG production from the corpus luteum (Gandara et al. 2007; Farage et al. 2009). It is important to note that inter- and intra-individual variations can exist across cycles, including occurrence of some nonovulatory cycles (Metcalf 1983; Metcalf et al. 1983).

The etiology of MRMDs is currently unknown; however, it has been suggested that some women may be differentially sensitive to changes in gonadal steroid fluctuations occurring during the ovarian cycle, increasing risk for the development of premenstrual symptoms (Schiller et al. 2014; Lentz et al. 2007). Research suggests that luteal phase changes in reproductive hormones, perhaps particularly their neuroactive steroid derivatives (of which allopregnanolone is the most widely studied), may trigger effective dysregulation in susceptible women (Schiller et al. 2014). It is also possible that sex steroid fluctuations across the ovarian cycle may modulate other neurobiological processes implicated in affective regulation including serotonin availability (Eriksson et al. 2008; Hindberg and Naesh 1992; Kikuchi et al. 2010), circadian rhythms (Parry et al. 2011; Shechter et al. 2012), neuronal growth factors such brain-derived neurotrophic factor (BDNF; Cubeddu et al. 2011; Pluchino et al. 2009), hypothalamic–pituitary-adrenal axis (HPA-axis) regulation (Crowley and Girdler 2014; Kirschbaum et al. 1999), and immune system function (Faas et al. 2000; Oertelt-Prigione 2012). Increased sensitivity to changes in the reproductive hormone environment, in some women, may stem from a complex interplay of genetic (Huo et al. 2007; Kendler et al. 1992), physiological (Masho et al. 2005), and psychosocial (e.g., early life adversity, chronic stress) factors (Bertone-Johnson et al. 2014).

Perinatal Depression

Perinatal depression, including antepartum depression (APD) and postpartum depression (PPD), describes a wide range of mood disorders that can affect women during pregnancy and after childbirth. Despite the classification of "perinatal depression," many women with the disorder experience symptoms of anxiety, mood lability, ruminative thoughts, panic attacks, and obsessive thoughts (particularly related to infant well-being; O'Hara and Wisner 2014; Wisner et al. 2013; Reck et al. 2008). The prevalence of APD is estimated at 10–20 % of childbearing women (Breedlove and Fryzelka 2011), and PPD is estimated to affect between 10 and 20 % of childbearing women (Gavin et al. 2005; O'Hara and McCabe 2013; O'Hara and Wisner 2014). Recently, the DSM-V restructured the definition of PPD (major depressive disorder with peripartum onset) as the onset of depressive symptoms during pregnancy or within 4 weeks of delivery (American Psychiatric Association 2013). However, the precise definition of PPD remains somewhat unclear (Wisner et al. 2010), and may, in part, reflect the difficulty in establishing the etiology of the disorder.

The DSM-V diagnosis of Major Depressive Disorder (MDD) with "peripartum" specifier (perinatal depression) requires the presentation of five of the following nine symptoms most of the day, nearly every day for at least a 2 week period: (1) depressed mood, (2) marked diminished interest or pleasure in all, or almost all, activities, (3) significant weight loss or weight gain, or a decrease or increase in appetite (4) insomnia or hypersomnia, (5) psychomotor agitation or psychomotor retardation, (6) fatigue or loss of energy, (7) feelings of worthlessness or excessive or inappropriate guilt, (8) cognitive difficulties such as diminished ability to think/concentrate, or indecisiveness, and (9) recurrent thoughts of death or recurrent suicidal ideation. To meet the diagnostic criteria for perinatal depression, the defining symptoms must represent a change from previous functioning and have had onset during pregnancy or within four weeks of delivery (American Psychiatric Association 2013). Despite these DSM-V criteria, many researchers and clinicians continue to define postpartum depression as occurring within the first year postpartum (Stuart-Parrigon and Stuart 2014).

The precise psychological, social, and biological factors which may help to identify and treat women with perinatal depression are still being understood. Several factors may be associated with increased risk for the development of depression and anxiety during pregnancy and the postpartum period, including a history of chronic stress, anxious and depressive symptoms during pregnancy, and low social support (O'Hara and Wisner 2014; Verreault et al. 2014; Falah-Hassani et al. 2016). In addition, disturbed sleep has been associated with both depressed mood (Okun et al. 2013; Okun 2015; Skouteris et al. 2008) and stress during pregnancy (Okun et al. 2013), and has also been shown to be a potential predictor of depressive mood postpartum (Okun et al. 2013; Goyal et al. 2009; Bei et al. 2010). Underlying biological processes which may be associated with these behavioral risk factors for perinatal depression include HPA-axis dysregulation, inflammatory processes, and genetic vulnerabilities (Crowley et al. 2016; Cox et al. 2015; Glynn et al. 2013; Garfield et al. 2015; Posillico and Schwarz 2016; Barth et al. 2015).

Due to the temporal association between the substantial and rapid changes in gonadal steroid hormone concentrations that occur during the perinatal period (particularly after delivery) and the onset of depressive and anxious symptoms (O'Hara et al. 1991), reproductive hormones (such as estrogen and PROG) have been implicated in the etiology and pathogenesis of perinatal depression. Indeed, both human and animal studies have suggested that gonadal steroid hormones, and/or their neuroactive steroid derivatives, may be linked to key physiological processes underlying affective regulation, including modulation of the HPA-axis, facilitation of neuroplasticity, and regulation of immune processes (McEwen 2002; Crowley et al. 2016; Pluchino et al. 2013; Morrow et al. 1995; Kipp et al. 2012). Whether the large and dramatic change in reproductive steroid hormones which occurs during the perinatal period might trigger dysregulation in susceptible women in one or more of these physiological processes remains to be established.

Depression During the Menopause Transition (Perimenopausal Depression)

There remains conflicting data regarding the increased incidence of depression and anxiety disorders during the menopause transition. Cross-sectional studies of midlife women indicate that women in the 40- to 55-year age group are more likely to report depressive symptoms than premenopausal and postmenopausal women (Soares and Almeida 2001; Avis et al. 2001; Dennerstein et al. 2004). Prevalence rates for mood disorders during the menopause transition are difficult to ascertain, in part due to the variability in how women biologically and psychosocially experience the menopause transition. Additionally, there is substantially less research in this area (compared to the investigation of PPD and PMDD). While it remains somewhat controversial whether there is increased risk for the development of mood and anxiety disorders during the menopause transition (Gordon et al. 2015), mood disturbances during this period are commonly reported (Burt et al. 1998) and often accompanied by increased irritability (Bromberger et al. 2003). Whether mood disturbances occurring during the menopause transition reflect new onset or recurrent depressive episodes is a matter of debate (Freeman 2015; Harlow et al. 2013).

Traditional views often suggested that mood disorders during the menopause transition were related to feelings of loss and sadness associated with mid-life (e.g., "empty nest syndrome") (Gibbs et al. 2012; Raup and Myers 1989). However, current research suggests that poor sleep, stressful or negative life events, lack of employment, higher body mass index (BMI), smoking, younger age, race (prevalence rates of depression during the menopause transition are substantially higher in African Americans) and a history of hormonally related mood disorders, may be associated with increased risk for the development of mood disturbances during the menopause transition (Gibbs et al. 2012; Gibbs and Kulkarni 2014). Evidence that women with a history of reproductive-related mood disorders (e.g., premenstrual syndrome, postpartum depression) are at elevated risk for the development of depression during the menopause transition suggests, at least in part, a hormonally mediated pathophysiology.

Typically occurring between the ages of 45–49, the menopause transition lasts an average of 5 years and is characterized by increased variability in menstrual cycles (with long cycles becoming more common as the menopause transition progresses), skipped cycles, and changes in hormone levels including estrogen, PROG, and FSH (Burger et al. 2001). It is important to note that there are substantial individual differences in hormone patterns during the menopause transition (Santoro et al. 2004). However, most women experience an increase in FSH levels; a decline in luteal-phase (prior to menses) PROG (Gordon et al. 2015); erratic changes in estradiol (the most prevalent endogenous estrogen) concentrations, including elevated estradiol (compared to premenopausal levels), which coincide with the increasing frequency of anovulatory cycles (O'Connor et al. 2009) and eventual estradiol and PROG production cessation (Schmidt and Rubinow 2009). Longitudinal studies have suggested that perimenopausal changes in reproductive function may be associated with an increased risk of depression in susceptible women (Freeman et al. 2014; Cohen et al. 2006; Schmidt et al. 2004).

Though the precise biological underpinnings of depression during the menopause transition are still under investigation, findings that depression prevalence appears to increase concurrent to changes in reproductive hormones (including elevated FSH and diminished estradiol and PROG) during the menopause transition (Schmidt et al. 2004), combined with the efficacy of estradiol therapy in the acute treatment of depression during this period (Schmidt et al. 2015; de Novaes Soares et al. 2001), suggests a hormonally driven event. It has been suggested that susceptible women may experience heightened sensitivity to environmental stressors during periods of hormonal fluctuation (including the menopause transition), thus increasing risk for the development of mood disorders during this time (Gordon et al. 2015, 2016). Additionally, endocrine events during the menopause transition have been associated with increased prevalence of somatic complaints including vasomotor symptoms (e.g., hot flushes, night sweats) and sleep disturbances (Brown et al. 2002; Dennerstein et al. 2000). Some evidence suggests these impairing somatic symptoms may precipitate or exacerbate affective disorders (Joffe et al. 2002; Gallicchio et al. 2007).

Physical Activity and Women's Reproductive-Related Mood Disorders

Regular participation in physical activity may offer women a non-pharmacological means to relieve depressive and anxious symptoms. Indeed, exercise training has been shown to have salutary effects on core symptoms of depression and anxiety disorders including sleep problems (Herring et al. 2015; Kline 2014), fatigue (Tomlinson et al. 2014), depressed mood (Da Costa et al. 2009; Lawlor and Hopker 2001; Mata et al. 2013), anxiety (Petruzzello et al. 1991), and cognitive difficulties (Hopkins et al. 2012; Bherer et al. 2013). While the mechanisms underlying the antidepressant and anxiolytic effects of exercise training are still under investigation, research suggests that the antidepressant effects of regular exercise training might be mediated through neurobiological adaptations (e.g., increased availability of neurotransmitters including serotonin and dopamine, positive effects on HPA-axis reactivity to stressors), which may be protective against the deleterious psychological effects of stress (Tsatsoulis and Fountoulakis 2006). Considering that reproductive hormone fluctuation may confer risk for the development of mood and anxiety disorders via increased sensitivity to environmental stressors, the potential for exercise to prevent or treat affective disorders during reproductive states might involve adaptations resulting from regular physical exercise training which also positively impact physiological adaptations to psychological stressors. Despite the potential positive impact of exercise training on affective regulation, symptoms associated with depression and anxiety disorders may impede the initiation and motivation to engage in physical activity in affected individuals (Leventhal 2012; McDevitt et al. 2006). This may be particularly salient to reproductive-related mood disorders, which are also associated with heightened somatic and pain-related symptoms (Bunevicius et al. 2013; Wang et al. 2003; Straneva et al. 2002; Joffe et al. 2002). Research investigating the influence of physiological and psychosocial factors related to women's reproductive mood disorders, and the initiation and maintenance of physical activity behavior during reproductive states is severely limited but may lend insight into the contribution of physical activity to women's psychological health during these life periods.

Relationships Among Physical Activity and Menstrually Related Mood Disorders

It has long been suggested that participation in exercise training may help to ameliorate premenstrual symptoms associated with MRMDs. Indeed, exercise is often recommended by healthcare providers for premenstrual symptom management (Kraemer and Kraemer 1998). However, epidemiological evidence supporting exercise for the treatment of premenstrual symptoms is mixed. Several studies have reported a reduction in premenstrual symptoms in physically active women, while other studies have reported either negative effects or no association (Aganoff and Boyle 1994; Choi and Salmon 1995; Freeman et al. 1988; Johnson et al. 1995; Rasheed and Al-Sowielem 2003; Samadi et al. 2013). Studies which have employed a physical activity-based intervention for the treatment of MRMDs have reported reductions in PMS-related symptomatology after participation in exercise training, though these studies have important methodical limitations, including small sample sizes and failure to control for important covariates (including BMI; Samadi et al. 2013; Steege and Blumenthal 1993; Stoddard et al. 2007).

The biopsychosocial mechanisms by which PA may be protective against the development of depression and anxiety not related to reproductive events may also confer protection against the development of MRMDs in susceptible women. For example, the notable central and peripheral physiological stress responses to exercise have led to the theory of "cross-stressor adaptation," which posits that physiological adaptations resulting from physical training may also result in physiological adaptations to psychological stressors (Sothmann et al. 1996). In line with this concept, some studies have shown physical training has resulted in decreased sympathetic nervous system (SNS) (Spalding et al. 2004; Anshel 1996; Rimmele et al. 2009) and HPA-axis activity (Rimmele et al. 2007, 2009) in response to psychological stressors. Considering the strong correlation between chronic stress and the development of MRMDs, and the potential for exercise training to positively modulate physiological stress reactivity, the plausibility of exercise training to prevent MRMDs may lie, in part, in its ability to attenuate the negative physiologic effects of stress. In addition, obesity (which is highly correlated with physical inactivity) has been associated with increased risk for the development of MRMDs (Masho et al. 2005). A large cross-sectional study by Masho et al. (2005) found that women with a BMI ≥ 30 had nearly a threefold increased risk for PMS than nonobese women [Odds Ratio (OR) = 2.8 (95% CI = 1.1–7.2)]. It is therefore possible that participation in regular physical activity may be protective against the development of MRMDs via its positive effects on body weight.

There are other plausible biological mechanisms by which exercise could reduce MRMD symptoms. For example, exercise training may influence levels of gonadal steroid hormones including estrogen and PROG (Kossman et al. 2011), positively modulate physiological responses to stress (Klaperski et al. 2014; Jackson and Dishman 2006; Rimmele et al. 2007), reduce the risk of obesity (which has been shown to be a risk factor for the development of MRMDs) (Slentz et al. 2004), and improve psychological well-being (Crowley et al. 2015b; Azar et al. 2008). The concept that exercise training may impact circulating steroid hormone levels in reproductive aged women, and in so doing, reduce the adverse cyclic symptoms associated with MRMDs is an intriguing, yet understudied phenomena. The plausibility of exercise training, through its modulatory effects on gonadal steroid hormones, to reduce depressive symptoms in women with MRMDs is supported by evidence which suggests that menstruating athletes with anovulatory menstrual cycles and low steroid hormone levels exhibit reduced menstrual cycle symptomatology (Shangold et al. 1990). Indeed, female athletes who participate in high volumes of vigorous exercise display menstrual cycle irregularities (including anovulatory cycles and/or amenorrhea), possibly due to the effects of strenuous exercise on steroid hormone levels (De Cree 1998). Shorter luteal phases during the menstrual cycle have been shown to correlate with low serum LH, FSH, estrogen, and PROG levels in female athletes (Shangold 1982; Prior et al. 1982; Shangold et al. 1979), and experimental evidence suggests that, in women with a history of PMDD, pharmacologically induced ovarian suppression eliminates PMDD symptoms while hormone (estradiol and progesterone) addback precipitates symptom return (Schmidt et al. 1998). Whether moderate exercise training may alleviate cyclic depressive symptoms in women via modulatory effects on reproductive steroid hormone levels has not yet been investigated, and findings have been mixed regarding whether an association exists between participation in moderate exercise training and reduction in circulating ovarian steroid hormone levels (Stoddard et al. 2007).

Though aerobic exercise may be effective at relieving symptoms of MRMDs, participation in exercise requires motivation to engage in physical activity during a period of time when MRMD symptoms run counter to engaging in physically active behaviors. As such, the initiation and maintenance of a physical activity program may be especially difficult for women with MRMDs. A recent study of 232 female collegiate athletes found that premenstrual symptoms such as difficulty concentrating and fatigue/lack of energy negatively impacted athletic performance (Takeda et al. 2015). More research is needed to determine whether the impairing symptoms of MRMDs adversely impact the ability to participate in exercise training.

Relationships Among Physical Activity and Perinatal Depression

Regular participation in physical activity (PA) has been shown to improve maternal cardiovascular fitness (Melzer et al. 2010; Nascimento et al. 2012), reduce adverse maternal obstetric complications and fetal/infant health outcomes (Joy et al. 2013; Currie et al. 2013), reduce postpartum weight retention (Joy et al. 2013), and improve maternal mood in euthymic women (Demissie et al. 2011; Takahasi et al. 2013). Non-pharmacological treatments (including exercise) for perinatal depression may be particularly favored by women who have concerns about possible adverse effects of antidepressant medications on the developing fetus or newborn. To date, however, little is known regarding the modality, intensity, or appropriate duration of PA interventions for the treatment of perinatal depression. Evidence suggests an inverse association between regular participation in PA (either prepregnancy or during pregnancy or postpartum) and the presence of postpartum depressive symptoms (Teychenne and York 2013). However, the majority of studies which have investigated physical activity interventions for the treatment of perinatal depression have been conducted on nonclinical samples (women without depression at study baseline) and many fail to report key components of PA interventions including intensity, modality, and/or duration of sessions (Teychenne and York 2013). For example, results from a recent systematic review and meta-analysis of six available studies indicate a low to moderate effect size for PA to significantly reduce depression scores, compared to matched controls, during pregnancy (SMD −0.46, 95 % CI −0.87 to −0.05, $P=0.03$) (Daley et al. 2015c). However, interpretations of these data warrant caution due to methodological limitations including the use of nonclinical samples, significant heterogeneity between studies, and large variability in outcome measures.

There is recent research which has investigated the efficacy of exercise training for postpartum depression, using an RCT study design, randomly assigning 94 participants who met the Edinburgh Postnatal Depression Scale (EPDS) score of 13+ (indicative of PPD; Cox et al. 1987) to 6 months of moderate intensity facilitated home-based aerobic exercise 3–5 days/week vs. usual care control (Daley et al. 2015b). In this latter study, Daley and colleagues found that significantly more women in the exercise training group exhibited EPDS scores indicative of recovery than women in the usual care condition; however, the magnitude of the difference in mean EPDS scores between the groups was moderate. The exercise intervention group in this study had higher social support scores at the 6 month measurement, despite the fact that substantially more usual-care participants were receiving psychological support at baseline and 6 months follow-up. The results of this randomized controlled trial (RCT) suggest that a facilitated exercise intervention with encouragement to exercise and to seek out social support may be an effective treatment for women with PPD; however, further research is warranted.

Current American College of Obstetricians and Gynecologists (ACOG) recommendations suggest that, in the absence of medical or obstetric complications, perinatal women can follow the current Centers for Disease Control and Prevention and American College of Sports Medicine recommendations for participation in moderate to vigorous physical activity (MVPA) for 30 min or more on most, if not all, days of the week (ACOG Committee opinion. Number 267, January 2002: exercise during pregnancy and the postpartum period 2002). However, epidemiological evidence suggests that ~70 % of pregnant women are inactive (Evenson et al. 2004) and that participation in PA declines across gestation (Hausenblas and Downs 2005; Schmidt et al. 2006) and the postpartum period (Pereira et al. 2007). Interestingly, this occurs even though the capacity to perform exercise at moderate to vigorous levels exist physiologically throughout gestation (Watson et al. 1991).

The biological mechanisms by which exercise may help to reduce or prevent perinatal depression have not yet been explored, but may involve similar physiological and psychological adaptations which have been shown to be beneficial for non-perinatal depression (for example, positive modulation of stress-responsive systems). Considering that exercise is also a physiologic and psychological stressor (Hackney 2006), and depression has been associated with disruption in stress-processing systems, examination of the safety and efficacy of PA interventions for women with perinatal depression may be particularly important. For example, research suggests that women exhibit different physiologic and psychological responses to stress across gestation (Christian 2012), and that these responses may be modified by the presence of a depressive or anxiety disorder (Evans et al. 2008). Therefore, in addition to exercise intensity, the timing of exercise initiation (e.g., prior to pregnancy or during certain gestational stages) may be an important consideration for women with perinatal depression.

Relationships Among Physical Activity and Affective Disorders During the Menopause Transition

There is a paucity of data regarding exercise as a treatment for depression during the menopausal transition. Several RCTs have investigated the efficacy of aerobic exercise training in improving mental health and quality of life in euthymic perimenopausal and postmenopausal women (Luoto et al. 2012; Reed et al. 2014; Mansikkamaki et al. 2012). Though these studies found that aerobic exercise training produced modest improvements in negative symptoms during mid-life (including mood swings, irritability, vasomotor symptoms, sleep difficulties, and depressed mood), the use of nonclinical samples and varied mid-life periods limits the ability to generalize these studies to women with mood and anxiety disorders during the menopause transition. A more recent population-based study of 2891 mid-life women participating in the Study of Women's Health Across the Nation (SWAN) investigated the prospective relationship between regular participation in physical activity [assessed via the Kaiser Physical Activity Survey, a self-administered questionnaire which asks about PA in the past year, and assesses PA in four domains: (1) sports/exercise, (2) active living, (3) occupational, and (4) household/caregiving] and the development of depressive symptoms [assessed via the 20-item Center for Epidemiological Studies Depression Scale (CES-D)] (Dugan et al. 2015). Dugan and colleagues found that participation in physical activity at the public health guidelines recommended dose of 150 min of moderate intensity PA weekly (Haskell et al. 2007) was associated with lower levels of depressive symptoms over a ten year period in mid-life women during the menopause transition. This study suggests a possible protective role for PA on the development of depression during the menopause transition.

The extent to which exercise may have a positive impact on vasomotor symptoms and subsequent mental health in women during the menopause transition is not known, although there are reasons for assuming that exercise may be beneficial. Recent RCTs have failed to find significant differences in vasomotor symptoms between mid-life women who participated in moderate-intensity aerobic exercise interventions and matched controls (Sternfeld et al. 2014; Daley et al. 2015a). To date, there is insufficient evidence that PA alleviates vasomotor symptoms in mid-life women. However, there is some limited evidence that exercise training may be beneficial for sleep disturbances (which are commonly associated with depression) in menopausal women (Mansikkamaki et al. 2012; Kline et al. 2012). Whether exercise training may help to alleviate the increased sleep disturbances occurring during the menopause transition remains to be explored.

Summary

The complex relationships among reproductive steroid hormones and the development and maintenance of affective disorders across the female life span are still being elucidated, and there remain many unanswered questions regarding the role of exercise in these associations. Physical activity may serve as a unique opportunity to help women cope with the multiple somatic, sleep-related, and mental health symptoms associated with fluctuating levels of reproductive steroid hormones. However, more research is needed in order to better understand the role of physical activity (and mechanisms underlying this role) in the prevention and treatment of women's reproductive-related mood and anxiety disorders. There has been limited study of the impact of reproductive-related affective disorders on the initiation and maintenance of regular participation in physical activity. Reproductive hormones play a major role in emotion regulation, arousal, cognition, and motivation. Therefore, it is also possible that reproductive steroid hormones may influence participation in physical activity during key life periods in women by indirectly influencing psychological and social risk factors for inactivity.

References

ACOG. ACOG Committee opinion Number 267, January 2002: exercise during pregnancy and the postpartum period. Obstet Gynecol. 2002;99(1):171–3.
Aganoff JA, Boyle GJ. Aerobic exercise, mood states and menstrual cycle symptoms. J Psychosom Res. 1994;38(3):183–92.
American Psychiatric Association. Diagnostic and statistical manual of mental disorders: DSM-5. Washington, DC: American Psychiatric Association; 2013.
Angst J, Vollrath M. The natural history of anxiety disorders. Acta Psychiatr Scand. 1991;84(5): 446–52.
Anshel MH. Effect of chronic aerobic exercise and progressive relaxation on motor performance and affect following acute stress. Behav Med (Washington, DC). 1996;21(4):186–96. doi:10.1 080/08964289.1996.9933757.
Avis NE, Stellato R, Crawford S, Bromberger J, Ganz P, Cain V, Kagawa-Singer M. Is there a menopausal syndrome? Menopausal status and symptoms across racial/ethnic groups. Soc Sci Med. 2001;52(3):345–56.
Azar D, Ball K, Salmon J, Cleland V. The association between physical activity and depressive symptoms in young women: a review. Ment Health Phys Act. 2008;1(2):82–8.

Barth C, Villringer A, Sacher J. Sex hormones affect neurotransmitters and shape the adult female brain during hormonal transition periods. Front Neurosci. 2015;9.

Bei B, Milgrom J, Ericksen J, Trinder J. Subjective perception of sleep, but not its objective quality, is associated with immediate postpartum mood disturbances in healthy women. Sleep. 2010; 33(4):531–8.

Bertone-Johnson ER, Whitcomb BW, Missmer SA, Manson JE, Hankinson SE, Rich-Edwards JW. Early life emotional, physical, and sexual abuse and the development of premenstrual syndrome: a longitudinal study. J Womens Health. 2014;23(9):729–39.

Bherer L, Erickson KI, Liu-Ambrose T. A review of the effects of physical activity and exercise on cognitive and brain functions in older adults. J Aging Res. 2013;2013.

Bloch M, Schmidt PJ, Rubinow DR. Premenstrual syndrome: evidence for symptom stability across cycles. Am J Psychiatry. 1997;154(12):1741–6. doi:10.1176/ajp.154.12.1741.

Breedlove G, Fryzelka D. Depression screening during pregnancy. J Midwifery Womens Health. 2011;56(1):18–25. doi:10.1111/j.1542-2011.2010.00002.x.

Breslau N, Schultz L, Peterson E. Sex differences in depression: a role for preexisting anxiety. Psychiatry Res. 1995;58(1):1–12.

Brilman EI, Ormel J. Life events, difficulties and onset of depressive episodes in later life. Psychol Med. 2001;31(5):859–69.

Bromberger JT, Assmann SF, Avis NE, Schocken M, Kravitz HM, Cordal A. Persistent mood symptoms in a multiethnic cohort of pre- and perimenopausal women. Am J Epidemiol. 2003; 158(4): 347-356.

Brown WJ, Mishra GD, Dobson A. Changes in physical symptoms during the menopause transition. Int J Behav Med. 2002;9(1):53–67.

Brown HE, Pearson N, Braithwaite RE, Brown WJ, Biddle SJ. Physical activity interventions and depression in children and adolescents. Sports Med. 2013;43(3):195–206.

Bunevicius A, Rubinow DR, Calhoun A, Leserman J, Richardson E, Rozanski K, Girdler SS. The association of migraine with menstrually related mood disorders and childhood sexual abuse. J Womens Health. 2013;22(10):871–6.

Burger HG, Dudley EC, Robertson DM, Dennerstein L. Hormonal changes in the menopause transition. Recent Prog Horm Res. 2001;57:257–75.

Burt VK, Altshuler LL, Rasgon N. Depressive symptoms in the perimenopause: prevalence, assessment, and guidelines for treatment. Harv Rev Psychiatry. 1998;6(3):121–32.

Byrne A, Byrne D. The effect of exercise on depression, anxiety and other mood states: a review. J Psychosom Res. 1993;37(6):565–74.

Choi PY, Salmon P. Symptom changes across the menstrual cycle in competitive sportswomen, exercisers and sedentary women. Br J Clin Psychol. 1995;34(3):447–60.

Christian LM. Physiological reactivity to psychological stress in human pregnancy: current knowledge and future directions. Prog Neurobiol. 2012;99(2):106–16. doi:10.1016/j.pneurobio.2012.07.003.

Cohen LS, Soares CN, Otto MW, Sweeney BH, Liberman RF, Harlow BL. Prevalence and predictors of premenstrual dysphoric disorder (PMDD) in older premenopausal women. The Harvard study of moods and cycles. J Affect Disord. 2002;70(2):125–32.

Cohen LS, Soares CN, Vitonis AF, Otto MW, Harlow BL. Risk for new onset of depression during the menopausal transition: the Harvard study of moods and cycles. Arch Gen Psychiatry. 2006; 63(4):385–90.

Cox JL, Holden JM, Sagovsky R. Detection of postnatal depression. Development of the 10-item Edinburgh Postnatal Depression Scale. Br J Psychiatry. 1987;150(6):782–6.

Cox EQ, Stuebe A, Pearson B, Grewen K, Rubinow D, Meltzer-Brody S. Oxytocin and HPA stress axis reactivity in postpartum women. Psychoneuroendocrinology. 2015;55:164–72. doi:10.1016/j.psyneuen.2015.02.009.

Crowley SK, Girdler SS. Neurosteroid, GABAergic and hypothalamic pituitary adrenal (HPA) axis regulation: what is the current state of knowledge in humans? Psychopharmacology (Berl). 2014;231(17):3619–34. doi:10.1007/s00213-014-3572-8.

Crowley SK, Pedersen CA, Leserman J, Girdler SS. The influence of early life sexual abuse on oxytocin concentrations and premenstrual symptomatology in women with a menstrually related mood disorder. Biol Psychol. 2015a;109:1–9. doi:10.1016/j.biopsycho.2015.04.003.

Crowley SK, Wilkinson LL, Wigfall LT, Reynolds AM, Muraca ST, Glover SH, Wooten NR, Sui X, Beets MW, Durstine JL, Newman-Norlund RD, Youngstedt SD. Physical fitness and depressive symptoms during army basic combat training. Med Sci Sports Exerc. 2015b;47(1):151–8. doi:10.1249/mss.0000000000000396.

Crowley SK, O'Buckley TK, Schiller CE, Stuebe A, Morrow AL, Girdler SS. Blunted neuroactive steroid and HPA axis responses to stress are associated with reduced sleep quality and negative affect in pregnancy: a pilot study. Psychopharmacology (Berl). 2016. doi:10.1007/s00213-016-4217-x.

Cubeddu A, Bucci F, Giannini A, Russo M, Daino D, Russo N, Merlini S, Pluchino N, Valentino V, Casarosa E. Brain-derived neurotrophic factor plasma variation during the different phases of the menstrual cycle in women with premenstrual syndrome. Psychoneuroendocrinology. 2011;36(4):523–30.

Currie LM, Blackman K, Clancy L, Levy DT. The effect of tobacco control policies on smoking prevalence and smoking-attributable deaths in Ireland using the IrelandSS simulation model. Tob Control. 2013;22(e1):e25–32. doi:10.1136/tobaccocontrol-2011-050248.

Da Costa D, Lowensteyn I, Abrahamowicz M, Ionescu-Ittu R, Dritsa M, Rippen N, Cervantes P, Khalifé S. A randomized clinical trial of exercise to alleviate postpartum depressed mood. J Psychosomat Obstetr Gynecol. 2009;30(3):191–200.

Daley A, Thomas A, Roalfe A, Stokes-Lampard H, Coleman S, Rees M, Hunter M, MacArthur C. The effectiveness of exercise as treatment for vasomotor menopausal symptoms: randomised controlled trial. BJOG. 2015a;122(4):565–75.

Daley AJ, Blamey RV, Jolly K, Roalfe AK, Turner KM, Coleman S, McGuinness M, Jones I, Sharp DJ, MacArthur C. A pragmatic randomized controlled trial to evaluate the effectiveness of a facilitated exercise intervention as a treatment for postnatal depression: the PAM-PeRS trial. Psychol Med. 2015b;45(11):2413–25. doi:10.1017/s0033291715000409.

Daley AJ, Foster L, Long G, Palmer C, Robinson O, Walmsley H, Ward R. The effectiveness of exercise for the prevention and treatment of antenatal depression: systematic review with meta-analysis. BJOG. 2015c;122(1):57–62. doi:10.1111/1471-0528.12909.

Daumit GL, Goldberg RW, Anthony C, Dickerson F, Brown CH, Kreyenbuhl J, Wohlheiter J, Dixon J. Physical activity patterns in adults with severe mental illness. J Nerv Ment Dis. 2005;193(10):641–6.

De Cree C. Sex steroid metabolism and menstrual irregularities in the exercising female. A review. Sports Med (Auckland, NZ). 1998;25(6):369–406.

de Novaes Soares C, Almeida OP, Joffe H, Cohen LS. Efficacy of estradiol for the treatment of depressive disorders in perimenopausal women: a double-blind, randomized, placebo-controlled trial. Arch Gen Psychiatry. 2001;58(6):529–34.

Demissie Z, Siega-Riz AM, Evenson KR, Herring AH, Dole N, Gaynes BN. Physical activity and depressive symptoms among pregnant women: the PIN3 study. Arch Womens Ment Health. 2011;14(2):145–57. doi:10.1007/s00737-010-0193-z.

Dennerstein L, Dudley EC, Hopper JL, Guthrie JR, Burger HG. A prospective population-based study of menopausal symptoms. Obstetr Gynecol. 2000;96(3):351–8.

Dennerstein L, Guthrie JR, Clark M, Lehert P, Henderson VW. A population-based study of depressed mood in middle-aged, Australian-born women. Menopause (New York, NY). 2004;11(5):563–8.

Dugan SA, Bromberger JT, Segawa E, Avery E, Sternfeld B. Association between physical activity and depressive symptoms: midlife women in SWAN. Med Sci Sports Exerc. 2015;47(2):335–42.

Dunn EC, Gilman SE, Willett JB, Slopen NB, Molnar BE. The impact of exposure to interpersonal violence on gender differences in adolescent-onset major depression: results from the National Comorbidity Survey Replication (NCS-R). Depress Anxiety. 2012;29(5):392–9. doi:10.1002/da.21916.

Eiland L, McEwen BS. Early life stress followed by subsequent adult chronic stress potentiates anxiety and blunts hippocampal structural remodeling. Hippocampus. 2012;22(1):82–91.

Ekholm UB, Backstrom T. Influence of premenstrual syndrome on family, social life, and work performance. Int J Health Serv. 1994;24(4):629–47.

Eriksson E, Ekman A, Sinclair S, Sorvik K, Ysander C, Mattson UB, Nissbrandt H. Escitalopram administered in the luteal phase exerts a marked and dose-dependent effect in premenstrual dysphoric disorder. J Clin Psychopharmacol. 2008;28(2):195–202. doi:10.1097/JCP.0b013e3181678a28.

Evans LM, Myers MM, Monk C. Pregnant women's cortisol is elevated with anxiety and depression—but only when comorbid. Arch Womens Ment Health. 2008;11(3):239–48. doi:10.1007/s00737-008-0019-4.

Evenson KR, Savitz DA, Huston SL. Leisure-time physical activity among pregnant women in the US. Paediatr Perinat Epidemiol. 2004;18(6):400–7. doi:10.1111/j.1365-3016.2004.00595.x.

Faas M, Bouman A, Moesa H, Heineman MJ, de Leij L, Schuiling G. The immune response during the luteal phase of the ovarian cycle: a Th2-type response? Fertil Steril. 2000;74(5):1008–13.

Falah-Hassani K, Shiri R, Dennis C-L. Prevalence and risk factors for comorbid postpartum depressive symptomatology and anxiety. J Affect Disord. 2016;198:142–7.

Farage MA, Neill S, MacLean AB. Physiological changes associated with the menstrual cycle: a review. Obstet Gynecol Surv. 2009;64(1):58–72. doi:10.1097/OGX.0b013e3181932a37.

Freeman EW. Premenstrual syndrome and premenstrual dysphoric disorder: definitions and diagnosis. Psychoneuroendocrinology. 2003;28:25–37.

Freeman EW. Depression in the menopause transition: risks in the changing hormone milieu as observed in the general population. Women Midlife Health. 2015;1(1):1.

Freeman EW, Sondheimer SJ. Premenstrual dysphoric disorder: recognition and treatment. Prim Care Companion J Clin Psychiatry. 2003;5(1):30–9.

Freeman EW, Sondheimer SJ, Rickels K. Effects of medical history factors on symptom severity in women meeting criteria for premenstrual syndrome. Obstet Gynecol. 1988;72(2):236–9.

Freeman EW, Sammel MD, Boorman DW, Zhang R. Longitudinal pattern of depressive symptoms around natural menopause. JAMA Psychiatry. 2014;71(1):36–43.

Gallicchio L, Schilling C, Miller SR, Zacur H, Flaws JA. Correlates of depressive symptoms among women undergoing the menopausal transition. J Psychosom Res. 2007;63(3):263–8.

Gandara BK, Leresche L, Mancl L. Patterns of salivary estradiol and progesterone across the menstrual cycle. Ann N Y Acad Sci. 2007;1098:446–50. doi:10.1196/annals.1384.022.

Garfield L, Mathews HL, Janusek LW. Inflammatory and epigenetic pathways for perinatal depression. Biol Res Nurs. 2015. doi:10.1177/1099800415614892.

Gavin NI, Gaynes BN, Lohr KN, Meltzer-Brody S, Gartlehner G, Swinson T. Perinatal depression: a systematic review of prevalence and incidence. Obstet Gynecol. 2005;106(5 Pt 1):1071–83. doi:10.1097/01.AOG.0000183597.31630.db.

Gibbs Z, Kulkarni J. Risk factors for depression during perimenopause. In: Barnes D, editor. Women's reproductive mental health across the lifespan. New, York, NY: Springer; 2014. p. 215–33.

Gibbs Z, Lee S, Kulkarni J. What factors determine whether a woman becomes depressed during the perimenopause? Arch Womens Ment Health. 2012;15(5):323–32. doi:10.1007/s00737-012-0304-0.

Girdler SS, Sherwood A, Hinderliter AL, Leserman J, Costello NL, Straneva PA, Pedersen CA, Light KC. Biological correlates of abuse in women with premenstrual dysphoric disorder and healthy controls. Psychosom Med. 2003;65(5):849–56.

Glynn LM, Davis EP, Sandman CA. New insights into the role of perinatal HPA-axis dysregulation in postpartum depression. Neuropeptides. 2013;47(6):363–70. doi:10.1016/j.npep.2013.10.007.

Goodwin RD. Association between physical activity and mental disorders among adults in the United States. Prev Med. 2003;36(6):698–703.

Gordon JL, Girdler SS, Meltzer-Brody SE, Stika CS, Thurston RC, Clark CT, Prairie BA, Moses-Kolko E, Joffe H, Wisner KL. Ovarian hormone fluctuation, neurosteroids, and HPA axis dysregulation in perimenopausal depression: a novel heuristic model. Am J Psychiatry. 2015;172(3):227–36. doi:10.1176/appi.ajp.2014.14070918.

Gordon JL, Rubinow DR, Eisenlohr-Moul TA, Leserman J, Girdler SS. Estradiol variability, stressful life events, and the emergence of depressive symptomatology during the menopausal transition. Menopause (New York, NY). 2016;23(3):257–66. doi:10.1097/gme.0000000000000528.

Goyal D, Gay C, Lee K. Fragmented maternal sleep is more strongly correlated with depressive symptoms than infant temperament at three months postpartum. Arch Womens Ment Health. 2009;12(4):229–37. doi:10.1007/s00737-009-0070-9.

Hackney AC. Exercise as a stressor to the human neuroendocrine system. Medicina (Kaunas). 2006;42(10):788–97.

Halbreich U, Borenstein J, Pearlstein T, Kahn LS. The prevalence, impairment, impact, and burden of premenstrual dysphoric disorder (PMS/PMDD). Psychoneuroendocrinology. 2003;28 Suppl 3:1–23.

Handa RJ, Burgess LH, Kerr JE, O'Keefe JA. Gonadal steroid hormone receptors and sex differences in the hypothalamo-pituitary-adrenal axis. Horm Behav. 1994;28(4):464–76.

Harlow BL, MacLehose RF, Smolenski DJ, Soares CN, Otto MW, Joffe H, Cohen LS. Disparate rates of new-onset depression during the menopausal transition in 2 community-based populations: real, or really wrong? Am J Epidemiol. 2013;177(10):1148–56.

Haskell WL, Lee IM, Pate RR, Powell KE, Blair SN, Franklin BA, Macera CA, Heath GW, Thompson PD, Bauman A. Physical activity and public health: updated recommendation for adults from the American College of Sports Medicine and the American Heart Association. Med Sci Sports Exerc. 2007;39(8):1423–34. doi:10.1249/mss.0b013e3180616b27.

Hausenblas HA, Downs DS. Prospective examination of leisure-time exercise behavior during pregnancy. J Appl Sport Psychol. 2005;17(3):240–6.

Herring MP, Kline CE, O'Connor PJ. Effects of exercise on sleep among young women with generalized anxiety disorder. Ment Health Phys Act. 2015;9:59–66. doi:10.1016/j.mhpa.2015.09.002.

Hindberg I, Naesh O. Serotonin concentrations in plasma and variations during the menstrual cycle. Clin Chem. 1992;38(10):2087–9.

Hopkins ME, Davis FC, VanTieghem MR, Whalen PJ, Bucci DJ. Differential effects of acute and regular physical exercise on cognition and affect. Neuroscience. 2012;215:59–68.

Howell HB, Brawman-Mintzer O, Monnier J, Yonkers KA. Generalized anxiety disorder in women. Psychiatr Clin North Am. 2001;24(1):165–78.

Huo L, Straub RE, Roca C, Schmidt PJ, Shi K, Vakkalanka R, Weinberger DR, Rubinow DR. Risk for premenstrual dysphoric disorder is associated with genetic variation in ESR1, the estrogen receptor alpha gene. Biol Psychiatry. 2007;62(8):925–33.

Jacka F, Pasco J, Williams L, Leslie E, Dodd S, Nicholson G, Kotowicz M, Berk M. Lower levels of physical activity in childhood associated with adult depression. J Sci Med Sport. 2011;14(3):222–6.

Jackson EM, Dishman RK. Cardiorespiratory fitness and laboratory stress: a meta-regression analysis. Psychophysiology. 2006;43(1):57–72. doi:10.1111/j.1469-8986.2006.00373.x.

Joffe H, Hall JE, Soares CN, Hennen J, Reilly CJ, Carlson K, Cohen LS. Vasomotor symptoms are associated with depression in perimenopausal women seeking primary care. Menopause (New York, NY). 2002;9(6):392–8.

Johnson WG, Carr-Nangle RE, Bergeron KC. Macronutrient intake, eating habits, and exercise as moderators of menstrual distress in healthy women. Psychosom Med. 1995;57(4):324–30.

Joy EA, Mottola MF, Chambliss H. Integrating exercise is medicine(R) into the care of pregnant women. Curr Sports Med Rep. 2013;12(4):245–7. doi:10.1249/JSR.0b013e31829a6f7e.

Kendler KS, Gardner CO. Sex differences in the pathways to major depression: a study of opposite-sex twin pairs. Am J Psychiatry. 2014;171(4):426–35. doi:10.1176/appi.ajp.2013.13101375.

Kendler K, Silberg J, Neale M, Kessler R, Heath A, Eaves L. Genetic and environmental factors in the aetiology of menstrual, premenstrual and neurotic symptoms: a population-based twin study. Psychol Med. 1992;22(01):85–100.

Kendler KS, Kuhn J, Prescott CA. The interrelationship of neuroticism, sex, and stressful life events in the prediction of episodes of major depression. Am J Psychiatry. 2004;161(4):631–6. doi:10.1176/appi.ajp.161.4.631.

Kessel B. Premenstrual syndrome: advances in diagnosis and treatment. Obstet Gynecol Clin North Am. 2000;27(3):625–39.

Kessler RC, McGonagle KA, Swartz M, Blazer DG, Nelson CB. Sex and depression in the National Comorbidity Survey. I: lifetime prevalence, chronicity and recurrence. J Affect Disord. 1993;29(2-3):85–96.

Kikuchi H, Nakatani Y, Seki Y, Yu X, Sekiyama T, Sato-Suzuki I, Arita H. Decreased blood serotonin in the premenstrual phase enhances negative mood in healthy women. J Psychosom Obstet Gynaecol. 2010;31(2):83–9. doi:10.3109/01674821003770606.

Kipp M, Berger K, Clarner T, Dang J, Beyer C. Sex steroids control neuroinflammatory processes in the brain: relevance for acute ischaemia and degenerative demyelination. J Neuroendocrinol. 2012;24(1):62–70. doi:10.1111/j.1365-2826.2011.02163.x.

Kirschbaum C, Kudielka BM, Gaab J, Schommer NC, Hellhammer DH. Impact of gender, menstrual cycle phase, and oral contraceptives on the activity of the hypothalamus-pituitary-adrenal axis. Psychosom Med. 1999;61(2):154–62.

Klaperski S, von Dawans B, Heinrichs M, Fuchs R. Effects of a 12-week endurance training program on the physiological response to psychosocial stress in men: a randomized controlled trial. J Behav Med. 2014;37(6):1118–33. doi:10.1007/s10865-014-9562-9.

Kline CE. The bidirectional relationship between exercise and sleep: implications for exercise adherence and sleep improvement. Am J Lifestyle Med. 2014;8(6):375–9. doi:10.1177/1559827614544437.

Kline CE, Sui X, Hall MH, Youngstedt SD, Blair SN, Earnest CP, Church TS. Dose-response effects of exercise training on the subjective sleep quality of postmenopausal women: exploratory analyses of a randomised controlled trial. BMJ Open. 2012;2(4):e001044. doi:10.1136/bmjopen-2012-001044.

Kossman DA, Williams NI, Domchek SM, Kurzer MS, Stopfer JE, Schmitz KH. Exercise lowers estrogen and progesterone levels in premenopausal women at high risk of breast cancer. J Appl Physiol. 2011;111(6):1687–93.

Kraemer GR, Kraemer RR. Premenstrual syndrome: diagnosis and treatment experiences. J Womens Health. 1998;7(7):893–907.

Kritz-Silverstein D, Barrett-Connor E, Corbeau C. Cross-sectional and prospective study of exercise and depressed mood in the elderly the Rancho Bernardo Study. Am J Epidemiol. 2001;153(6):596–603.

Lawlor DA, Hopker SW. The effectiveness of exercise as an intervention in the management of depression: systematic review and meta-regression analysis of randomised controlled trials. BMJ. 2001;322(7289):763.

Lentz MJ, Woods N, Heitkemper M, Mitchell E, Henker R, Shaver J. Ovarian steroids and premenstrual symptoms: a comparison of group differences and intra-individual patterns. Res Nurs Health. 2007;30(3):238–49. doi:10.1002/nur.20188.

Leventhal AM. Relations between anhedonia and physical activity. Am J Health Behav. 2012;36(6):860–72. doi:10.5993/ajhb.36.6.12.

Luoto R, Moilanen J, Heinonen R, Mikkola T, Raitanen J, Tomas E, Ojala K, Mansikkamaki K, Nygard CH. Effect of aerobic training on hot flushes and quality of life – a randomized controlled trial. Ann Med. 2012;44(6):616–26. doi:10.3109/07853890.2011.583674.

Mansikkamaki K, Raitanen J, Nygard CH, Heinonen R, Mikkola T, EijaTomas Luoto R. Sleep quality and aerobic training among menopausal women – a randomized controlled trial. Maturitas. 2012;72(4):339–45. doi:10.1016/j.maturitas.2012.05.003.

Masho SW, Adera T, South-Paul J. Obesity as a risk factor for premenstrual syndrome. J Psychosomat Obstetr Gynecol. 2005;26(1):33–9.

Mata J, Hogan CL, Joormann J, Waugh CE, Gotlib IH. Acute exercise attenuates negative affect following repeated sad mood inductions in persons who have recovered from depression. J Abnorm Psychol. 2013;122(1):45.

Matud MP. Gender differences in stress and coping styles. Personal Individ Differ. 2004;37(7):1401–15.

McDevitt J, Snyder M, Miller A, Wilbur J. Perceptions of barriers and benefits to physical activity among outpatients in psychiatric rehabilitation. J Nurs Scholarsh. 2006;38(1):50–5.

McEwen B. Estrogen actions throughout the brain. Recent Prog Horm Res. 2002;57:357–84.

McHichi alami K, Tahiri SM, Moussaoui D, Kadri N. [Assessment of premenstrual dysphoric disorder symptoms: population of women in Casablanca]. Encéphale. 2002;28(6 Pt 1):525–30.

Mead GE, Morley W, Campbell P, Greig CA, McMurdo M, Lawlor DA. Exercise for depression. Cochrane Database Syst Rev. 2009;3.

Melzer K, Schutz Y, Soehnchen N, Othenin-Girard V, Martinez de Tejada B, Irion O, Boulvain M, Kayser B. Effects of recommended levels of physical activity on pregnancy outcomes. Am J Obstet Gynecol. 2010;202(3):261–6. doi:10.1016/j.ajog.2009.10.876.

Metcalf MG. Incidence of ovulation from the menarche to the menopause: observations of 622 New Zealand women. N Z Med J. 1983;96(738):645–8.

Metcalf MG, Skidmore DS, Lowry GF, Mackenzie JA. Incidence of ovulation in the years after the menarche. J Endocrinol. 1983;97(2):213–9.

Morrow AL, Devaud LL, Purdy RH, Paul SM. Neuroactive steroid modulators of the stress response. Ann N Y Acad Sci. 1995;771:257–72.

Mundy EA, Weber M, Rauch SL, Killgore WD, Simon NM, Pollack MH, Rosso IM. Adult anxiety disorders in relation to trait anxiety and perceived stress in childhood. Psychol Rep. 2015;117(2):473–89. doi:10.2466/02.10.PR0.117c17z6.

Nascimento SL, Surita FG, Cecatti JG. Physical exercise during pregnancy: a systematic review. Curr Opin Obstet Gynecol. 2012;24(6):387–94. doi:10.1097/GCO.0b013e328359f131.

O'Brien PMS, Bäckström T, Brown C, Dennerstein L, Endicott J, Epperson CN, Eriksson E, Freeman E, Halbreich U, Ismail KM. Towards a consensus on diagnostic criteria, measurement and trial design of the premenstrual disorders: the ISPMD Montreal consensus. Arch Womens Ment Health. 2011;14(1):13–21.

O'Connor KA, Ferrell R, Brindle E, Trumble B, Shofer J, Holman DJ, Weinstein m. Progesterone and ovulation across stages of the transition to menopause. Menopause (New York, NY). 2009;16(6):1178–87. doi:10.1097/gme.0b013e3181aa192d.

Oertelt-Prigione S. Immunology and the menstrual cycle. Autoimmun Rev. 2012;11(6):A486–92.

O'Hara MW, McCabe JE. Postpartum depression: current status and future directions. Annu Rev Clin Psychol. 2013;9:379–407. doi:10.1146/annurev-clinpsy-050212-185612.

O'Hara MW, Wisner KL. Perinatal mental illness: definition, description and aetiology. Best Pract Res Clin Obstet Gynaecol. 2014;28(1):3–12. doi:10.1016/j.bpobgyn.2013.09.002.

O'Hara MW, Schlechte JA, Lewis DA, Varner MW. Controlled prospective study of postpartum mood disorders: psychological, environmental, and hormonal variables. J Abnorm Psychol. 1991;100(1):63–73.

Okun ML. Sleep and postpartum depression. Curr Opin Psychiatry. 2015;28(6):490–6. doi:10.1097/yco.0000000000000206.

Okun ML, Kline CE, Roberts JM, Wettlaufer B, Glover K, Hall M. Prevalence of sleep deficiency in early gestation and its associations with stress and depressive symptoms. J Womens Health (Larchmt). 2013;22(12):1028–37. doi:10.1089/jwh.2013.4331.

Parry BL, Meliska CJ, Sorenson DL, Martinez LF, Lopez AM, Elliott JA, Hauger RL. Reduced phase-advance of plasma melatonin after bright morning light in the luteal, but not follicular, menstrual cycle phase in premenstrual dysphoric disorder: an extended study. Chronobiol Int. 2011;28(5):415–24. doi:10.3109/07420528.2011.567365.

Pereira MA, Rifas-Shiman SL, Kleinman KP, Rich-Edwards JW, Peterson KE, Gillman MW. Predictors of change in physical activity during and after pregnancy: project viva. Am J Prev Med. 2007;32(4):312–9. doi:10.1016/j.amepre.2006.12.017.

Petruzzello SJ, Landers DM, Hatfield BD, Kubitz KA, Salazar W. A meta-analysis on the anxiety-reducing effects of acute and chronic exercise. Sports Med. 1991;11(3):143–82.

Pluchino N, Cubeddu A, Begliuomini S, Merlini S, Giannini A, Bucci F, Casarosa E, Luisi M, Cela V, Genazzani A. Daily variation of brain-derived neurotrophic factor and cortisol in women with normal menstrual cycles, undergoing oral contraception and in postmenopause. Hum Reprod. 2009;24(9):2303–9.

Pluchino N, Russo M, Santoro AN, Litta P, Cela V, Genazzani AR. Steroid hormones and BDNF. Neuroscience. 2013;239:271–9. doi:10.1016/j.neuroscience.2013.01.025.

Posillico CK, Schwarz JM. An investigation into the effects of antenatal stressors on the postpartum neuroimmune profile and depressive-like behaviors. Behav Brain Res. 2016;298(Pt B):218–28. doi:10.1016/j.bbr.2015.11.011.

Prior JC, Yuen BH, Clement P, Bowie L, Thomas J. Reversible luteal phase changes and infertility associated with marathon training. Lancet (Lond). 1982;2(8292):269–70.

Rasheed P, Al-Sowielem LS. Prevalence and predictors of premenstrual syndrome among college-aged women in Saudi Arabia. Ann Saudi Med. 2003;23(6):381–7.

Raup JL, Myers JE. The empty nest syndrome: myth or reality. J Counsel Dev. 1989;68(2):180–3.

Reck C, Struben K, Backenstrass M, Stefenelli U, Reinig K, Fuchs T, Sohn C, Mundt C. Prevalence, onset and comorbidity of postpartum anxiety and depressive disorders. Acta Psychiatr Scand. 2008;118(6):459–68. doi:10.1111/j.1600-0447.2008.01264.x.

Reed SD, Guthrie KA, Newton KM, Anderson GL, Booth-LaForce C, Caan B, Carpenter JS, Cohen LS, Dunn AL, Ensrud KE, Freeman EW, Hunt JR, Joffe H, Larson JC, Learman LA, Rothenberg R, Seguin RA, Sherman KJ, Sternfeld BS, LaCroix AZ. Menopausal quality of life: RCT of yoga, exercise, and omega-3 supplements. Am J Obstet Gynecol. 2014;210(3):241–4. doi:10.1016/j.ajog.2013.11.016.

Rimmele U, Zellweger BC, Marti B, Seiler R, Mohiyeddini C, Ehlert U, Heinrichs M. Trained men show lower cortisol, heart rate and psychological responses to psychosocial stress compared with untrained men. Psychoneuroendocrinology. 2007;32(6):627–35.

Rimmele U, Seiler R, Marti B, Wirtz PH, Ehlert U, Heinrichs M. The level of physical activity affects adrenal and cardiovascular reactivity to psychosocial stress. Psychoneuroendocrinology. 2009;34(2):190–8. doi:10.1016/j.psyneuen.2008.08.023.

Rothon C, Edwards P, Bhui K, Viner RM, Taylor S, Stansfeld SA. Physical activity and depressive symptoms in adolescents: a prospective study. BMC Med. 2010;8(1):1.

Samadi Z, Taghian F, Valiani M. The effects of 8 weeks of regular aerobic exercise on the symptoms of premenstrual syndrome in non-athlete girls. Iran J Nurs Midwif Res. 2013;18(1).

Santoro N, Lasley B, McConnell D, Allsworth J, Crawford S, Gold EB, Finkelstein JS, Greendale GA, Kelsey J, Korenman S, Luborsky JL, Matthews K, Midgley R, Powell L, Sabatine J, Schocken M, Sowers MF, Weiss G. Body size and ethnicity are associated with menstrual cycle alterations in women in the early menopausal transition: the study of women's health across the nation (SWAN) daily hormone study. J Clin Endocrinol Metab. 2004;89(6):2622–31. doi:10.1210/jc.2003-031578.

Schiller CE, Schmidt PJ, Rubinow DR. Allopregnanolone as a mediator of affective switching in reproductive mood disorders. Psychopharmacology (Berl). 2014;231(17):3557–67. doi:10.1007/s00213-014-3599-x.

Schiller CE, Meltzer-Brody S, Rubinow DR. The role of reproductive hormones in postpartum depression. CNS Spectr. 2015;20(1):48–59. doi:10.1017/s1092852914000480.

Schmidt PJ, Rubinow DR. Sex hormones and mood in the perimenopause. Ann N Y Acad Sci. 2009;1179:70–85. doi:10.1111/j.1749-6632.2009.04982.x.

Schmidt PJ, Nieman LK, Danaceau MA, Adams LF, Rubinow DR. Differential behavioral effects of gonadal steroids in women with and in those without premenstrual syndrome. N Engl J Med. 1998;338(4):209–16. doi:10.1056/nejm199801223380401.

Schmidt PJ, Haq N, Rubinow DR. A longitudinal evaluation of the relationship between reproductive status and mood in perimenopausal women. Am J Psychiatry. 2004;161(12):2238–44.

Schmidt MD, Pekow P, Freedson PS, Markenson G, Chasan-Taber L. Physical activity patterns during pregnancy in a diverse population of women. J Womens Health (Larchmt). 2006;15(8):909–18. doi:10.1089/jwh.2006.15.909.

Schmidt PJ, Ben Dor R, Martinez PE, Guerrieri GM, Harsh VL, Thompson K, Koziol DE, Nieman LK, Rubinow DR. Effects of estradiol withdrawal on mood in women with past perimenopausal depression: a randomized clinical trial. JAMA Psychiatry. 2015;72(7):714–26. doi:10.1001/jamapsychiatry.2015.0111.

Shangold MM. Menstrual irregularity in athletes: basic principles, evaluation, and treatment. Can J Appl Sport Sci. 1982;7(2):68–73.

Shangold M, Freeman R, Thysen B, Gatz M. The relationship between long-distance running, plasma progesterone, and luteal phase length. Fertil Steril. 1979;31(2):130–3.

Shangold M, Rebar RW, Wentz AC, Schiff I. Evaluation and management of menstrual dysfunction in athletes. JAMA. 1990;263(12):1665–9.

Shechter A, Lespérance P, Kin NNY, Boivin DB. Pilot investigation of the circadian plasma melatonin rhythm across the menstrual cycle in a small group of women with premenstrual dysphoric disorder. PLoS One. 2012;7(12), e51929.

Skouteris H, Germano C, Wertheim EH, Paxton SJ, Milgrom J. Sleep quality and depression during pregnancy: a prospective study. J Sleep Res. 2008;17(2):217–20. doi:10.1111/j.1365-2869.2008.00655.x.

Slentz CA, Duscha BD, Johnson JL, Ketchum K, Aiken LB, Samsa GP, Houmard JA, Bales CW, Kraus WE. Effects of the amount of exercise on body weight, body composition, and measures of central obesity: STRRIDE—a randomized controlled study. Arch Intern Med. 2004;164(1):31–9.

Soares CN, Almeida OP. Depression during the perimenopause. Arch Gen Psychiatry. 2001;58(3):306.

Soares CN, Zitek B. Reproductive hormone sensitivity and risk for depression across the female life cycle: a continuum of vulnerability? J Psychiatry Neurosci. 2008;33(4):331–43.

Sothmann MS, Buckworth J, Claytor RP, Cox RH, White-Welkley JE, Dishman RK. Exercise training and the cross-stressor adaptation hypothesis. Exerc Sport Sci Rev. 1996;24:267–87.

Spalding TW, Lyon LA, Steel DH, Hatfield BD. Aerobic exercise training and cardiovascular reactivity to psychological stress in sedentary young normotensive men and women. Psychophysiology. 2004;41(4):552–62. doi:10.1111/j.1469-8986.2004.00184.x.

Steege JF, Blumenthal JA. The effects of aerobic exercise on premenstrual symptoms in middle-aged women: a preliminary study. J Psychosom Res. 1993;37(2):127–33.

Sternfeld B, Guthrie KA, Ensrud KE, LaCroix AZ, Larson JC, Dunn AL, Anderson GL, Seguin RA, Carpenter JS, Newton KM. Efficacy of exercise for menopausal symptoms: a randomized controlled trial. Menopause (New York, NY). 2014;21(4):330.

Stoddard JL, Dent CW, Shames L, Bernstein L. Exercise training effects on premenstrual distress and ovarian steroid hormones. Eur J Appl Physiol. 2007;99(1):27–37. doi:10.1007/s00421-006-0313-7.

Straneva PA, Maixner W, Light KC, Pedersen CA, Costello NL, Girdler SS. Menstrual cycle, beta-endorphins, and pain sensitivity in premenstrual dysphoric disorder. Health Psychol. 2002;21(4):358.

Stuart-Parrigon K, Stuart S. Perinatal depression: an update and overview. Curr Psychiatry Rep. 2014;16(9):468. doi:10.1007/s11920-014-0468-6.

Takahasi EH, Alves MT, Alves GS, Silva AA, Batista RF, Simoes VM, Del-Ben CM, Barbieri MA. Mental health and physical inactivity during pregnancy: a cross-sectional study nested in the BRISA cohort study. Cad Saude Publica. 2013;29(8):1583–94.

Takeda T, Imoto Y, Nagasawa H, Muroya M, Shiina M. Premenstrual syndrome and premenstrual dysphoric disorder in Japanese collegiate athletes. J Pediatr Adolesc Gynecol. 2015;28(4):215–8.

Teychenne M, York R. Physical activity, sedentary behavior, and postnatal depressive symptoms: a review. Am J Prev Med. 2013;45(2):217–27. doi:10.1016/j.amepre.2013.04.004.

Teychenne M, Costigan SA, Parker K. The association between sedentary behaviour and risk of anxiety: a systematic review. BMC Public Health. 2015;15:513. doi:10.1186/s12889-015-1843-x.

Tomlinson D, Diorio C, Beyene J, Sung L. Effect of exercise on cancer-related fatigue: a meta-analysis. Am J Phys Med Rehabil. 2014;93(8):675–86.

Tsatsoulis A, Fountoulakis S. The protective role of exercise on stress system dysregulation and comorbidities. Ann N Y Acad Sci. 2006;1083:196–213. doi:10.1196/annals.1367.020.

Verreault N, Da Costa D, Marchand A, Ireland K, Dritsa M, Khalife S. Rates and risk factors associated with depressive symptoms during pregnancy and with postpartum onset. J Psychosom Obstet Gynaecol. 2014;35(3):84–91. doi:10.3109/0167482x.2014.947953.

Wang SJ, Fuh JL, Lu SR, Juang KD, Wang PH. Migraine prevalence during menopausal transition. Headache. 2003;43(5):470–8.

Watson WJ, Katz VL, Hackney AC, Gall MM, McMurray RG. Fetal responses to maximal swimming and cycling exercise during pregnancy. Obstet Gynecol. 1991;77(3):382–6.

Wisner KL, Moses-Kolko EL, Sit DK. Postpartum depression: a disorder in search of a definition. Arch Womens Ment Health. 2010;13(1):37–40. doi:10.1007/s00737-009-0119-9.

Wisner KL, Sit DK, McShea MC, Rizzo DM, Zoretich RA, Hughes CL, Eng HF, Luther JF, Wisniewski SR, Costantino ML, Confer AL, Moses-Kolko EL, Famy CS, Hanusa BH. Onset timing, thoughts of self-harm, and diagnoses in postpartum women with screen-positive depression findings. JAMA Psychiatry. 2013;70(5):490–8. doi:10.1001/jamapsychiatry.2013.87.

Yonkers KA. Anxiety symptoms and anxiety disorders: how are they related to premenstrual disorders? J Clin Psychiatry. 1997;58 Suppl 3:62–7. discussion 68-69.

Young LJ, Pfaff DW. Sex differences in neurological and psychiatric disorders. Front Neuroendocrinol. 2014;35(3):253–4. doi:10.1016/j.yfrne.2014.05.005.

Chapter 11
Stress Reactivity and Exercise in Women

Tinna Traustadóttir

Introduction

Stress reactivity can be defined as any physiological response to a perturbation to homeostasis and generally includes both the response and recovery to a stressor. More broadly, in addition to the physiological response, it can include behavioral, subjective, and cognitive response to stress (Schlotz 2013). It is important to note that a robust response can be more beneficial than a lower response, as long as recovery is optimized after removal of the stressor and not prolonged. In the context of this chapter, the literature on stress reactivity is limited to cardiovascular and neuroendocrine responses to acute mental or physical challenges. Cardiovascular responses include heart rate and blood pressure responses to a stimulus and are driven by activation of the sympathetic nervous system. The neuroendocrine response is most often represented by measures of cortisol (salivary or plasma) as an indicator of hypothalamic–pituitary–adrenal (HPA) axis activity.

Stress Reactivity and Health

Assessing stress reactivity can have implications for future disease risk. One example is heart rate recovery in the first minute after a maximal graded exercise test; individuals who recover less than 12 bpm in the first minute of recovery have a fourfold increase in mortality compared to individuals who recover faster, regardless of the maximal heart rate response during the test (Cole et al. 1999; Gupta 2005). Similarly,

---

T. Traustadóttir, Ph.D. (✉)
Department of Biological Sciences, Northern Arizona University,
Flagstaff, AZ 86011, USA
e-mail: tinna.traustadottir@nau.edu

blood pressure response and recovery after a laboratory stressor are associated with greater risk for future hypertension (Stewart et al. 2006; Trivedi et al. 2008; Carroll et al. 2012). Cortisol response to a psychosocial or mental laboratory challenge is associated with risk for coronary heart disease and future risk of depression (Hamer et al. 2012; Morris et al. 2012). There are important differences between the effects of acute and chronic stress on the organism and these effects are also mediated by the stress reactivity of an individual. Evolutionary speaking, the activation of the HPA axis in response to acute stress can be considered beneficial since it helps the individual survive a challenge by mobilizing fuel for energy, inhibiting reproductive behavior, and increase arousal and vigilance. However, when the system is chronically challenged, either continuously or too frequently to allow for recovery and adaptation, the stress response becomes maladaptive and leads to an increased risk for diseases such as cardiovascular disease, diabetes, hypertension, and osteoporosis (McEwen 1998; McEwen 2007; Lazzarino et al. 2013; Nagaraja et al. 2016).

Methods for Testing Stress Reactivity

There are several established protocols for evaluating stress reactivity under standard laboratory conditions. By far the one most commonly used is the *Trier Social Stress Test* (TSST), a psychosocial laboratory challenge established by investigators at the University of Trier (Kirschbaum et al. 1993). The test has a few variations but typically consists of an anticipatory period, a 5-min free speech and 5-min mental arithmetic task of serial subtraction, performed in front of a panel of evaluators (sometimes videotaping is added as well) (Birkett 2011). For additional information on the TSST the reader is referred to some excellent previously published reviews (e.g., Dickerson and Kemeny 2004; Foley and Kirschbaum 2010; Allen et al. 2014).

The *Montreal Imaging Stress Task* (MIST) is a challenge that is specifically used in conjunction with imaging such as functional magnetic resonance imaging (fMRI) and positron emission tomography (PET) and uses a series of computerized arithmetic challenges along with social evaluative threat components presented within the program or by an investigator (Dedovic et al. 2005).

The *Matt Stress Reactivity Protocol* (MSRP) is another laboratory challenge which consists of a series of stressors in a set order: Stroop color-word task, mental arithmetic, anagram task, a cold pressor test, and an interpersonal interview about a particularly stressful event in the person's life (Traustadóttir et al. 2005; Bosch et al. 2009). Other studies have used driving simulation challenge (Seeman et al. 1995) or a combination of cognitive tests such as Stroop color-word task and mirror tracing task (Gotthardt et al. 1995; Seeman et al. 2001).

These laboratory challenges are all designed to elicit a stress response as demonstrated by increases in cardiovascular and HPA axis activity. The latter is usually assessed by changes in plasma and/or salivary cortisol. Recently, other measures including markers of sympathetic nervous system activity such as salivary alpha-amylase (sAA) and heart rate variability are also being included in studies on stress reactivity (Allen et al. 2014).

Are There Gender Differences in Stress Reactivity?

Since this chapter and book focuses on studies in women it is important to establish that there are in fact gender differences—otherwise it would not be necessary to differentiate the discussion based on gender. Numerous studies have shown significant differences in the HPA axis response to psychosocial or mental stressors between men and women. However, the results have not always been consistent in regard to which gender is more stress reactive, with some finding greater responses in men (Kirschbaum et al. 1992; Earle et al. 1999; Kirschbaum et al. 1999; Kudielka et al. 1999; Seeman et al. 2001; Traustadóttir et al. 2003; Uhart et al. 2006) and other in women (Seeman et al. 1995; Ahwal et al. 1997), and some showing an interaction with age (Seeman et al. 2001; Kudielka et al. 2004). One potential explanation for the unequivocal results may be due to different stressors used. To this effect, it has been shown that women have a greater cortisol response to a stressor invoking social rejection while men are more reactive to achievement-related stressors (Stroud et al. 2002). Other explanations may be due to not controlling for potential confounding variables such as menstrual cycle phase, fitness levels, or mental conditions that could influence the HPA axis response such as depression, anxiety, or other psychiatric disorders (Allen et al. 2014). Nevertheless, these studies illustrate that gender definitely has an effect on psychosocial stress reactivity and data from men and women should not be lumped together in analyses.

A recent study, however, by Stephens et al. (Stephens et al. 2016) may have put the question of 'which gender is more stress reactive' finally to rest. They had a much larger sample size than any of the previous studies, with a total of 282 subjects who underwent the TSST. The women were tested in the early follicular phase. Their results show equivocally that men had greater HPA axis response to the psychosocial stressor as measured by plasma ACTH, serum cortisol, and salivary cortisol (see Fig. 11.1), analyzed by the change across time points, overall response (area-under-the-response-curve), as well as slopes of baseline-to-peak and peak-to-end.

It is worth noting that the results from psychosocial stressors do not extend to other stimuli of the HPA axis such as pharmacological challenges where women tend to have a more pronounced response (Greenspan et al. 1993; Heuser et al. 1994; Born et al. 1995) or exhibit blunted negative feedback sensitivity (Wilkinson et al. 1997) and acute exercise where the responses in men and women are similar (Kraemer et al. 1993; Sandoval and Matt 2002; Szivak et al. 2013). However, the gender differences in responses to psychosocial or mental stress may contribute to differences in morbidity and mortality of diseases that have distinct differences in prevalence between men and women such as cardiovascular disease (prior to menopause) and autoimmune diseases (Stoney et al. 1987; Sternberg et al. 1990; Bjorntorp 1997). One reason for the discrepancies in results of studies using pharmacological challenges versus psychosocial challenges may be related to where they stimulate the HPA axis. Many of the pharmacological challenges, such as infusion of corticotropin release hormone (CRH), stimulate the axis at the level of the pituitary. Psychosocial challenges, however, require the stressor to be processed in the brain and therefore acts as a suprapituitary stimulus, activating the HPA axis response by

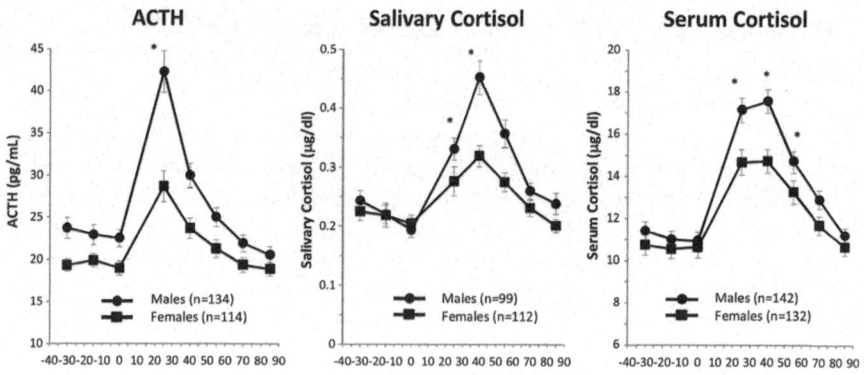

Fig. 11.1 Mean HPA-axis hormone levels (means ± SE) in response to the TSST for men ($n=147$) and women in the follicular phase of the menstrual cycle ($n=135$). Times prior to the test are shown as negative values on the *x*-axis (time). *Significant interaction with gender ($p<0.05$). Reprinted from Stephens et al. (2016) with permission from Elsevier

stimulating the paraventricular nucleus (PVN) through the limbic system (prefrontal cortex, hippocampus, amygdala) whereas physiological stressors have a more direct pathway to the PVN (Herman and Cullinan 1997).

A general consensus from the literature is that men exhibit greater cardiovascular and HPA axis responses to psychological stress than women when compared between puberty and menopause whereas gender differences are smaller when compared in individuals before puberty or after menopause (Kajantie and Phillips 2006).

Effects of Estrogen on Stress Reactivity

Sex hormones, particularly estrogen, have been shown to influence the HPA axis response in both animal and human studies. Animal studies where estrogen levels are decreased by removing the ovaries and increased with estrogen replacement show that the effect of estrogen is an enhanced HPA axis response (Lesniewska et al. 1990a; Lesniewska et al. 1990b). The same finding was shown in young men treated with an estrogen-patch or a placebo for 24-48 h before being exposed to the TSST (Kirschbaum et al. 1996). The estrogen treated group had significantly higher ACTH and cortisol response as compared to the placebo group.

Menstrual Cycle Phases

The question is whether these results from extreme differences in estrogen extend to normal estrogen fluctuations across the menstrual cycle. Based on the fact that estrogen levels are higher in the mid-luteal phase compared to early follicular phase it would be predicted that stress reactivity would be greater in the luteal phase. This prediction is supported by many studies (Tersman et al. 1991; Kirschbaum et al. 1999; Sato and Miyake 2004; Lustyk et al. 2010) but there are also number of studies who have not found significant differences in stress reactivity between follicular and luteal phases (Choi and Salmon 1995; Pico-Alfonso et al. 2007; Veldhuijzen van Zanten et al. 2009; Shenoy et al. 2014). Using exercise as a stimulus to induce a cortisol response, Boisseau et al. (Boisseau et al. 2013), found no differences in salivary or urinary cortisol response in women tested in the follicular and luteal phase of the menstrual cycle. In contrast, one study found that the effect of menstrual cycle on neuroendocrine activation to Stroop test and handgrip exercise depended on trait anxiety where women who had high trait anxiety had greater responses in the follicular phase versus luteal phase (Hlavacova et al. 2008). One caveat in many of these studies is that the comparison is not made in the same subjects across the different phases of the menstrual cycles but compares two different cohorts. The reason for this is because an important component of psychosocial stressors such as the TSST is the "element of surprise" and therefore these tests do not lend themselves to repeated measures. However, comparing within-subjects as opposed to between-subjects would be a much stronger research design to get at this question properly. One such study, that did not use a challenge, compared heart rate and blood pressure responses in everyday working life of women who reported their perceived stress (Pollard et al. 2007). They found that heart rate response to perceived stress was greater in the luteal phase but blood pressure was unaffected (Pollard et al. 2007). A recent study tested cardiovascular and epinephrine reactivity to the TSST in women in the early follicular, late follicular, and luteal phase using a within-subject design (Gordon and Girdler 2014). Their results were in agreement with the previously discussed study and showed that the autonomic stress reactivity in response to the TSST was significantly greater in the luteal phase. In contrast to most other studies, the TSST did not elicit a significant increase in cortisol in this cohort. However, this is probably related to their methodology where the only sampling times for plasma cortisol were at baseline and at the end of the recovery period.

How does the potential effect of menstrual cycle phase translate to female athletes and exercise performance? To my knowledge athletes do not schedule their races or tournaments around their menstrual cycle. However, it would be interesting to evaluate performance in female athletes who compete in sports where *control* of stress reactivity is of particular importance such as archery, biathlons, and shooting. A PubMed search revealed that no such studies have been conducted and hence this is an area in need of future research.

Oral Contraceptives

It is well known that basal cortisol levels are increased in women who take oral contraceptives (Burke 1969). This increase is seen in free and total cortisol and there is increased production of cortisol-binding-globulin (CBG). CBG levels have been shown to be negatively correlated with salivary cortisol response to the TSST in women (Kumsta et al. 2007). Perhaps not surprising then is that women on oral contraceptives exhibit a blunted cortisol response to stress reactivity challenges, particularly when measured in saliva (free cortisol) (Kirschbaum et al. 1995; Kirschbaum et al. 1999; Rohleder et al. 2003). These results are corroborated in studies using exercise as the HPA axis stimulus (Bonen et al. 1991; Boisseau et al. 2013). However, when cortisol response was measured in elite female athletes to heavy training sessions and competitions there were no differences between oral contraceptive users and nonusers suggesting that high-intensity and competition stress overrides the effects of oral contraceptives (Crewther et al. 2015).

Taken together, the data from comparison between menstrual cycle phases and oral contraceptives suggest that estrogen may modulate the effects on cardiovascular and neuroendocrine stress response in premenopausal women but it is dependent on the type of stressor and potentially an interaction with other factors such as trait anxiety.

Effects of Aging on Stress Reactivity in Women

General HPA axis function is altered with aging and these changes appear to be more extensive in women (Wilkinson et al. 1997; Luisi et al. 1998). These changes include increases in 24-h mean cortisol concentrations, decreased diurnal variability, and blunting of negative feedback sensitivity (Van Cauter et al. 1996; Deuschle et al. 1997; Traustadóttir et al. 2004; Nater et al. 2013). Maximal response of the axis appears to be maintained with aging while the response to a submaximal challenge is often greater in older women.

The literature on the effects of aging on psychosocial stress reactivity in women is still surprisingly sparse. Traustadóttir et al. (Traustadóttir et al. 2005) used the MSRP to induce a cardiovascular and HPA axis response in young and older women. The older women exhibited a significantly greater plasma cortisol response to the challenge (see Fig. 11.2). Markers of cardiovascular reactivity were divided with the young exhibiting a significantly higher heart rate response and the older women having a significantly greater increase in systolic blood pressure in response to the challenge. Interestingly, the age-related increase in cortisol reactivity was attenuated in age-matched older women who were physically fit (the effects of fitness are discussed further in section 5.2). Similar results were found using the TSST where older women had significantly greater plasma cortisol response, however, there were no age-related differences in the response of salivary cortisol (Kudielka et al. 2004). A recent study also reported greater cardiovascular reactivity in postmenopausal women compared to premenopausal women as indicated by systolic blood pressure and heart rate variability (Hirokawa et al. 2014).

The specific role of estrogen in the age-related changes in stress reactivity in women has not been well elucidated. Postmenopausal women on hormone replacement therapy had higher baseline levels of cortisol compared to age-matched women not on hormone replacement therapy but there were no differences in the cortisol response to a psychological stressor between the groups (Burleson et al. 1998). Similarly, another study that compared postmenopausal women treated with

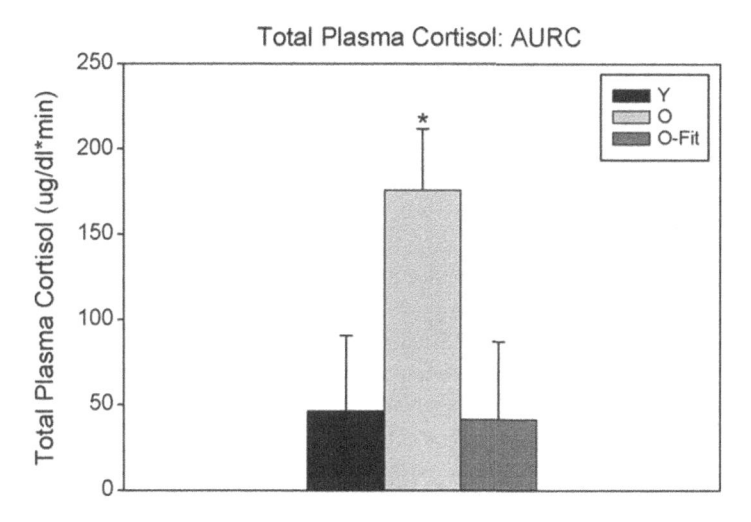

Fig. 11.2 Plasma cortisol response to a psychological challenge, calculated as area-under-the-response-curve (AURC) in young (*black bar*, $n=10$), older (*light-grey bar*, $n=12$), and older-fit (*dark-grey bar*, $n=11$) women. The cortisol response was significantly greater in the older women compared to young and older-fit ($p<0.05$). Reprinted from Traustadóttir et al. (2005) with permission from Elsevier

estrogen or a placebo for 2 weeks prior to undergoing the TSST found no significant differences in ACTH, cortisol (plasma or salivary), or heart responses between these groups (Kudielka et al. 1999). This study also included a group of premenopausal women as a control but there were no reported differences between the young and older women in contrast to a subsequent study from the same laboratory (Kudielka et al. 2004). The discrepancy between these two studies may potentially be due to the way the data were analyzed in the earlier study which treated the baseline values as a covariate, essentially losing the initial response of the challenge.

Effects of Exercise on Stress Reactivity in Women

Acute exercise is a potent stimulus of the neuroendocrine system, including catecholamines and the HPA axis response, with the magnitude of response related to intensity and duration of the exercise bout (Hackney 2006; Hill et al. 2008). There appears to be a critical threshold of relative intensity of 50-60 % of maximal aerobic capacity ($VO_{2\,max}$) that must be exceeded before a rise in cortisol occurs (Davies and Few 1973; Farrell et al. 1983). The main effect of repeated bouts of exercise, as in regular training, in terms of the stress response is that the threshold of activation is higher (Buono et al. 1987). In other words, the work required to stimulate the same response after training as before is greater and comparing an exercise response at the same absolute intensity pre- to post-training shows a lower response after an exercise intervention (Galbo 2001; Eliakim et al. 2013). These adaptations to training occur to a similar extent in older individuals (Korkushko et al. 1995).

Acute Exercise

A single bout of acute exercise leads to improved insulin sensitivity and greater resistance to oxidative stress, even 16-h after acute exercise (Weiss et al. 2008; Nordin et al. 2014). A related question of importance for understanding the beneficial effects of exercise on lowering risk for chronic diseases is whether acute exercise leads to increased psychosocial stress resilience for a period after the exercise session. Rejeski et al. (Rejeski et al. 1992) studied premenopausal women who were low to moderately fit. Subjects completed a psychosocial challenge comprised of Stroop color-word task and public speech on two occasions; with a 40-min exercise session at 70% of age-predicted maximal heart rate preceding the stress challenge and a non-exercising control condition. The outcome variables were limited to heart rate and blood pressure measurements. The acute exercise elicited significantly lower blood pressure responses to the psychosocial stressor but there were no differences in heart rate reactivity (Rejeski et al. 1992). A meta-analysis specifically on blood pressure responses to psychosocial stressors also concluded that acute exercise provided protection in form of lower hemodynamic reactivity (Hamer et al. 2006). A recent study designed around this same research question included measures of salivary cortisol and sAA although the study cohort was limited to highly trained and sedentary young men (Zschucke et al. 2015). Due to the paucity of information on the effect of acute exercise, the results of this study are included here and the reader can ponder whether these data would translate to women. The stress challenge used in this study was the MIST and the response was tested approximately 90 min after an exercise bout that was performed at 60–70% of their maximal aerobic capacity for 30-min and compared to a non-exercise control condition. The acute exercise elicited a significantly lower cortisol response as compared to the control trial in support of the hypothesis that acute exercise can act as a stress-buffer. There were no differences in sAA responses between trials (Zschucke et al. 2015). Additionally, the effects of acute exercise on subsequent response to a psychosocial stressor may be dependent on intensity of exercise and the time frame between the exercise bout and the administration of the stress challenge (Alderman et al. 2007).

In summary, there are limited data available to make a definitive conclusion on the effect of acute exercise on lowering subsequent stress reactivity and the mechanisms are unclear. Certainly this appears to be an area that warrants further studying.

Regular Exercise

Regular exercise or training results in physiological adaptations where tolerance to an acute exercise stimulus is increased due to greater capacity. In the context of the HPA axis response these adaptations manifest in a lower pituitary–adrenal response at a given absolute workload (Buono et al. 1987; Galbo 2001; Eliakim et al. 2013). In addition, the maximal capacity of the adrenal gland is also increased with training, allowing for a greater response when appropriate such as very high intensity exercise or prolonged duration (Luger et al. 1987; Kjaer 1992). Regular lifelong physical activity is associated with many health benefits and recent data support that habitual exercise may protect older individuals from changes in diurnal endocrine rhythms and increased cortisol levels during periods of high stress (Heaney et al. 2014).

The early studies on whether physical fitness is associated with lower response to psychosocial stress were almost all designed around measuring cardiovascular and hemodynamic reactivity. The data demonstrate that physical fitness (measured by VO_{2max}, physical activity questionnaires, or activity monitoring) is generally associated with a blunted heart rate and blood pressure response to laboratory stress challenges. These studies have been reviewed extensively elsewhere and the reader is referred to the following narrative and meta-analytic reviews: (Crews and Landers 1987; Forcier et al. 2006; Huang et al. 2013).

The studies that have been designed to test this hypothesis around measures of HPA axis response have reported either a significant effect of fitness on attenuating the response or no difference between groups of different levels of physical fitness. Of these studies, only two have been conducted on women. Two other studies included both men and women but did not report separate analyses based on gender. These studies are reviewed in further detail below.

Studies on Women

Traustadóttir et al. (Traustadóttir et al. 2005) was one of the first studies to show a significant effect of physical fitness on psychosocial stress resilience as demonstrated by significantly lower plasma cortisol response in older women who were physically fit (as measured by VO_{2max}) compared to age-matched unfit controls (see Fig. 11.2) in response to the MSRP. In contrast, Jayasinghe et al. (2016) found no differences in plasma cortisol or catecholamine responses to the TSST between fit and unfit women. Aside from the different challenges used in these studies, the cohorts differed in age. The former study compared postmenopausal women that were not on hormone replacement therapy (mean age 66 years) while the latter study compared premenopausal women (mean age 38–40 years) tested in the mid-follicular phase.

Studies on Men and Women Combined

Two studies that analyzed men and women grouped together found no effect of fitness on the HPA axis response to psychosocial stress. One of those studies assessed physical activity levels through a questionnaire and defined exercisers as those who reported exercising ≥1×/week (Childs and de Wit 2014). They found no differences in salivary cortisol responses between the two groups who were comprised of young individuals (mean age 22 years). It could be argued that their definition of physical fitness is not rigorous enough and that may have minimized the chance of seeing differences between the groups. Another study assessed fitness levels by measuring VO_{2peak} and found no correlation with plasma ACTH or cortisol responses to the TSST (Arvidson and Jonsdottir 2015). Subjects in this study ranged in age between 20 and 50 years.

Interestingly, children who were more physically active as measured with an activity monitor exhibited lower salivary cortisol response to the TSST compared to their peers who were less physically active (Martikainen et al. 2013).

Studies on Men

Rimmele et al. (2007) and colleagues completed two similar studies, one compared elite athletes to untrained while the other compared three groups of young men; elite athletes, amateur athletes, and untrained (Rimmele et al. 2009). Salivary cortisol response to the TSST was significantly lower in the elite athletes in both studies and in the latter the other two groups did not differ. These data suggest that perhaps the effects of fitness on increasing stress resilience in young individuals is only seen in very high levels of fitness such as in elite athletes. In contrast, Zschucke et al. (2015) did not find differences between trained and sedentary in their salivary cortisol response to the MIST. They did however find a significant negative correlation between VO_{2max} levels and the cortisol reactivity, supporting the idea of greater fitness leading to lower stress reactivity. It is worth noting that the average VO_{2max} levels reported for their sedentary group was 47.5 mL/kg/min which despite being significantly lower than their fit group would not be considered sedentary according to any norms.

Summary of Studies on Regular Exercise

Taken together, there are a few things that surface as possibilities of explaining the discrepancies in results. One explanation could be related to the age of the subjects. It is likely that the effects of fitness would be greater in individuals that have compromised stress resilience and therefore the effects would be more readily seen when fitness is layered onto aging. This is analogous to the effect of exercise training on blood pressure. Exercise training lowers blood pressure, but only in individuals with hypertension and not in normotensive individuals. If we consider healthy young individuals to have appropriate or normal stress responses then there is no reason to expect physical fitness to change the response. Alternatively, there may be a higher threshold of fitness needed in the young to actually see an effect, as seen by the differences in elite athletes versus fit young men (Rimmele et al. 2009). Third, as men generally show greater stress reactivity to a psychosocial stressor such as the TSST compared to women, the effects of fitness may be more pronounced in men than women—although this has not been compared to date.

Conclusions and Future Directions

Stress reactivity is clinically relevant because of the association with risk for many chronic diseases such as cardiovascular disease, diabetes, osteoporosis, and Alzheimer's disease. Stress-related cortisol secretion is positively correlated with risk factors for these diseases such as visceral obesity, metabolic dysregulation, hypertension, and cognitive dysfunction (Stoney et al. 1987; Brindley and Rolland 1989; Bjorntorp 1997; 1999; Rosmond et al. 1998). While the understanding of factors that affect stress reactivity and stress resilience has increased and the studies have become more standardized in terms of challenges used and outcome variables measured, there is still much work to be done especially on whether lowering of stress reactivity translates to lower disease risk. There is need for more studies on women, in particular in older women. It also would be beneficial if more studies would employ specific analyses of recovery after a peak response as that may be more informative regarding the stress resilience and therefore more relevant to health.

In order to really understand whether exercise increases psychosocial stress resilience we need randomized controlled trials (RCT) with successful exercise interventions and comparison to non-exercising control groups. The obstacle has been that psychosocial laboratory stressors often are not conducible for repeated testing due to habituation or desensitization. To my knowledge there has only been one exercise intervention study completed that measured cortisol responses to a laboratory stressor (Klaperski et al. 2014). This study used a version of the TSST adapted for groups (von Dawans et al. 2011) and the challenge stimulated a significant increase in salivary cortisol and heart rate at both measurement times, before and after a 12-week intervention. Cortisol reactivity was attenuated in both the endurance training group as well as the relaxation group, while there was no change in the control group (Klaperski et al. 2014). These results are promising for future studies and need to be replicated in women.

References

Ahwal WN, Mills PJ, Kalshan DA, Nelesen RA. Effects of race and sex on blood pressure and hemodynamic stress response as a function of the menstrual cycle. Blood Press Monit. 1997;2(4):161–7.

Alderman BL, Arent SM, Landers DM, Rogers TJ. Aerobic exercise intensity and time of stressor administration influence cardiovascular responses to psychological stress. Psychophysiology. 2007;44(5):759–66.

Allen AP, Kennedy PJ, Cryan JF, Dinan TG, Clarke G. Biological and psychological markers of stress in humans: Focus on the Trier Social Stress Test. Neurosci Biobeh Rev. 2014;38:94–124.

Arvidson E, Jonsdottir IH. The relationship between HPA-axis response, perceived stress and peak aerobic capacity. Psychoneuroendocrinology. 2015;61:71.

Birkett MA. The Trier Social Stress Test protocol for inducing psychological stress. J Vis Exp. 2011;56.

Bjorntorp P. Stress and cardiovascular disease. Acta Physiol Scand Suppl. 1997;640:144–8.

Bjorntorp P. Neuroendocrine perturbations as a cause of insulin resistance. Diabetes Metab Res Rev. 1999;15(6):427–41.

Boisseau N, Enea C, Diaz V, Dugue B, Corcuff JB, Duclos M. Oral contraception but not menstrual cycle phase is associated with increased free cortisol levels and low hypothalamo-pituitary-adrenal axis reactivity. J Endocrinol Invest. 2013;36(11):955–64.

Bonen A, Haynes FW, Graham TE. Substrate and hormonal responses to exercise in women using oral contraceptives. J Appl Physiol (1985). 1991;70(5):1917–27.

Born J, Ditschuneit I, Schreiber M, Dodt C, Fehm HL. Effects of age and gender on pituitary-adrenocortical responsiveness in humans. Eur J Endocrinol. 1995;132(6):705–11.

Bosch PR, Traustadottir T, Howard P, Matt KS. Functional and physiological effects of yoga in women with rheumatoid arthritis: a pilot study. Altern Ther Health Med. 2009;15(4):24–31.

Brindley DN, Rolland Y. Possible connections between stress, diabetes, obesity, hypertension and altered lipoprotein metabolism that may result in atherosclerosis. Clin Sci (Lond). 1989;77(5):453–61.

Buono MJ, Yeager JE, Sucec AA. Effect of aerobic training on the plasma ACTH response to exercise. J Appl Physiol (1985). 1987;63(6):2499–501.

Burke CW. Biologically active cortisol in plasma of oestrogen-treated and normal subjects. Br Med J. 1969;2(5660):798–800.

Burleson MH, Malarkey WB, Cacioppo JT, Poehlmann KM, Kiecolt-Glaser JK, Berntson GG, Glaser R. Postmenopausal hormone replacement: effects on autonomic, neuroendocrine, and immune reactivity to brief psychological stressors. Psychosom Med. 1998;60(1):17–25.

Carroll D, Ginty AT, Painter RC, Roseboom TJ, Phillips AC, de Rooij SR. Systolic blood pressure reactions to acute stress are associated with future hypertension status in the Dutch Famine Birth Cohort Study. Int J Psychophysiol. 2012;85(2):270–3.

Childs E, de Wit H. Regular exercise is associated with emotional resilience to acute stress in healthy adults. Front Physiol. 2014;5:161.

Choi PY, Salmon P. Stress responsivity in exercisers and non-exercisers during different phases of the menstrual cycle. Soc Sci Med. 1995;41(6):769–77.

Cole CR, Blackstone EH, Pashkow FJ, Snader CE, Lauer MS. Heart-rate recovery immediately after exercise as a predictor of mortality. N Engl J Med. 1999;341(18):1351–7.

Crews DJ, Landers DM. A meta-analytic review of aerobic fitness and reactivity to psychosocial stressors. Med Sci Sports Exerc. 1987;19(5 Suppl):S114–20.

Crewther BT, Hamilton D, Casto K, Kilduff LP, Cook CJ. Effects of oral contraceptive use on the salivary testosterone and cortisol responses to training sessions and competitions in elite women athletes. Physiol Behav. 2015;147:84–90.

Davies CT, Few JD. Effects of exercise on adrenocortical function. J Appl Physiol. 1973;35(6):887–91.

Dedovic K, Renwick R, Mahani NK, Engert V, Lupien SJ, Pruessner JC. The Montreal Imaging Stress Task: using functional imaging to investigate the effects of perceiving and processing psychosocial stress in the human brain. J Psychiatry Neurosci. 2005;30(5):319–25.

Deuschle M, Gotthardt U, Schweiger U, Weber B, Korner A, Schmider J, Standhardt H, Lammers CH, Heuser I. With aging in humans the activity of the hypothalamus-pituitary-adrenal system increases and its diurnal amplitude flattens. Life Sci. 1997;61(22):2239–46.

Dickerson SS, Kemeny ME. Acute stressors and cortisol responses: a theoretical integration and synthesis of laboratory research. Psychol Bull. 2004;130(3):355–91.

Earle TL, Linden W, Weinberg J. Differential effects of harassment on cardiovascular and salivary cortisol stress reactivity and recovery in women and men. J Psychosom Res. 1999;46(2):125–41.

Eliakim A, Portal S, Zadik Z, Meckel Y, Nemet D. Training reduces catabolic and inflammatory response to a single practice in female volleyball players. J Strength Cond Res. 2013;27(11):3110–5.

Farrell PA, Garthwaite TL, Gustafson AB. Plasma adrenocorticotropin and cortisol responses to submaximal and exhaustive exercise. J Appl Physiol Respir Environ Exerc Physiol. 1983;55(5):1441–4.

Foley P, Kirschbaum C. Human hypothalamus-pituitary-adrenal axis responses to acute psychosocial stress in laboratory settings. Neurosci Biobehav Rev. 2010;35(1):91–6.

Forcier K, Stroud LR, Papandonatos GD, Hitsman B, Reiches M, Krishnamoorthy J, Niaura R. Links between physical fitness and cardiovascular reactivity and recovery to psychological stressors: a meta-analysis. Health Psychol. 2006;25(6):723–39.

Galbo H. Influence of aging and exercise on endocrine function. Int J Sport Nutr Exerc Metab. 2001;11(Suppl):S49–57.

Gordon JL, Girdler SS. Mechanisms underlying hemodynamic and neuroendocrine stress reactivity at different phases of the menstrual cycle. Psychophysiology. 2014;51(4):309–18.

Gotthardt U, Schweiger U, Fahrenberg J, Lauer CJ, Holsboer F, Heuser I. Cortisol, ACTH, and cardiovascular response to a cognitive challenge paradigm in aging and depression. Am J Physiol. 1995;268(4 Pt 2):R865–73.

Greenspan SL, Rowe JW, Maitland LA, McAloon-Dyke M, Elahi D. The pituitary-adrenal glucocorticoid response is altered by gender and disease. J Gerontol. 1993;48(3):M72–7.

Gupta SB. Exercise ECG testing—is it obsolete? J Assoc Physicians India. 2005;53:615–8.

Hackney AC. Exercise as a stressor to the human neuroendocrine system. Medicina (Kaunas). 2006;42(10):788–97.

Hamer M, Taylor A, Steptoe A. The effect of acute aerobic exercise on stress related blood pressure responses: a systematic review and meta-analysis. Biol Psychol. 2006;71(2):183–90.

Hamer M, Endrighi R, Venuraju SM, Lahiri A, Steptoe A. Cortisol responses to mental stress and the progression of coronary artery calcification in healthy men and women. PLoS One. 2012;7(2):31356.

Heaney JL, Carroll D, Phillips AC. Physical activity, life events stress, cortisol, and DHEA: preliminary findings that physical activity may buffer against the negative effects of stress. J Aging Phys Act. 2014;22(4):465–73.

Herman JP, Cullinan WE. Neurocircuitry of stress: central control of the hypothalamo-pituitary-adrenocortical axis. Trends Neurosci. 1997;20(2):78–84.

Heuser IJ, Gotthardt U, Schweiger U, Schmider J, Lammers CH, Dettling M, Holsboer F. Age-associated changes of pituitary-adrenocortical hormone regulation in humans: importance of gender. Neurobiol Aging. 1994;15(2):227–31.

Hill EE, Zack E, Battaglini C, Viru M, Viru A, Hackney AC. Exercise and circulating cortisol levels: the intensity threshold effect. J Endocrinol Invest. 2008;31(7):587–91.

Hirokawa K, Nagayoshi M, Ohira T, Kajiura M, Kitamura A, Kiyama M, Okada T, Iso H. Menopausal status in relation to cardiovascular stress reactivity in healthy Japanese participants. Psychosom Med. 2014;76(9):701–8.

Hlavacova N, Wawruch M, Tisonova J, Jezova D. Neuroendocrine activation during combined mental and physical stress in women depends on trait anxiety and the phase of the menstrual cycle. Ann N Y Acad Sci. 2008;1148:520–5.

Huang CJ, Webb HE, Zourdos MC, Acevedo EO. Cardiovascular reactivity, stress, and physical activity. Front Physiol. 2013;4:314.

Jayasinghe SU, Lambert GW, Torres SJ, Fraser SF, Eikelis N, Turner AI. Hypothalamo-pituitary adrenal axis and sympatho-adrenal medullary system responses to psychological stress were not attenuated in women with elevated physical fitness levels. Endocrine. 2016;51(2):369–79.

Kajantie E, Phillips DI. The effects of sex and hormonal status on the physiological response to acute psychosocial stress. Psychoneuroendocrinology. 2006;31(2):151–78.

Kirschbaum C, Wust S, Hellhammer D. Consistent sex differences in cortisol responses to psychological stress. Psychosom Med. 1992;54(6):648–57.

Kirschbaum C, Pirke KM, Hellhammer DH. The 'Trier Social Stress Test'—a tool for investigating psychobiological stress responses in a laboratory setting. Neuropsychobiology. 1993;28(1-2):76–81.

Kirschbaum C, Pirke KM, Hellhammer DH. Preliminary evidence for reduced cortisol responsivity to psychological stress in women using oral contraceptive medication. Psychoneuroendocrinology. 1995;20(5):509–14.

Kirschbaum C, Schommer N, Federenko I, Gaab J, Neumann O, Oellers M, Rohleder N, Untiedt A, Hanker J, Pirke KM, Hellhammer DH. Short-term estradiol treatment enhances pituitary-adrenal axis and sympathetic responses to psychosocial stress in healthy young men. J Clin Endocrinol Metab. 1996;81(10):3639–43.

Kirschbaum C, Kudielka BM, Gaab J, Schommer NC, Hellhammer DH. Impact of gender, menstrual cycle phase, and oral contraceptives on the activity of the hypothalamus-pituitary-adrenal axis. Psychosom Med. 1999;61(2):154–62.

Kjaer M. Regulation of hormonal and metabolic responses during exercise in humans. Exerc Sport Sci Rev. 1992;20:161–84.

Klaperski S, von Dawans B, Heinrichs M, Fuchs R. Effects of a 12-week endurance training program on the physiological response to psychosocial stress in men: a randomized controlled trial. J Behav Med. 2014;37(6):1118-33.

Korkushko OV, Frolkis MV, Shatilo VB. Reaction of pituitary-adrenal and autonomic nervous systems to stress in trained and untrained elderly people. J Auton Nerv Syst. 1995;54(1):27-32.

Kraemer WJ, Fleck SJ, Dziados JE, Harman EA, Marchitelli LJ, Gordon SE, Mello R, Frykman PN, Koziris LP, Triplett NT. Changes in hormonal concentrations after different heavy-resistance exercise protocols in women. J Appl Physiol (1985). 1993;75(2):594-604.

Kudielka BM, Schmidt-Reinwald AK, Hellhammer DH, Kirschbaum C. Psychological and endocrine responses to psychosocial stress and dexamethasone/corticotropin-releasing hormone in healthy postmenopausal women and young controls: the impact of age and a two-week estradiol treatment. Neuroendocrinology. 1999;70(6):422-30.

Kudielka BM, Buske-Kirschbaum A, Hellhammer DH, Kirschbaum C. HPA axis responses to laboratory psychosocial stress in healthy elderly adults, younger adults, and children: impact of age and gender. Psychoneuroendocrinology. 2004;29(1):83-98.

Kumsta R, Entringer S, Hellhammer DH, Wust S. Cortisol and ACTH responses to psychosocial stress are modulated by corticosteroid binding globulin levels. Psychoneuroendocrinology. 2007;32(8-10):1153-7.

Lazzarino AI, Hamer M, Gaze D, Collinson P, Steptoe A. The association between cortisol response to mental stress and high-sensitivity cardiac troponin T plasma concentration in healthy adults. J Am Coll Cardiol. 2013;62(18):1694-701.

Lesniewska B, Miskowiak B, Nowak M, Malendowicz LK. Sex differences in adrenocortical structure and function. XXVII. The effect of ether stress on ACTH and corticosterone in intact, gonadectomized, and testosterone- or estradiol-replaced rats. Res Exp Med (Berl). 1990a;190(2):95-103.

Lesniewska B, Nowak M, Malendowicz LK. Sex differences in adrenocortical structure and function. XXVIII. ACTH and corticosterone in intact, gonadectomised and gonadal hormone replaced rats. Horm Metab Res. 1990b;22(7):378-81.

Luger A, Deuster PA, Kyle SB, Gallucci WT, Montgomery LC, Gold PW, Loriaux DL, Chrousos GP. Acute hypothalamic-pituitary-adrenal responses to the stress of treadmill exercise. Physiologic adaptations to physical training. N Engl J Med. 1987;316(21):1309-15.

Luisi S, Tonetti A, Bernardi F, Casarosa E, Florio P, Monteleone P, Gemignani R, Petraglia F, Luisi M, Genazzani AR. Effect of acute corticotropin releasing factor on pituitary-adrenocortical responsiveness in elderly women and men. J Endocrinol Invest. 1998;21(7):449-53.

Lustyk MK, Olson KC, Gerrish WG, Holder A, Widman L. Psychophysiological and neuroendocrine responses to laboratory stressors in women: implications of menstrual cycle phase and stressor type. Biol Psychol. 2010;83(2):84-92.

Martikainen S, Pesonen AK, Lahti J, Heinonen K, Feldt K, Pyhala R, Tammelin T, Kajantie E, Eriksson JG, Strandberg TE, Raikkonen K. Higher levels of physical activity are associated with lower hypothalamic-pituitary-adrenocortical axis reactivity to psychosocial stress in children. J Clin Endocrinol Metab. 2013;98(4):E619-27.

McEwen BS. Protective and damaging effects of stress mediators. N Engl J Med. 1998;338(3):171-9.

McEwen BS. Physiology and neurobiology of stress and adaptation: central role of the brain. Physiol Rev. 2007;87(3):873-904.

Morris MC, Rao U, Garber J. Cortisol responses to psychosocial stress predict depression trajectories: social-evaluative threat and prior depressive episodes as moderators. J Affect Disord. 2012;143(1-3):223-30.

Nagaraja AS, Sadaoui NC, Dorniak PL, Lutgendorf SK, Sood AK. SnapShot: stress and disease. Cell Metab. 2016;23(2):388.e1.

Nater UM, Hoppmann CA, Scott SB. Diurnal profiles of salivary cortisol and alpha-amylase change across the adult lifespan: evidence from repeated daily life assessments. Psychoneuroendocrinology. 2013;38(12):3167-71.

Nordin TC, Done AJ, Traustadottir T. Acute exercise increases resistance to oxidative stress in young but not older adults. Age (Dordr). 2014;36(6):9727.

Pico-Alfonso MA, Mastorci F, Ceresini G, Ceda GP, Manghi M, Pino O, Troisi A, Sgoifo A. Acute psychosocial challenge and cardiac autonomic response in women: the role of estrogens, corticosteroids, and behavioral coping styles. Psychoneuroendocrinology. 2007;32(5):451–63.

Pollard TM, Pearce KL, Rousham EK, Schwartz JE. Do blood pressure and heart rate responses to perceived stress vary according to endogenous estrogen level in women? Am J Phys Anthropol. 2007;132(1):151–7.

Rejeski WJ, Thompson A, Brubaker PH, Miller HS. Acute exercise: buffering psychosocial stress responses in women. Health Psychol. 1992;11(6):355–62.

Rimmele U, Zellweger BC, Marti B, Seiler R, Mohiyeddini C, Ehlert U, Heinrichs M. Trained men show lower cortisol, heart rate and psychological responses to psychosocial stress compared with untrained men. Psychoneuroendocrinology. 2007;32(6):627–35.

Rimmele U, Seiler R, Marti B, Wirtz PH, Ehlert U, Heinrichs M. The level of physical activity affects adrenal and cardiovascular reactivity to psychosocial stress. Psychoneuroendocrinology. 2009;34(2):190–8.

Rohleder N, Wolf JM, Piel M, Kirschbaum C. Impact of oral contraceptive use on glucocorticoid sensitivity of pro-inflammatory cytokine production after psychosocial stress. Psychoneuroendocrinology. 2003;28(3):261–73.

Rosmond R, Dallman MF, Bjorntorp P. Stress-related cortisol secretion in men: relationships with abdominal obesity and endocrine, metabolic and hemodynamic abnormalities. J Clin Endocrinol Metab. 1998;83(6):1853–9.

Sandoval DA, Matt KS. Gender differences in the endocrine and metabolic responses to hypoxic exercise. J Appl Physiol (1985). 2002;92(2):504–12.

Sato N, Miyake S. Cardiovascular reactivity to mental stress: relationship with menstrual cycle and gender. J Physiol Anthropol Appl Human Sci. 2004;23(6):215–23.

Schlotz W. Stress Reactivity. In: Gellman MD, Turner JR, editors. Encyclopedia of behavioral medicine. New York, NY: Springer; 2013. p. 1891–4.

Seeman TE, Singer B, Charpentier P. Gender differences in patterns of HPA axis response to challenge: MacArthur studies of successful aging. Psychoneuroendocrinology. 1995;20(7):711–25.

Seeman TE, Singer B, Wilkinson CW, McEwen B. Gender differences in age-related changes in HPA axis reactivity. Psychoneuroendocrinology. 2001;26(3):225–40.

Shenoy JP, Pa S, Shivakumar J. Study of cardiovascular reactivity to mental stress in different phases of menstrual cycle. J Clin Diagn Res. 2014;8(6):BC01–4.

Stephens MA, Mahon PB, McCaul ME, Wand GS. Hypothalamic-pituitary-adrenal axis response to acute psychosocial stress: effects of biological sex and circulating sex hormones. Psychoneuroendocrinology. 2016;66:47–55.

Sternberg EM, Wilder RL, Gold PW, Chrousos GP. A defect in the central component of the immune system—hypothalamic-pituitary-adrenal axis feedback loop is associated with susceptibility to experimental arthritis and other inflammatory diseases. Ann N Y Acad Sci. 1990;594:289–92.

Stewart JC, Janicki DL, Kamarck TW. Cardiovascular reactivity to and recovery from psychological challenge as predictors of 3-year change in blood pressure. Health Psychol. 2006;25(1):111–8.

Stoney CM, Davis MC, Matthews KA. Sex differences in physiological responses to stress and in coronary heart disease: a causal link? Psychophysiology. 1987;24(2):127–31.

Stroud LR, Salovey P, Epel ES. Sex differences in stress responses: social rejection versus achievement stress. Biol Psychiatry. 2002;52(4):318–27.

Szivak TK, Hooper DR, Dunn-Lewis C, Comstock BA, Kupchak BR, Apicella JM, Saenz C, Maresh CM, Denegar CR, Kraemer WJ. Adrenal cortical responses to high-intensity, short rest, resistance exercise in men and women. J Strength Cond Res. 2013;27(3):748–60.

Tersman Z, Collins A, Eneroth P. Cardiovascular responses to psychological and physiological stressors during the menstrual cycle. Psychosom Med. 1991;53(2):185–97.

Traustadóttir T, Bosch PR, Matt KS. Gender differences in cardiovascular and hypothalamic-pituitary-adrenal axis responses to psychological stress in healthy older adult men and women. Stress. 2003;6(2):133–40.

Traustadóttir T, Bosch PR, Cantu T, Matt KS. Hypothalamic-pituitary-adrenal axis response and recovery from high-intensity exercise in women: effects of aging and fitness. J Clin Endocrinol Metab. 2004;89(7):3248–54.

Traustadóttir T, Bosch PR, Matt KS. The HPA axis response to stress in women: effects of aging and fitness. Psychoneuroendocrinology. 2005;30(4):392–402.

Trivedi R, Sherwood A, Strauman TJ, Blumenthal JA. Laboratory-based blood pressure recovery is a predictor of ambulatory blood pressure. Biol Psychol. 2008;77(3):317–23.

Uhart M, Chong RY, Oswald L, Lin PI, Wand GS. Gender differences in hypothalamic-pituitary-adrenal (HPA) axis reactivity. Psychoneuroendocrinology. 2006;31(5):642–52.

Van Cauter E, Leproult R, Kupfer DJ. Effects of gender and age on the levels and circadian rhythmicity of plasma cortisol. J Clin Endocrinol Metab. 1996;81(7):2468–73.

Veldhuijzen van Zanten JJ, Carroll D, Ring C. Mental stress-induced haemoconcentration in women: effects of menstrual cycle phase. Br J Health Psychol. 2009;14(Pt 4):805–16.

von Dawans B, Kirschbaum C, Heinrichs M. The Trier Social Stress Test for Groups (TSST-G): a new research tool for controlled simultaneous social stress exposure in a group format. Psychoneuroendocrinology. 2011;36(4):514–22.

Weiss EP, Arif H, Villareal DT, Marzetti E, Holloszy JO. Endothelial function after high-sugar-food ingestion improves with endurance exercise performed on the previous day. Am J Clin Nutr. 2008;88(1):51–7.

Wilkinson CW, Peskind ER, Raskind MA. Decreased hypothalamic-pituitary-adrenal axis sensitivity to cortisol feedback inhibition in human aging. Neuroendocrinology. 1997;65(1):79–90.

Zschucke E, Renneberg B, Dimeo F, Wustenberg T, Strohle A. The stress-buffering effect of acute exercise: evidence for HPA axis negative feedback. Psychoneuroendocrinology. 2015;51:414–25.

Chapter 12
Sex Hormones, Cancer and Exercise Training in Women

Kristin L. Campbell

Introduction

Higher levels of circulating sex hormones are linked to risk of several sex-hormone related cancers in women, specifically breast and endometrial cancers (Brown and Hankinson 2015). It is proposed that sex hormones can have a mitotic effect on target tissues, by promoting greater cellular proliferation, inhibiting apoptosis and increasing DNA damage (Henderson and Feigelson 2000; Yue et al. 2013; Caldon 2014). Therefore it is suggested that cancer risk could be altered by reducing cumulative lifetime exposure to sex hormones, particularly estrogens. Early age of menarche (before age 12), later age of menopause, and late age at first birth or nulliparity, and lack of lactation are all reproductive factors that are linked to an increased risk of breast cancer (Henderson and Feigelson 2000; Hoffman-Goetz et al. 1998). Postmenopausal hormone therapy use and higher postmenopausal body mass index are proposed to increase cumulative sex hormone exposure and in turn, increase breast cancer risk (Henderson and Feigelson 2000; Morimoto et al. 2002).

In pooled analysis of nine prospective studies, postmenopausal women with elevated levels of endogenous estrogens (estradiol, free estradiol, estrone, estrone sulfate) and androgens (androstenedione, dehydroepiandrosterone (DHEA), dehydroepiandrosterone sulfate (DHEAS), and testosterone) had an increased risk of developing postmenopausal breast cancer, with a relative risk 2.0 (95 % CI 1.47–2.71) comparing lowest

---

K.L. Campbell, P.T., M.Sc., Ph.D. (✉)
Department of Physical Therapy, Faculty of Medicine, University of British Columbia, 212 Friedman Building, 2177 Wesbrook Mall, Vancouver, BC, Canada V6T 1Z3

Centre of Excellence in Cancer Prevention, School of Population and Public Health, Faculty of Medicine, University of British Columbia, 2206 East Mall, Vancouver, BC, Canada V6T 1Z3
e-mail: kristin.campbell@ubc.ca

to highest quintile of estradiol (Endogenous Hormones und Breast Cancer Collaborative Group 2002). The risk was reduced with increasing levels of sex hormone binding globulin (SHBG) (Endogenous Hormones und Breast Cancer Collaborative Group 2002). For premenopausal cancer, the association appears to be similar. In pooled analysis of seven prospective studies of premenopausal women, risk of premenopausal breast cancer was positively associated with level of circulating estrogens (estradiol, free estradiol, estrone) and androgens (androstenedione, DHEAS and testosterone), with an odds ratio of 1.19 (95 % CI 1.06–1.35) for doubling of estradiol levels. However, no association between premenopausal breast cancer risk and SHBG was observed.

For endometrial cancer, there is consistent evidence from three available prospective studies that women with elevated estrogen levels (estradiol, free estradiol, and estrone) are at an increased risk for postmenopausal endometrial cancer (Allen et al. 2008; Lukanova et al. 2004; Zeleniuch-Jacquotte et al. 2001). A less consistent, but positive, association with androgens levels has also been observed, specifically elevated androstenedione (Lukanova et al. 2004) and free testosterone (Allen et al. 2008). To date, the relationship between estradiol levels and endometrial cancer risk in premenopausal women has not been studied with sufficient numbers to develop definitive conclusions (Brown and Hankinson 2015). The purpose of this chapter is to provide an overview of the impact of physical activity or structured exercise training on risk of sex hormone-related cancers, namely breast cancer and endometrial cancer. The chapter first outlines the epidemiological evidence and potential mechanisms. This is followed by a summary of the impact of exercise training on sex hormones at key reproductive timepoints, namely prepuberty, between puberty and menopause, and post-menopause. The impact of exercise training on sex hormones for women at higher risk of sex hormone-related cancers is also outlined.

Epidemiology of Physical Activity and Sex Hormone-Related Cancer Risk

There is now a wealth of available epidemiologic evidence for the association between higher physical activity levels and reduced risk of postmenopausal breast cancer and endometrial cancer (Friedenreich and Orenstein 2002; Lee 2003). For postmenopausal breast cancer the average risk reduction is reported as 25 % among the most physically active women compared to the least physically activity women. The association is strongest for physical activity that is recreational or house-hold activities, and for physical activity either sustained over the lifetime or engaged in after menopause (Friedenreich et al. 2010a). Furthermore, breast cancer is a heterogeneous disease, most commonly defined by hormone receptor status. Tumors can be estrogen receptor (ER) and progesterone receptor (PR) positive or negative. The observational evidence for an effect modification of hormone receptor status on the association between exercise and breast cancer risk is mixed and remains unclear (Lynch et al. 2011; Steindorf et al. 2013). The current public health recommendations for breast cancer risk reduction are for all women to engage in at least 4–7 h per week of moderate to vigorous-intensity physical activity (World Cancer Research Fund 2007; Physical Activity Guidelines for Americans: Department of Health und Human Services 2008).

For endometrial cancer, a risk reduction of 20–30 % is reported among the most physically active women compared to the least physically activity women (Cust et al. 2007; Voskuil et al. 2007; Du et al. 2014; Schmid et al. 2015). However, there is emerging data that this effect may be limited to women who are overweight or obese (Du et al. 2014; Schmid et al. 2015). While there is less available data regarding the benefits of physical activity done in different age periods across the life span, a stronger effect for recent or lifetime physical activity has been observed (Friedenreich et al. 2010a). Based on the available studies, engaging at least moderate-intensity activity for 1 hour daily appears to reduce risk of endometrial cancer (Friedenreich et al. 2010a).

Studying the association between an important exposure, such as physical activity, and a cancer diagnosis is a challenge. Observational studies are reliant on self-reported physical activity, where reporting error can be introduced, and the long latency of cancer development, means that prospective cohorts must be followed for many year. To date a randomized controlled trial of physical activity with risk of pre or postmenopausal breast cancer as the outcome has not been undertaken, as there are several logistical considerations that make such a trial different to undertake (Ballard-Barbash et al. 2009). Therefore, in order to generate a better understanding of how exercise influences cancer risk researchers have focused on examining the effect of exercise on biomarkers, such sex hormones, as surrogate outcomes rather than on development of cancer as the outcome (Ballard-Barbash et al. 2009). Biomarkers are biological factors thought to be involved in the causal pathway between exposure and cancer development (Rundle 2005). Therefore, researchers have undertaken randomized controlled trial to prospectively test the effect supervised exercise interventions on proposed biomarkers of sex hormone-related cancer risk.

Proposed Mechanisms for Sex Hormone-Related Cancer Risk Reduction Due to Exercise

The effect of exercise on age at menarche, menstrual cycle function, and level of circulating endogenous sex steroid hormone levels in girls and women are often cited as potential mechanisms for reduced breast and endometrial cancer risk (Bernstein et al. 1994). In premenopausal women the hypothalamic–pituitary–gonadal axis, which is responsible for key reproductive hormones, may be disrupted with stress or energy availability, namely by disrupting gonadotropin-releasing hormone (GnRH) pulsatility. This can result in primary amenorrhea (a delay on onset of menarche), oligomenorrhea (irregular menstrual cycles), or secondary amenorrhea (loss of menstrual cycle). (Borer 2003). These alterations would in turn, reduce cumulative lifestyle exposure to sex hormones and are proposed to in turn reduce the risk of sex hormone related cancers.

In postmenopausal women, the beneficial effect of physical activity is closely linked to body composition. After menopause, the production of estrogen is no longer under feedback regulation as it is in premenopausal women. A higher risk of postmenopausal breast cancer is observed for postmenopausal women who are overweight or obese. This is attributed primarily to greater amounts of adipose tissue, where estrogens are produced via aromatization of other sex hormone precursors (Morimoto et al. 2002). Postmenopausal women who are obese have up to twofold higher serum concentrations of estradiol than lean postmenopausal women (Key et al. 2001). Increasing BMI is also associated with a drop in SHBG, resulting in a notable increase in levels of free estradiol in women (Key et al. 2001). Therefore, one way exercise is proposed to lower postmenopausal breast cancer risk by assisting with reduction of body fat or with maintenance of lower body fat. Furthermore, engaging in higher levels of physical activity may be able to counteract some of the increased risk associated with obesity through other mechanisms, such as improving metabolic function (i.e., hyperinsulinemia, insulin resistance), reducing systemic inflammation (i.e., prostaglandin, C-reactive protein), reducing oxidative stress (i.e., reactive oxygen species), and improving immune surveillance (i.e., natural killer cells, leukocytes, t helper cells). Exercise has the potential to affect all of these biological pathways and their contribution may overlap or be synergistic (Campbell and McTiernan 2007). The discussion of these potential interactions is beyond the scope of this chapter.

In addition exercise is proposed to alter how estrogens are metabolized in the body, namely to favorably alter metabolism toward 2-hydroxyestrone (2-OHE1), which has little or no estrogenic effect rather than toward 16α-hydroxyestrone (16α-OHE1), which has an estrogenic effect (Campbell et al. 2007). Prospective cohort studies have reported a nonstatistically significant reduction in breast cancer risk among women with higher ratios of 2-OHE1 to 16α-OHE1, especially premenopausal women (Meilahn et al. 1998; Muti et al. 2000; Wellejus et al. 2005) and emerging data on measures of estrogen metabolism using a more comprehensive panel of estrogen metabolites through liquid chromatography–tandem mass spectrometry (LC–MS/MS) may shed new light onto the association of estrogen metabolism and cancer risk (Ziegler et al. 2015).

Exercise Effect: Prepuberty

Observational research points to an association between regular strenuous exercise such as ballet dancing, gymnastics, and running, and a delay in onset of menses (Bernstein et al. 1987; Frisch et al. 1981; Warren 1980). In one observational study, Frisch et al. (1981) reported that each year of training before menarche delayed menarche by 5 months. Exercise around the time of menarche may also delay establishment of truly ovulatory menstrual cycles, thus reducing subsequent exposure to sex hormones (Bernstein et al. 1987). However, there is a potential issue of bias in the available observational studies, which used cross-sectional or retrospective study designs. Later maturation may favor athletic ability and therefore girls who are later in maturing may be more likely to engaged in sports, rather than vice versa (Loucks 1990). Body weight, height, and body mass index are also strongly correlated with age of menarche

(Karapanou and Papadimitriou 2010). So energy availability may play an important role in age of menarche, rather than specifically exercise levels per se (Loucks 1990).

Exercise Effect: Puberty to Menopause

Exercise may cause minor shifts in the hormonal milieu of premenopausal women, which is proposed to play a role in reducing cumulative exposure to sex hormones and subsequent sex hormone-related cancer risk (Bullen et al. 1984; Keizer et al. 1987). Originally, it was proposed that exercise of significant frequency and intensity was needed to induce menstrual dysfunction sufficient to result in significantly decreased exposure to sex-steroid hormones (Bullen et al. 1985). In premenopausal women, observational research points to a continuum of menstrual dysfunction (i.e., amenorrhea, anovular cycles, luteal phase deficiency), longer menstrual cycles, and lower progesterone and estradiol levels in athletes compared with control subjects (Broocks et al. 1990; De Souza et al. 1998; Baker and Demers 1988; Pirke et al. 1990; Schweiger et al. 1988; Ronkainen 1985; Ellison and Lager 1986). However, this has been harder to document with prospective intervention studies and the few available prospective intervention studies are hampered by small samples sizes and mixed results. Two studies found that a moderate-intensity running intervention did not disrupt reproductive function (Bonen 1992; Rogol et al. 1992), while two other studies reported minor changes in measures of reproductive function (Bullen et al. 1984; Keizer et al. 1987), and one study documented menstrual dysfunction with significant exercise frequency and intensity, namely daily 10 mile run in addition to 3.5 h of sports at a moderate exercise intensity (Bullen et al. 1985).

The more modern prospective intervention studies that followed this early work have demonstrated that exercise and other stressors have little or no disruptive effect on reproductive function beyond that of their energy cost on energy availability (Loucks 2003; Loucks and Redman 2004; Williams et al. 2001). Recently Williams et al. demonstrated experimentally that there is a dose-response relationship between the magnitude of energy deficiency and the frequency of menstrual disturbances (Williams et al. 2015). Participants were randomly assigned to one of four groups: (1) Exercise Control (15 % energy deficit with exercise but calories added back to diet to remain in energy balance); (2) Energy Deficit 1 (15 % energy deficit with exercise; mean −162 kcal/day); (3) Energy Deficit 2 (30 % energy deficit with combination of exercise and reduced dietary intake; mean −470 kcal/day); and (4) Energy Deficit 3 (60 % energy deficit with combination of exercise (30 % deficit) and reduced dietary intake (30 % deficit); mean −813 kcal/day). Luteal phase defects, anovulation, and oligomenorrhea were observed to a greater degree in the two highest energy deficit groups and the main predictor of these disturbances was percent energy deficit (Williams et al. 2015).

The issue of menstrual dysfunction in athletes has been explored extensively under the umbrella of the female athlete triad, defined as a combination of: (1) low energy availability, with or without disordered eating; (2) menstrual dysfunction; and (3) low bone mineral density (Nattiv et al. 2007). One of the key effects of menstrual dysfunction is a subsequently lower level of circulating estrogens, which in turn has a negative impact on bone health and increases the risk of stress fractures. There are now consensus guidelines to address the treatment of the female athlete trial and return to play (Joy et al. 2014). Therefore, relative to the prevention of sex hormone-related cancers, the proposed goal is a balance between lowering estrogen exposure by encouraging mild shifts in menstrual cycle function (i.e., subtle luteal phase defects that could in turn lengthen the menstrual cycle and reduce the total number of cycles per year or across a lifetime), while at the same time maintaining sufficient estrogen levels to maintain bone health. How best to strike this balance has not been established.

To add to the complexity, for premenopausal women, being overweight or obese lowers risk of breast cancer, possibly because overweight and obesity is linked to a higher frequency of anovular menstrual cycles (Friedenreich 2001; Carmichael and Bates 2004). This may result in less exposure to estrogens, which may subsequently reduce risk of premenopausal breast cancer risk. However, overweight or obesity also results in lower progesterone levels, which may play a key role in the increased endometrial cancer risk for overweight or obese premenopausal women because of exposure to unopposed estrogens (Key et al. 2001).

The largest prospective intervention study to date to examine the impact of exercise training on sex hormone levels in premenopausal women is the WISER (Women In Steady Exercise Research) study. In this study 391 previously sedentary, premenopausal women, age 18–30 years with regular menstrual cycles (24–35 days) were randomized to either 150 min per week of supervised moderate-intensity aerobic exercise (30 min/day, 5 days per week) for 16 weeks or usual lifestyle control. Despite high adherence to the exercise intervention, no differences in sex hormones or SHBG levels were noted between groups (Smith et al. 2011). The intervention group improved fitness, and while there was no change in body weight in either group, the intervention group had significant reductions in body fat (mean reduction of 1 %) and increases in lean mass (mean increase of 0.5 kg). The authors concluded that favorable effects of moderate-intensity exercise on breast cancer risk may be operating through other biological pathways than sex hormones in the absence of significant deficit in energy availability or weight loss.

Specific to estrogen metabolites, observational studies in premenopausal women have reported higher ratios of 2-OHE1 to 16α-OHE1 in athletes compared with control subjects (Russell et al. 1984a); with high-intensity training that also resulted in the development of menstrual dysfunction (Russell et al. 1984a, b; Snow et al. 1989); with higher self-reported daily physical activity (Bentz et al. 2005; Matthews et al. 2004); and with higher aerobic fitness (VO_2max) (Campbell et al. 2005). However, these associations may be related to body composition, with a less favorable patterns seen with higher BMI (Bentz et al. 2005; Matthews et al. 2004; Campbell et al. 2005). In two recent prospective interventions studies in premenopausal women, the exercise group in the 16-week aerobic exercise intervention in the WISER study had a statistically significant favorable increase in 24-hour urinary 2-OHE1/16α-OHE1 ratio, consistent with a reduction in estrogen exposure (Smith et al. 2013), while Campbell et al. (2007) reported no change in first morning urinary estrogen metabolism pattern with a 12-week aerobic exercise training intervention versus delayed exercise control in a similar population of 32 previously sedentary, premenopausal women, with regular menstrual cycles. Interestingly, an increase in lean body mass was associated with a favorable change in 2-OHE1 to 16alpha-OHE1 ratio ($r=0.43$; $p=0.015$).

Effect of Exercise: After menopause

In postmenopausal women, increased physical activity is associated with decreased serum concentrations of estradiol, estrone, and androgens after adjustment for BMI in some (Cauley et al. 1989; McTiernan et al. 2008) but not other studies (Verkasalo et al. 2001). In a random subsample of women in the Women's Health Initiative Dietary Modification Trial (Howard et al. 2006), women with a high BMI and low self-reported physical activity had higher levels of estrone, estradiol, and free estradiol and lower levels of SHBG than women with a similar BMI who were active or with low BMI in either activity category (McTiernan et al. 2008) (Fig. 12.1). To date, six published randomized controlled trials have examined the effect of physical activity on biomarkers of breast cancer risk (Table 12.1). All trials enrolled previously sedentary, overweight, postmenopausal women.

The Physical Activity and Total Health Trial is a 2-arm trial in 173 women that examined the effect of a 12-month moderate-intensity aerobic exercise (45 min/day, 5 days/week) versus usual lifestyle control. The exercise group had a reduction in body weight, total body fat, intraabdominal fat, and subcutaneous fat compared with the control group, and a significant dose response for greater body fat loss was observed with increasing duration of exercise (Irwin et al. 2003). A significant decrease in estradiol, estrone, and free estradiol was seen from baseline to 3 months with an attenuation of the effect at 12 months (McTiernan et al. 2004a). However, in women who lost body fat, the exercise intervention resulted in a statistically significant decrease in these

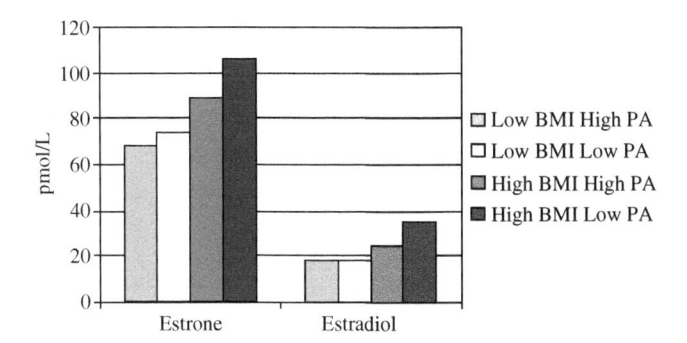

Fig. 12.1 Associations of BMI and physical activity with serum estrogens in postmenopausal women: Women's Health Initiative ($n=267$) (McTiernan et al. 2006). Low BMI<29.0; high BMI≥29.0; low physical activity ≤6.5 MET-hours per week; high physical activity >6.5 MET-hours per week

Table 12.1 Change in estradiol, estrone and sex hormone binding globulin in randomized controlled trials of lifestyle interventions focused on biomarkers of postmenopausal breast cancer risk in inactive, overweight, postmenopausal women

Study	Location	N	Duration	Intervention	Outcome (% change from baseline)
Physical activity and total health (PI: McTiernan) (McTiernan et al. 2004a)	USA	173	12 month	2-arm 1. Aerobic (225 min/wk) 2. Control	Estradiol: 1. −4.4 (NS) 2. −0.6 Estrone 1. −1.8 (NS) 2. +3.9 SHBG: 1. +8.8 (NS) 2. +2.5
ALPHA (PI: Friedenreich) (Friedenreich et al. 2010b)	Canada	320	12 month	2-arm 1. Aerobic (225 min/week) 2. Control	Estradiol: 1. −14* 2. −2.9 Estrone 1. −6.4 (NS) 2. −2.2 SHBG: 1. +4.0* 2. +0.8
SHAPE (PI: Monninkhof) (Monninkhof et al. 2009)	Netherlands	189	12 month	2-arm 1. Combined aerobic and resistance (150 min/week) 2. Control	Estradiol: 1. −8.0 (NS) 2. −10.1 Estrone: 1. −13.9 (NS) 2. −7.4 SHBG: 1. −0.7 (NS) 2. −3.3

(continued)

12 Sex Hormones, Cancer and Exercise Training in Women

Table 12.1 (continued)

Study	Location	N	Duration	Intervention	Outcome (% change from baseline)
NEW (PI: McTiernan) (Campbell et al. 2012)	USA	439	12 month	4-arm: 1. Reduced calorie diet (−10% BW) 2. Aerobic exercise (225 min/week) 3. Combined reduced calorie diet and aerobic exercise (−10% BW and 225 min/week) 4. Control	Estrone: 1. −9.6* 2. −5.5 (NS) 3. −11.1* 4. +8.1 Estradiol: 1. −16.2* 2. −4.9 (NS) 3. −20.3* 4. +4.9 SHBG 1. +22.4* 2. −0.7 (NS) 3. +25.8* 4. −2.7
BETA (PI: Friedenreich) (Friedenreich et al. 2015)	Canada	400	12 months	2-arm 1. Aerobic— moderate volume (150 min/week) 2. Aerobic— high volume (300 min/week)	Estradiol: 1. −4.5 2. −3.6 (NS) Estrone: 1. −3.2 2. 0.1 (NS) SHBG: 1. 9.6 2. 6.4 (NS)
SHAPE II (PI: Monninkhof) (van Gemert et al. 2015)	Netherlands	243	16-weeks	Three-arm 1. Reduced Calorie Diet (−5 to 6 kg) 2. Combined aerobic and RT intervention (240 min/week) with slight reduction in calorie intake (with goal to reduce 5–6 kg) 3. Control	Estradiol: 1. −13.8* 2. −12.7* 3. +3.1 Estrone: 1. −1.3 (NS) 2. −6.7 (NS) 3. +1.5 SHBG: 1. +12.6* 2. +19.0* 3. −8.3

Legend: *statistically significant compared to control group; *BW* body weight, *NS* not statistically significant compared to control group or comparison group (moderate intensity) in BETA Trial, *SHBG* sex hormone binding globulin

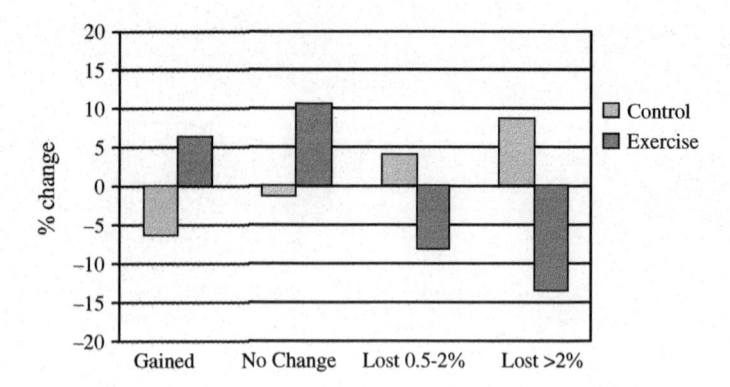

Fig. 12.2 Percent change in estradiol by percent change in body fat in a randomized controlled trial of 1-year moderate-intensity exercise in postmenopausal women (McTiernan et al. 2004a). Statistical significant difference in estradiol level in exercisers who lost 0.5–2 % body fat ($p=0.02$) and for those who lost >2 % body fat ($p=0.008$)

estrogens (McTiernan et al. 2004a) (Fig. 12.2) and a statistically significant decrease in testosterone and free testosterone at 3 and 12 months (McTiernan et al. 2004b).

The ALPHA Trial (Alberta Physical Activity and Breast Cancer Prevention Trial) is a 2-arm trial in 320 women that examined the effect of a 12-month aerobic exercise intervention (45 min/day, 5 days/week) compared with usual lifestyle control (Friedenreich et al. 2010b). A significant reduction in estradiol and free estradiol, and increase in SHBG was observed in the intervention group compared the control group at 12-months, suggesting that women that engaged in at least 150 min per week of moderate-intensity aerobic exercise could lower exposure to estradiol levels (Friedenreich et al. 2010b). Change in sex hormone levels by amount of weight loss was not reported.

The SHAPE Trial (Sex Hormones And Physical Exercise) is a 2-arm trial in 189 women that examined the effect of a 12-month combined aerobic (20–30 min per session) and resistance intervention (25 min per session) compared to usual lifestyle control (Monninkhof et al. 2009). The intervention was two supervised sessions per week of the combined intervention and one-home-based session of 30 min of brisk walking. There were no differences in sex hormones between groups at 12-months. In women who lost >2 % of baseline body weight, regardless of group assignment, there was a significant reduction in testosterone, free testosterone and androstenedione in the exercise group compared to control (Monninkhof et al. 2009). The authors suggest these findings confirm that weight loss may be key in altering sex hormone levels in postmenopausal women, but that exercise may also play a role in favorably altering sex hormone levels.

The NEW Trial (Nutrition and Exercise for Women) is a 4-arm trial examining in 439 women that examined the effects of a 12-month intervention of dietary weight loss alone, exercise alone, dietary weight loss plus exercise, or usual lifestyle control (Campbell et al. 2012; Foster-Schubert et al. 2012). The dietary weight loss intervention was a reduced calorie diet with a goal of 10 % reduction from baseline body weight. The exercise intervention was 45 min of moderate-intensity aerobic exercise 5 days per week (with three of the session supervised). The combined group undertook both interventions. A reduction in estrone compared to control was seen in all three intervention groups. However, a reduction in estradiol, free estradiol, and free testosterone was only noted in the dietary weight loss alone or dietary weight loss plus exercise groups, and not in the exercise alone group. A similar pattern of increase in SHBG only in the dietary weight loss alone and dietary weight loss group plus exercise groups (Campbell et al. 2012). The control group lost −0.6 kg, while the exercise group lost −3.3 kg, dietary weight loss group alone group lost −10.8 kg and the dietary weight loss group plus exercise lost −11.9 kg (Foster-Schubert et al. 2012). The authors concluded that greater weight loss produced greater changes in estrogens and SHBG, and therefore, the findings supported weight loss as a risk reduction strategy for postmenopausal breast cancer by lower exposure to biomarkers of risk (Campbell et al. 2012).

The BETA Trial (Breast Cancer and Exercise Trial in Alberta) is a 2-arm trial in 400 women that examined the effects of a 12-month intervention of moderate volume of aerobic exercise (150 min/week) and high volume of aerobic exercise (300 min/week) (Friedenreich et al. 2015). Adherence to the intervention resulted in a median of 137 min/week performed by the moderate volume group and a median of 253 min/week performed by the high volume group. At 12-months there were similar reductions in estrone, estradiol and free estradiol and similar increases in SHBG in both groups, with no difference between groups. While greater decreases in estradiol and free estradiol were borderline significant in the high volume group, the authors suggested that the lack of observed difference may be due to the fact that the volume of exercise achieved between the groups may not have been sufficiently different. A dose effect was observed more so for obese women, and amount of time spend in vigorous intensity aerobic exercise, as compared with more moderate intensity (Friedenreich et al. 2015).

The SHAPE-2 Trial (Sex Hormones And Physical Exercise-2) is a three-arm trial in 243 women that examined the effects of a 12-month reduced calorie diet with a weight loss goal of 5–6 kg from baseline body weight, an exercise intervention which was a combined aerobic and resistance program with a small calorie deficit with the same weight loss goal of 5–6 kg, and a usual lifestyle control group. There was no change in body weight in the control group (van Gemert et al. 2015). Both intervention groups reached the body weight loss target at 12 months, with a statistically significantly greater reduction in the exercise group compared to the reduced calorie diet group (−5.5 kg vs. −4.9 kg, $p<0.001$). At 12 months, the only difference between groups was a reduction in free testosterone in the mainly exercise group compared to control, and an increase in SHBG in both intervention groups compared to control. After adjustment for changes in body fat, intervention effects were attenuated or disappeared (van Gemert et al. 2015). The authors suggest that the beneficial effect of exercise on sex hormones may be through promoting greater weight loss and greater reductions in body fat when combined with reduced calorie diets versus dietary weight loss alone.

Specific to estrogen metabolism, the only trial to measure this is the Physical Activity and Total Health Trial. No significant effect of the aerobic exercise intervention on 2-OHE1, 16-alpha-OHE1, or their ratio was observed (Atkinson et al. 2004).

Overall these findings suggest that physical activity alone can result in some favorable changes in sex hormones. However, weight loss appears to have a larger impact on sex hormones and the role of exercise in efforts to lower risk of postmenopausal breast cancer risk may be to support weight loss efforts undertaken with reduced calorie diet.

Exercise Effect: High Risk Groups

Only 5–10 % of sex hormone-related cancers are linked to genetic factors (Easton et al. 1995; Wooster et al. 1995). Mutations in two breast cancer susceptibility genes (BReast CAncer or BRCA1 and BCRA2), which are tumor suppressor genes, are strongly linked to risk of hereditary breast and ovarian cancer, with carriers having a 40–85 % chance of developing breast cancer in their lifetime, along with a higher risk of developing ovarian cancer (25–65 % in BCRA1 carriers and 15–10 % in BRCA2 carriers) (King et al. 2003; Antoniou et al. 2006). Currently treatment involves several medical options to reduce hormone exposure, including prophylactic oophorectomy, which can lower breast cancer risk by 50–70 % or use of Selective Estrogen Receptor Modulators (SERMS, e.g., tamoxifen and raloxifene) which can lower breast cancer risk by 50 %. Prophylactic mastectomy is another option, which can reduce risk by 90–95 %(Pruthi et al. 2010).

One randomized controlled trial has been conducted in women at high risk of breast cancer (i.e., BRCA 1 or 2 mutation, first degree relative with breast cancer diagnosis, and/or Claus or Gail model risk of 18 %). The WISER Sister study is a three-arm trial of 150 min/week of aerobic exercise, 300 min/week of aerobic exercise or usual lifestyle control for five menstrual cycles. Using measures of urinary hormones in daily first morning urines in menstrual cycle 1 and 2 for baseline and menstrual cycles 6 and 7 for post intervention, the control group had an 11.6 % increase in area under the curve for follicular phase estrogen, compared to a −2.1 and a 0.2 % change in the low- and high-dose groups, respectively. There was no difference in luteal phase. In looking at the dose-response relationship, every 100 min of exercise was associated with 3.6 % lower follicular phase estrogen (Schmitz et al. 2015). A particularly unique aspect of this study was that the impact of the intervention directly on breast tissue. The amount of glandular breast tissue, the constituent of breast tissue that is hormone responsive, was measured using parenchymal enhancement magnetic resonance imaging. Every 100 min of exercise was associated with a 9.7 % decrease in background parenchymal enhancement (Schmitz et al. 2015; Brown et al. 2016). The authors conclude that these results offer support for physical activity as an additional options for women at high risk of breast cancer to blunt exposure levels of estrogen (Brown et al. 2016).

Future Directions

Future exercise interventions should expand on current knowledge by testing different types of exercise (i.e., resistance and aerobic) and different volumes of exercise (i.e., other intensities and durations of exercise) in different populations and in persons at different risk of developing cancer. Further research should also be undertaken to confirm that proposed biomarkers do indeed lie on the causal pathway between physical activity and sex hormone related cancer development and examine the role of genetic polymorphisms related to biomarkers of interest.

Summary

Moderate-intensity physical activity has biological effects that may reduce risk of postmenopausal breast and endometrial cancer risk. However, both prior to and following menopause energy balance and body weight may play a significant role in the relationship between physical activity and sex steroid hormone levels. This suggests the need for future trials to examine the independent and combined effects of physical activity and diet in support of weight management and weight loss to reduce the risk of sex hormone related cancers.

References

Allen NE, Key TJ, Dossus L, Rinaldi S, Cust A, Lukanova A, et al. Endogenous sex hormones and endometrial cancer risk in women in the European Prospective Investigation into Cancer and Nutrition (EPIC). Endocr Relat Cancer. 2008;15(2):485–97.

Antoniou AC, Pharoah PD, Easton DF, Evans DG. BRCA1 and BRCA2 cancer risks. J Clin Oncol. 2006;24(20):3312–3. author reply 3–4.

Atkinson C, Lampe JW, Tworoger SS, Ulrich CM, Bowen D, Irwin ML, et al. Effects of a moderate intensity exercise intervention on estrogen metabolism in postmenopausal women. Cancer Epidemiol Biomarkers Prev. 2004;13(5):868–74.

Baker E, Demers L. Menstrual status in female athletes: correlation with reproductive hormones and bone density. Obstet Gynecol. 1988;72(5):683–7.

Ballard-Barbash R, Hunsberger S, Alciati MH, Blair SN, Goodwin PJ, McTiernan A, et al. Physical activity, weight control, and breast cancer risk and survival: clinical trial rationale and design considerations. J Natl Cancer Inst. 2009;101(9):630–43.

Bentz AT, Schneider CM, Westerlind KC. The relationship between physical activity and 2-hydroxyestrone, 16alpha-hydroxyestrone, and the 2/16 ratio in premenopausal women (United States). Cancer Causes Control. 2005;16(4):455–61.

Bernstein L, Ross R, Lobo RA, Hanisch R, Krailo MD, Henderson BE. The effects of moderate physical activity on menstrual cycle patterns in adolescence: Implications for breast cancer prevention. Br J Cancer. 1987;55:681–5.

Bernstein L, Henderston BE, Hanisch R, Sullivan-Halley J, Ross RK. Physical exercise and reduced risk of breast cancer in young women. J Natl Cancer Inst. 1994;86(18):1403–8.

Bonen A. Recreational exercise does not impair menstrual cycles: A prospective study. Int J Sports Med. 1992;13:110–20.

Borer K. Exercise endocrinology. Champaign, IL: Human Kinetics; 2003.
Broocks A, Pirke KM, Schweiger U, Tuschl RJ, Laessle RG, Strowitzki T, et al. Cyclic ovarian function in recreational athletes. J Appl Physiol. 1990;68(5):2083–6.
Brown SB, Hankinson SE. Endogenous estrogens and the risk of breast, endometrial, and ovarian cancers. Steroids. 2015;99:8–10.
Brown JC, Kontos D, Schnall M, Wu S, Schmitz KH. The Dose-Response Effects of Aerobic Exercise on Body Composition and Breast Tissue among Women at High Risk for Breast Cancer: A Randomized Trial. Cancer Prev Res (Phila). 2016.
Bullen BA, Skrinar GS, Beitins IZ, Carr DB, Reppert SM, Dotson CO, et al. Endurance training effects on plasma hormonal responsiveness and sex hormone excretion. J Appl Physiol. 1984;56(6):1453–63.
Bullen BA, Skrinar GS, Beitins IZ, Von Mering G, Turnbull BA, McArthur JW. Induction of menstrual disorders by strenuous exercise in untrained women. N Engl J Med. 1985;312:1349–53.
Caldon CE. Estrogen signaling and the DNA damage response in hormone dependent breast cancers. Front Oncol. 2014;4:106.
Campbell KL, McTiernan A. Exercise and biomarkers for cancer prevention studies. J Nutr. 2007;137(1):161S–9.
Campbell KL, Westerlind KC, Harber VJ, Friedenreich CM, Courneya KS. Associations between aerobic fitness and estrogen metabolites in premenopausal women. Med Sci Sports Exerc. 2005;37(4):585–92.
Campbell KL, Westerlind KC, Harber VJ, Bell GJ, Mackey JR, Courneya KS. Effects of aerobic exercise training on estrogen metabolism in premenopausal women: a randomized controlled trial. Cancer Epidemiol Biomarkers Prev. 2007;16(4):731–9.
Campbell KL, Foster-Schubert KE, Alfano CM, Wang CC, Wang CY, Duggan CR, et al. Reduced-Calorie Dietary Weight Loss, Exercise, and Sex Hormones in Postmenopausal Women: Randomized Controlled Trial. J Clin Oncol. 2012;30(19):2314–26.
Carmichael AR, Bates T. Obesity and breast cancer: a review of the literature. Breast. 2004;13(2):85–92.
Cauley JA, Gutai JP, Kuller LH, LeDonne D, Powell JG. The epidemiology of serum sex hormones in postmenopausal women. Am J Epidemiol. 1989;129(6):1120–31.
Cust AE, Armstrong BK, Friedenreich CM, Slimani N, Bauman A. Physical activity and endometrial cancer risk: a review of the current evidence, biologic mechanisms and the quality of physical activity assessment methods. Cancer Causes Control. 2007;18(3):243–58.
De Souza MJ, Miller BE, Loucks AB, Luciano AA, Pescatello LS, Campbell CG, et al. High frequency of luteal phase deficiency and anovulation in recreational women runners: Blunted elevation in follicle-stimulating hormone observed during luteal-follicular transition. J Clin Endocrinol Metab. 1998;83(12):4220–32.
Du M, Kraft P, Eliassen AH, Giovannucci E, Hankinson SE, De Vivo I. Physical activity and risk of endometrial adenocarcinoma in the Nurses' Health Study. [Research Support, N.I.H., Extramural]. Int J Cancer. 2014;134(11):2707–16.
Easton DF, Ford D, Bishop DT. Breast and ovarian cancer incidence in BRCA1-mutation carriers. Breast cancer linkage consortium. Am J Hum Genet. 1995;56(1):265–71.
Ellison PT, Lager C. Moderate recreational running is associated with lowered saliva progesterone profiles in women. Am J Obstet Gynecol. 1986;154(5):1000–3.
Endogenous Hormones and Breast Cancer Collaborative Group. Endogenous sex hormones and breast cancer in postmenopausal women: reanalysis of nine prospective studies. J Natl Cancer Inst. 2002;94:606–16.
Foster-Schubert KE, Alfano CM, Duggan CR, Xiao L, Campbell KL, Kong A, et al. Effect of Diet and Exercise, Alone or Combined, on Weight and Body Composition in Overweight-to-Obese Postmenopausal Women. Obesity. 2012;20(8):1628–38.
Friedenreich CM. Review of anthropometric factors and breast cancer risk. Eur J Cancer Prev. 2001;10:15–32.
Friedenreich CM, Orenstein MR. Physical activity and cancer prevention: etiologic evidence and biological mechanisms. J Nutr. 2002;132(11):3456S–64.

Friedenreich CM, Neilson HK, Lynch BM. State of the epidemiological evidence on physical activity and cancer prevention. Eur J Cancer. 2010a;46(14):2593–604.

Friedenreich CM, Woolcott CG, McTiernan A, Ballard-Barbash R, Brant RF, Stanczyk FZ, et al. The Alberta Physical Activity and Breast Cancer Prevention Trial: Sex Hormone Changes in a Year-Long Exercise Intervention Among Postmenopausal Women. J Clin Oncol. 2010b;28(9):1458–66.

Friedenreich CM, Neilson HK, Wang Q, Stanczyk FZ, Yasui Y, Duha A, et al. Effects of exercise dose on endogenous estrogens in postmenopausal women: a randomized trial. Endocr Relat Cancer. 2015;22(5):863–76.

Frisch RE, Gotz-Welbergen AV, McArthur JW, Albright T, Witschi J, Bullen B, et al. Delayed menarche and amenorrhea of college athletes in relation to age of onset of training. J Am Med Assoc. 1981;246(14):1559–63.

Henderson BE, Feigelson HS. Hormonal carcinogenesis. Carcinogenesis. 2000;21(3):427–33.

Hoffman-Goetz L, Apter D, Demark-Wahnefried W, Goran M, McTiernan A, Reichman M. Possible mechanisms mediating an association between physical activity and breast cancer. Cancer. 1998;83(3 Suppl):621–8.

Howard BV, Manson JE, Stefanick ML, Beresford SA, Frank G, Jones B, et al. Low-fat dietary pattern and weight change over 7 years: the Women's Health Initiative Dietary Modification Trial. JAMA. 2006;295(1):39–49.

Irwin ML, Yasui Y, Ulrich CM, Bowen D, Rudolph RE, Schwartz RS, et al. Effect of exercise on total and intra-abdominal body fat in postmenopausal women: a randomized controlled trial. JAMA. 2003;289(3):323–30.

Joy E, De Souza MJ, Nattiv A, Misra M, Williams NI, Mallinson RJ, et al. 2014 female athlete triad coalition consensus statement on treatment and return to play of the female athlete triad. Curr Sports Med Rep. 2014;13(4):219–32.

Karapanou O, Papadimitriou A. Determinants of menarche. Reprod Biol Endocrinol. 2010;8:115.

Keizer HA, Kuipers H, de Haan J, Janssen GM, Beckers E, Habets L, et al. Effect of a 3-month endurance training program on metabolic and multiple hormonal responses to exercise. Int J Sports Med. 1987;8 Suppl 3:154–60.

Key TJ, Allen NE, Verkasalo PK, Banks E. Energy balance and cancer: the role of sex hormones. Proc Nutr Soc. 2001;60(1):81–9.

King MC, Marks JH, Mandell JB. Breast and ovarian cancer risks due to inherited mutations in BRCA1 and BRCA2. Science. 2003;302(5645):643–6.

Lee IM. Physical activity and cancer prevention--data from epidemiologic studies. Med Sci Sports Exerc. 2003;35(11):1823–7.

Loucks AB. Effects of exercise training on the menstrual cycle: existence and mechanisms. Med Sci Sports Exerc. 1990;22(3):275–80.

Loucks AB. Energy availability, not body fatness, regulated reproductive function in women. Exerc Sport Sci Rev. 2003;31(3):144–8.

Loucks AB, Redman LM. The effect of stress on menstrual function. Trends Endocrinol Metab. 2004;15(10):466–71.

Lukanova A, Lundin E, Micheli A, Arslan A, Ferrari P, Rinaldi S, et al. Circulating levels of sex steroid hormones and risk of endometrial cancer in postmenopausal women. Int J Cancer. 2004;108(3):425–32.

Lynch BM, Neilson HK, Friedenreich CM. Physical activity and breast cancer prevention. Recent Results Cancer Res. 2011;186:13–42.

Matthews CE, Fowke JH, Dai Q, Bradlow HL, Jin F, Shu XO, et al. Physical activity, body size, and estrogen metabolism in women. Cancer Causes Control. 2004;15(5):473–81.

McTiernan A, Tworoger SS, Ulrich CM, Yasui Y, Irwin ML, Rajan KB, et al. Effect of exercise on serum estrogens in postmenopausal women: a 12-month randomized clinical trial. Cancer Res. 2004a;64(8):2923–8.

McTiernan A, Tworoger SS, Rajan KB, Yasui Y, Sorenson B, Ulrich CM, et al. Effect of exercise on serum androgens in postmenopausal women: a 12-month randomized clinical trial. Cancer Epidemiol Biomarkers Prev. 2004b;13(7):1099–105.

McTiernan A, Wu L, Chen C, Chlebowski R, Mossavar-Rahmani Y, Modugno F, et al. Relation of BMI and physical activity to sex hormones in postmenopausal women. Obesity (Silver Spring). 2006;14(9):1662–77.

McTiernan A, Wu L, Barnabei VM, Chen C, Hendrix S, Modugno F, et al. Relation of demographic factors, menstrual history, reproduction and medication use to sex hormone levels in postmenopausal women. Breast Cancer Res Treat. 2008;108(2):217–31.

Meilahn EN, De Stavola B, Allen DS, Fentiman I, Bradlow HL, Sepkovic DW, Kuller LH. Do urinary oestrogen metabolites predict breast cancer? Br J Cancer. 1998;78:1250–5.

Monninkhof EM, Velthuis MJ, Peeters PH, Twisk JW, Schuit AJ. Effect of exercise on postmenopausal sex hormone levels and role of body fat: a randomized controlled trial. J Clin Oncol. 2009;27(27):4492–9.

Morimoto LM, White E, Chen Z, Chlebowski RT, Hays J, Kuller L, et al. Obesity, body size, and risk of postmenopausal breast cancer: the Women's Health Initiative (United States). Cancer Causes Control. 2002;13(8):741–51.

Muti P, Bradlow HL, Micheli A, Krogh V, Freudenheim JL, Schunemann HJ, et al. Estrogen metabolism and risk of breast cancer: a prospective study of 2:16alpha hydroxyestrone ratio in premenopausal and postmenopausal women. Epidemiology. 2000;11:635–40.

Nattiv A, Loucks AB, Manore MM, Sanborn CF, Sundgot-Borgen J, Warren MP. American College of Sports Medicine position stand. The female athlete triad. Med Sci Sports Exerc. 2007;39(10):1867–82.

Physical Activity Guidelines for Americans: Department of Health and Human Services; 2008.

Pirke KM, Schweiger U, Broocks A, Tuschl RJ, Laessle RG. Luteinizing hormone and follicle stimulating hormone secretion patterns in female athletes with and without menstrual disturbances. Clin Endocrinol (Oxf). 1990;33(3):345–53.

Pruthi S, Gostout BS, Lindor NM. Identification and management of women with BRCA mutations or hereditary predisposition for breast and ovarian cancer. Mayo Clin Proc. 2010;85(12):1111–20.

Rogol AD, Weltman A, Weltman JY, Seip RL, Snead DB, Levine S, et al. Durability of the reproductive axis in eumenorrheic women during 1 yr of endurance training. J Appl Physiol. 1992;72(4):1571–80.

Ronkainen H. Depressed follicle-stimulating hormone, luteinizing hormone, and prolactin responses to the luteinizing hormone-releasing hormone thyrotropin-releasing hormone, and metoclopramide test in endurance runners in the hard-training season. Fertil Steril. 1985;44(6):755–9.

Rundle A. Molecular epidemiology of physical activity and cancer. Cancer Epidemiol Biomarkers Prev. 2005;14(1):227–36.

Russell JB, Mitchell DE, Musey PI, Collins DC. The relationship of exercise to anovluatory cycles in female athletes: hormonal and physical characteristics. Obstet Gynecol. 1984a;63:452–6.

Russell JB, Mitchell DE, Musey PI, Collins DC. The role of beta-endorphins and catechol estrogens on the hypothalamic-pituitary axis in female athletes. Fertil Steril. 1984b;42(5):690–5.

Schmid D, Behrens G, Keimling M, Jochem C, Ricci C, Leitzmann M. A systematic review and meta-analysis of physical activity and endometrial cancer risk. Eur J Epidemiol. 2015;30(5):397–412.

Schmitz KH, Williams NI, Kontos D, Domchek S, Morales KH, Hwang WT, et al. Dose-response effects of aerobic exercise on estrogen among women at high risk for breast cancer: a randomized controlled trial. Breast Cancer Res Treat. 2015;154(2):309–18.

Schweiger U, Laessle R, Schweiger M, Herrmann F, Riedel W, Pirke KM. Caloric intake, stress, and menstrual function in athletes. Fertil Steril. 1988;49(3):447–50.

Smith AJ, Phipps WR, Arikawa AY, O'Dougherty M, Kaufman B, Thomas W, et al. Effects of aerobic exercise on premenopausal sex hormone levels: results of the WISER study, a randomized clinical trial in healthy, sedentary, eumenorrheic women. Cancer Epidemiol Biomarkers Prev. 2011;20(6):1098–106.

Smith AJ, Phipps WR, Thomas W, Schmitz KH, Kurzer MS. The effects of aerobic exercise on estrogen metabolism in healthy premenopausal women. Cancer Epidemiol Biomarkers Prev. 2013;22(5):756–64.

Snow RC, Barbiebi RL, Frisch RE. Estrogen 2-hydroxylase oxidation and menstrual function among elite oarswomen. J Clin Endocrinol Metab. 1989;69(2):369–76.

Steindorf K, Ritte R, Eomois PP, Lukanova A, Tjonneland A, Johnsen NF, et al. Physical activity and risk of breast cancer overall and by hormone receptor status: the European prospective investigation into cancer and nutrition. Int J Cancer. 2013;132(7):1667–78.

van Gemert WA, Schuit AJ, van der Palen J, May AM, Iestra JA, Wittink H, et al. Effect of weight loss, with or without exercise, on body composition and sex hormones in postmenopausal women: the SHAPE-2 trial. Breast Cancer Res. 2015;17:120.

Verkasalo PK, Thomas HV, Appleby PN, Davey GK, Key TJ. Circulating levels of sex hormones and their relation to risk factors for breast cancer: a cross-sectional study in 1092 pre- and postmenopausal women. Cancer Causes Control. 2001;12:47–59.

Voskuil DW, Monninkhof EM, Elias SG, Vlems FA, van Leeuwen FE. Physical activity and endometrial cancer risk, a systematic review of current evidence. Cancer Epidemiol Biomarkers Prev. 2007;16(4):639–48.

Warren MP. The effects of exercise on pubertal progression and reproductive function in girls. J Clin Endocrinol Metab. 1980;51(5):1150–7.

Wellejus A, Olsen A, Tjonneland A, Thomsen BL, Overvad K, Loft S. Urinary hydroxyestrogens and breast cancer risk among postmenopausal women: a prospective study. Cancer Epidemiol Biomarkers Prev. 2005;14(9):2137–42.

Williams NI, Helmreich DL, Parfitt DB, Caston-Balderrama A, Cameron JL. Evidence for a causal role of low energy availability in the induction of menstrual cycle disturbances during strenuous exercise training. J Clin Endocrinol Metab. 2001;86:5184–93.

Williams NI, Leidy HJ, Hill BR, Lieberman JL, Legro RS, De Souza MJ. Magnitude of daily energy deficit predicts frequency but not severity of menstrual disturbances associated with exercise and caloric restriction. Am J Physiol Endocrinol Metab. 2015;308(1):29–39.

Wooster R, Bignell G, Lancaster J, Swift S, Seal S, Mangion J, et al. Identification of the breast cancer susceptibility gene BRCA2. Nature. 1995;378(6559):789–92.

World Cancer Research Fund. Food, nutrition, physical activity, and the prevention of cancer: a global perspective. Washington, DC: AICR; 2007.

Yue W, Yager JD, Wang JP, Jupe ER, Santen RJ. Estrogen receptor-dependent and independent mechanisms of breast cancer carcinogenesis. Steroids. 2013;78(2):161–70.

Zeleniuch-Jacquotte A, Akhmedkhanov A, Kato I, Koenig KL, Shore RE, Kim MY, et al. Postmenopausal endogenous oestrogens and risk of endometrial cancer: results of a prospective study. Br J Cancer. 2001;84(7):975–81.

Ziegler RG, Fuhrman BJ, Moore SC, Matthews CE. Epidemiologic studies of estrogen metabolism and breast cancer. Steroids. 2015;99:67–75.

Chapter 13
The Effects of Acute Exercise on Physiological Sexual Arousal in Women

Cindy M. Meston and Amelia M. Stanton

Introduction

Over the past two decades, research has demonstrated a strong link between acute exercise and physiological (i.e., genital) sexual arousal in women. In this chapter we provide a summary of the laboratory studies that have examined the effects of acute exercise on sexual arousal in women, and provide a potential explanation for the mechanisms of action underlying this relationship. In the latter part of this chapter we provide a discussion of the clinical and treatment implications for the facilitatory effect of exercise on women's sexual response.

Physiological Sexual Arousal in Women

Physiological sexual arousal results from genital vasocongestion, which occurs with increased blood flow to the genitals. When blood begins to pool in the vaginal walls, the increase in blood volume leads to increased pressure inside the capillaries, which subsequently triggers lubricated plasma to transcend the vaginal epithelium onto the surface of the vagina (Levin, 1980). These platelets form droplets, creating the lubricative film that typically covers the vaginal walls during sexual activity. Increased blood flow also leads the clitoris and the vestibular bulbs to protrude and become engorged (Berman, 2005), and well-oxygenated blood is also supplied to the skin and the breasts (Levin, 2002). In addition to increased blood flow, sexual arousal causes relaxation of the smooth muscles in the vaginal wall, which allows the vagina to lengthen and dilate.

C.M. Meston, Ph.D. (✉) • A.M. Stanton, B.A.
Department of Psychology, The University of Texas at Austin, 108 E. Dean Keeton, Stop A8000, Austin, TX 78712, USA
e-mail: mestoncm@gmail.com

A certain level of arousal is required for orgasm, and that level differs by individual. Stimulation by friction and pressure activates specialized nerve endings in the genitals (Krantz, 1958), which generates impulses to the spinal cord and possibly to the vagus nerve (Komisaruk et al., 1997). According to Levin (2002), researchers do not fully understand how the signals from the nerve endings are converted into sexual pleasure and ultimately to orgasm, but it is known that the afferent impulses of these nerve endings not only create the spinal reflexes that influence genital blood flow, but they also ascend the spinal cord, via the spinothalamic and spinoreticular tracts, to the brain for processing.

Physiological sexual arousal in women is most commonly measured in laboratory studies using a vaginal photoplethysmograph (Sintchak & Geer, 1975). The vaginal photoplethysmograph is a clear acrylic, tampon-shaped device that contains either an incandescent light source, or an infrared light-emitting diode as a light source, and a photosensitive light detector. The light source illuminates the capillary bed of the vaginal wall, and the phototransistor detects the light that is reflected back from the vaginal wall and the blood circulating within it. The amount of back-scattered light is in direct relation to the transparency of engorged and unengorged tissue and thus serves as an indirect measure of vasoengorgement. Simply stated, the greater the back-scattering signal the more blood is assumed to be in the vessels (Levin, 1992). The vaginal probe was designed to be easily inserted by the participant. A positioning shield can be placed on the probe's cable in order to standardize the depth of insertion between uses.

There are two components of the signal that can be derived from the photoplethysmograph. When the signal is coupled to a Direct Current (DC) amplifier, a measure of vaginal blood volume (VBV) is obtained. VBV is believed to reflect slow changes in the pooling of blood in the vaginal tissue (Hatch, 1979). The DC signal is used at low sensitivity and the standard dependent variable is change from levels of VBV at baseline. Because there is no discernible zero point with VBV, absolute measures of blood volume cannot be detected, hence the need to measure in units of blood volume change. When the signal is AC-coupled (alternating current), a measure of vaginal pulse amplitude (VPA) is obtained. VPA is believed to reflect phasic changes in vaginal engorgement with each heartbeat; higher amplitudes indicate higher levels of blood flow (e.g., Geer, Morokoff, & Greenwood, 1974). The dependent variable typically used is the amplitude of the pulse signal, which is measured from the bottom to the top of the pulse wave. As there is no absolute zero point with VPA, analyses are conducted by either averaging across specific stimulus presentations, across the highest 20–30 s of arousal, or across selected time periods. The change in mean genital arousal is typically calculated by subtracting the mean VPA to the neutral film from the mean VPA to the erotic film for each set of films in a given study. These values are then standardized within subjects and compared between stimulus categories.

Effect of Acute Exercise on Physiological Sexual Response

In a series of laboratory studies, Meston and colleagues examined the direct effects of acute exercise on female sexual function. The first of these studies required sexually functional participants to engage in 20 min of intense exercise (stationary cycling) prior to viewing a nonsexual and erotic film sequence (Meston & Gorzalka, 1995). The procedure consisted of an orientation screening and questionnaire session, a 20-min bicycle ergometer fitness test, and then two counterbalanced experimental sessions (Exercise, No-exercise) that took place on different days. During the fitness test, the experimenters determined each participant's maximum volume of oxygen uptake so that they could have the participants cycle at a constant 70% of their estimated maximum volume during the exercise session. By ensuring that all participants worked at equivalent levels of their maximum volume of oxygen uptake, differences in physiological responses resulting from variations in fitness levels were minimized. In the exercise experimental session, participants cycled for 20 min on the stationary bicycle then after the cessation of exercise they inserted the vaginal photoplethysmograph and watched a nonsexual film followed by an erotic film while their vaginal pulse amplitude was measured. From the cessation of exercise to the onset of the erotic film, approximately 15 min had passed. In the no-exercise condition, participants sat for 20 min, inserted the vaginal photoplethysmograph and viewed a second nonsexual and erotic film sequence. The results revealed that VPA was significantly higher during the presentation of the erotic film after exercise than it was during the erotic film in the no-exercise condition. There were no significant differences between conditions in VPA responses during the nonsexual film indicating that exercise did not simply increase blood flow to the genitals but, rather, it prepared the woman's body for sexual arousal so that when she was in a sexual context (e.g., viewing the erotic film) her body responded more intensely. This was the first finding to provide support for a facilitatory effect of acute exercise on physiological sexual arousal in women.

In a follow-up study, Meston and Gorzalka (1996) examined the effect of timing on the relationship between exercise and increased sexual arousal in women by measuring physiological arousal in response to erotic films at either 5, 15, or 30 min post-exercise. Each condition consisted of an experimental exercise session and a no-exercise control session. The results revealed that at both 15 and 30 min post-exercise there was a significant increase in genital arousal (VPA) to the erotic films compared to the no-exercise control condition. The finding of a significant facilitatory effect at 15 min post-exercise replicated Meston and Goralka's earlier study (1995). However, in contrast to the facilitation noted at 15 and 30 min post-exercise, acute exercise inhibited physiological sexual arousal when measured immediately following exercise. The authors noted that, during and immediately following exercise, a decrease in vascular resistance of the working muscles causes a significant increase in blood flow to those muscles (Christensen & Galbo, 1983). Therefore, blood flow may have shifted away from the genital region to temporarily help restore the working muscles. The finding that exercise inhibited genital arousal immediately following exercise but facilitated at 15 and 30 min post-exercise led the authors to speculate an optimal time for sexual activity following exercise.

To further explore whether an optimal level of sympathetic nervous system (SNS) activation from exercise may exist for facilitating sexual arousal in women (Lorenz, Harte, Hamilton, and Meston, 2012) performed a secondary analysis of participants from the control conditions of three previously published studies (Hamilton, Fogle, & Meston, 2008; Harte & Meston, 2008; Harte & Meston, 2007). Sympathetic nervous system activity was assessed using heart rate variability, which refers to the degree of variability in the lengths of time between successive heartbeats, and is a useful noninvasive index of autonomic activity. The degree of variability in the lengths of time between successive heartbeats (HRV) provides important information about the relative balance of sympathetic and parasympathetic forces acting on the heart (Thayer et al., 2010). Participants in all three studies were sexually healthy women. The methodology of each study involved having the participants watch a nonsexual and erotic film sequence while their VPA responses were recorded. As predicted, the results revealed a curvilinear relationship between SNS activity and women's physiological sexual arousal. That is, moderate increases in SNS activity were associated with greater physiological sexual arousal responses, while low and high SNS activation were associated with lower physiological sexual arousal. These results provide support for the notion that there is an optimal level of SNS activity from acute exercise for the facilitation of genital sexual arousal in women.

Mechanism of Action for the Facilitation of Physiological Sexual Arousal with Exercise

Acute exercise influences a number of bodily systems that could feasibly impact women's sexual function. Exercise has been shown to affect a variety of hormones such as cortisol (e.g., Hill et al., 2008), estrogen (e.g., Smith, Phipps, Thomas, Schmitz, & Kurzer, 2013), prolactin (e.g., Rojas Vega, Hollmann, & Strüder, 2012), oxytocin (e.g., Hew-Butler, Noakes, Soldin, & Verbalis, 2008), and testosterone (for reviews, see Hackney, 1996; Vingren et al., 2012), all of which have been linked to sexual arousal in women. In a recent study, high levels of cortisol and chronic stress were related to low levels of genital sexual arousal in women (Hamilton & Meston, 2013). Reductions in estradiol during menopause and lactation have been associated with reduced blood flow, vasocongestion, and subsequently lubrication (e.g., Simon, 2011). With respect to testosterone, some studies have concluded that moderate levels of exercise increase free or total testosterone (e.g., Vingren et al., 2009), while others have found no change in testosterone from pre- to post-exercise (e.g., Linnamo, Pakarinen, Komi, Kraemer, & Hakkinen, 2005). In women, testosterone is most often linked to increased sexual desire, but it may also affect the genital tissues. One study demonstrated that women treated with exogenous androgens exhibited increases in genital arousal

(Heard-Davison et al., 2007). Clinically high levels of prolactin have been associated with sexual arousal dysfunction in women, specifically decreased vaginal lubrication, as well as with other sexual problems, including decreased desire, atrophic vaginitis, and anorgasmia (Smith, 2003). Finally, plasma oxytocin levels have been associated with genital sexual arousal; specifically, plasma oxytocin was significantly correlated with vaginal lubrication during the luteal phase of the menstrual cycle, and there was a trend toward statistical significance during the follicular phase (Salonia et al., 2005).

To examine whether changes in testosterone may, in part, account for the increases in genital arousal with exercise, Hamilton, Fogle, and Meston (2008) assessed salivary measures of testosterone at multiple time points during a no-exercise and exercise experimental session. The study methodology was similar to the exercise studies described earlier, with the exception that testing was done between 2:00 pm and 6:00 pm on days 5 through 10 of the woman's menstrual cycle in order to control for diurnal and menstrual cycle fluctuations in testosterone. Saliva samples were taken at the start of each session to provide a baseline sample, again 10 min after the 20-min period of vigorous exercise (during the exercise session) and 10 min after the pre-testing rest period of the no-exercise session. The findings indicated that testosterone did not increase in response to either exercise or the erotic film. In fact, testosterone remained stable during both the exercise session and the no-exercise session, and there were no differences in testosterone between the two sessions. This suggests that testosterone is not likely the mechanism of action associated with increased genital arousal post-exercise.

It is feasible that SNS activation may be driving the association between acute exercise and increased physiological sexual arousal in women. Biochemical and physiologic research indicates diffuse SNS discharge occurs during the later stages of sexual arousal in women (Jovanovic, 1971) with marked increases in heart rate and blood pressure occurring during orgasm (Fox & Fox, 1969). Increases in plasma norepinephrine, a sensitive index of SNS activity, have also been shown to accompany increases in sexual arousal during intercourse (Wiedeking et al., 1979).

Laboratory research that specifically manipulated SNS activity supports the mechanistic role that it may play in female sexual arousal. In one such study 20 sexually functional women participated in two counterbalanced conditions in which they received either placebo or ephedrine sulfate (50 mg), a sympathomimetic amine that stimulates the adrenergic receptor system by increasing the activity of norepinephrine, before viewing a nonsexual and erotic film sequence (Meston & Heiman, 1998). Norepinephrine is considered to be the dominant neurotransmitter through which the SNS exerts its effects. As in the prior studies described, physiological sexual responses to the films were measured using vaginal photoplethysmography (VPA). The results revealed ephedrine significantly increased VPA responses to the erotic film compared to placebo, but there were no differences in VPA responses to the nonsexual film with ephedrine. As was the case with exercise, these results suggest that ephedrine did not simply facilitate physiological responses through a general increase in peripheral resistance, but, rather, it selectively prepared the body for genital response.

If SNS activation increases sexual arousal, as suggested by the previous study, it is likely that drugs that decrease SNS activity would also decrease sexual arousal. Moreover, if exercise increases genital arousal via SNS activation, then blocking SNS arousal during exercise would be expected to diminish the enhancing influence of exercise on VPA responses. To test this hypothesis, Meston and colleagues (1997) administered either 0.2 mg of clonidine or placebo to 30 sexually functional women in two counterbalanced sessions where they viewed a nonsexual and erotic film sequence. The researchers chose the antihypertensive medication clonidine because it acts centrally as a norepinephrine antagonist and peripherally as an inhibitor of sympathetic outflow. Before viewing the experimental films, half of the participants engaged in 20 min of exercise in order to elicit significant SNS activation, and the other half did not exercise. Following heightened SNS activation (via acute exercise), there was a significant decrease in VPA responses to the erotic film in the clonidine compared to placebo condition. Among the participants who did not engage in exercise prior to viewing the film sequence, clonidine showed a nonsignificant trend toward decreasing VPA responses compared with placebo. Because clonidine has both central and peripheral properties, it is unclear at which level clonidine acted to influence sexual responding (Meston et al., 1997). Centrally, clonidine may have suppressed sexual responses indirectly via changes in neurohypophyseal hormone release, or directly by activating central sites that are responsible for the inhibition of sexual reflexes (Riley, 1995). Peripherally, clonidine may have suppressed sexual arousal by direct inhibition of sympathetic outflow. Support for the latter explanation is provided by the finding that clonidine significantly inhibited sexual responding only when participants were in a state of heightened SNS activity. The fact that clonidine has been reported to significantly inhibit SNS, but not hormonal, responses to exercise (Engelman et al., 1989) is consistent with the suggestion that clonidine acted to inhibit sexual responding via suppressed SNS activity.

Research on sexual function in women following spinal cord injury provides additional support for the relationship between SNS activation and physiological sexual arousal in women. In one study, Sipski and colleagues (2001) assessed the impact of spinal cord injury on genital sexual arousal in women by comparing premenopausal women with spinal cord injuries to able-bodied, age-matched controls. They found that preservation of sensory function in the T11-L2 level of the spinal cord was associated with genital sexual arousal. As sympathetic pathways controlling genital function originate at this level of the spinal cord (Hancock & Peveto, 1979; Neuhber, 1982; Nadelhaft & McKenna, 1987), the authors noted that their findings were consistent with those of Meston and colleagues, who showed that activation of the SNS via exercise (Meston & Gorzalka, 1995; Meston & Gorzalka, 1996) and ephedrine (Meston & Heiman, 1998) led to increases in genital sexual arousal. Building upon their findings, Sipski and colleagues (2004) assessed the effects of sympathetic stimulation on sexual arousal in women with spinal cord injuries. Because of the physical limitations of the population, the authors used anxiety-eliciting videos, which have been shown to increase genital arousal in sexually dysfunctional women (Palace & Gorzalka, 1990), instead of exercise in order to elicit sympathetic arousal. In women with greater sensory function in the T11-L2 level of the spinal cord, where the sympathetic nerve fibers to the genitals arise, there was a significant effect of the anxiety-inducing film on genital responsiveness; this was not the case for women with low sensory function at the T11-L2 level. The authors interpreted their findings as further evidence for the role of the sympathetic nervous system in the regulation of genital vasocongestion.

Clinical Implications: Exercise and Sexual Arousal in Women with a History of Childhood Sexual Abuse

Several clinical populations of women may be directly affected by the observed relationship between acute exercise and increased physiological sexual arousal. One such population is women with histories of childhood sexual abuse (CSA), specifically those who meet diagnostic criteria for posttraumatic stress disorder (PTSD). Individuals with both CSA histories and PTSD diagnoses have increased levels of baseline SNS activity (e.g., Yehuda, 2003). Given the evidence that there may be an optimal level of SNS activity for the facilitation of sexual arousal in women, Rellini and Meston (2006) investigated the possibility that activating the SNS before sexual arousal in women with a history of CSA and PTSD, who already have high baseline SNS activity, may have a negative impact on their physiological sexual arousal response. The same methodology used in the earlier exercise studies was applied to three groups of women: women with both a CSA history and a PTSD diagnosis, women with a CSA history and no PTSD diagnosis, and a control group of women with no history of CSA or PTSD. As in previous studies (e.g., Meston & Gorzalka, 1995, 1996), exercise had a significant facilitatory effect on physiological sexual arousal in the control group of women with no history of CSA. However, this effect did not hold for the women who had histories of CSA either with or without coexistent PTSD. In these women, there was no additional increase in physiological sexual arousal to the erotic videos during the exercise visit; to the contrary, there was a nonsignificant inhibition of sexual arousal responding. The authors speculated that, given these women had elevated baseline SNS activity, increasing SNS activity further, as was the case with exercise, may have put them beyond the optimal level of SNS activation for the facilitation of sexual arousal. The authors suggested that women with a history of CSA and/or PTSD who are experiencing problems with physiological sexual arousal may benefit from treatment that focuses on decreasing, rather than increasing, SNS activity during sexual activity. This might entail engaging in relaxation exercises prior to engaging in sexual activity.

Clinical Implications: Exercise and Sexual Arousal in Women Who Have Undergone Hysterectomy

Hysterectomy is the most frequently performed gynecological surgery in many world nations. In the USA, 80% of hysterectomies are intended to treat benign conditions (Merrill, 2008). Reports of positive outcomes of hysterectomies include the cessation of abnormal uterine bleeding, relief from menstrual symptoms and pelvic pain, and decreases in depression and anxiety (for review, see Farquhar & Steiner, 2002). However, some women experience negative symptoms post-hysterectomy, including depression, fatigue, urinary incontinence, constipation, early ovarian failure, and sexual dysfunction (e.g., Thakar, Ayers, Clarkson, Stanton, & Manyonda, 2002). Up to 40% of women report a decrease in their sex life following the surgery (e.g., Dennerstein, Wood, & Burrows, 1977), including lack of vaginal lubrication, loss of libido, and sexual pain. The uterine supporting ligaments contain sympathetic, parasympathetic, sensory, and sensory-motor nerve types and are considered a major pathway for autonomic nerves to the pelvic organs. It is feasible that the negative sexual outcomes following a hysterectomy are a result of the pelvic autonomic nervous being affected through excision of the cervix and separation of the uterus from the cardinal and uterosacral ligaments (Thakar et al., 1997).

If sexual arousal processes are negatively impacted by hysterectomy, and this is associated with autonomic innervation, differences between women who have and have not undergone hysterectomy may emerge under conditions of heightened autonomic arousal. To test this hypothesis, Meston (2003) examined subjective and physiological sexual arousal processes in women with a history of benign uterine fibroids who had or had not undergone hysterectomy using the same study methodology as in the prior exercise studies. Based on research that the uterine supporting ligaments are transected in hysterectomy (Butler-Manuel et al., 2002) and on research indicating that autonomic innervation is important for physiological sexual arousal (Giuliano et al., 2001), Meston (2004) expected that women who have undergone hysterectomy would have an impaired vasocongestive response to erotic stimuli, and that this would be most apparent during the exercise condition. The results revealed that, contrary to Meston's hypothesis, exercise significantly increased VPA responses in women who had undergone hysterectomy. Meston suggested that epinephrine and/or norepinephrine may have been responsible for the findings. Epinephrine and norepinephrine are released from the adrenal medulla during exercise, and they could have feasibly facilitated physiological arousal. Exercise could also have induced changes in endocrine factors, neuromediators, or substances released by endothelial cells (Guiliano, Rampin O, Allard J, 2002). Regardless of the mechanisms that may have been involved, it is clinically relevant that exercise facilitated physiological sexual arousal in women who had undergone hysterectomy. As such, exercise may serve as a noninvasive way to enhance sexual responding in women who experience sexual arousal difficulties post-hysterectomy.

Clinical Implications: Exercise and Sexual Arousal in Women Experiencing Antidepressant-Induced Sexual Dysfunction

Women compared to men are at twice the risk for mood and anxiety disorders, and are twice as likely to be prescribed antidepressants for their complaints (Thiels et al., 2005). In the USA, an estimated one in six women has been prescribed an antidepressant (Paulose-Ram et al., 2007), the most commonly prescribed antidepressants being selective serotonin reuptake inhibitors (SSRIs) and selective norepinephrine reuptake inhibitors (SNRIs). The vast majority of women taking antidepressants (96%) report at least one sexual side effect (Clayton et al., 2006), most commonly decreased desire, decreased arousal, and impaired orgasm. Both SSRIs and SNRIs are associated with these sexual problems, though SNRIs have been shown to have lower rates of arousal and orgasm side effects compared to SSRIs (Serretti & Chiesa, 2009).

The sexual side effects of SSRIs are most likely linked to peripheral nervous system adrenergic pathways (Montejo & Rico-Villademoros, 2008), particularly to changes in SNS activity (Serretti & Chiesa, 2009). Antidepressants, specifically SSRIs, inhibit serotonin (5HT) reuptake via antagonism of the serotonin transporter, which increases synaptic serotonin (Stahl, 1998). It is generally accepted that serotonin diminishes sexual function (e.g., Stahl, 2001), likely due to its inhibitory effect on norepinephrine (Millan et al., 2000), which is associated with sympathetically controlled blood vessels (Gothert et al., 1995) and other peripheral nervous system outputs (e.g., Hull, Muschamp, & Sato, 2004). In other words, SSRIs likely suppress SNS activity through norepinephrine release (Shores et al., 2001) and through sympathetic muscle and vascular nerve firing (Barton et al., 2007). Unlike SSRIs, SNRIs may counter the inhibition of norepinephrine, which occurs due to increased serotonin, by facilitating an increase in the availability of norepinephrine (Licht et al., 2009). Given that moderate SNS activity, compared to very high or very low SNS activity, is associated with increased genital arousal, it follows that SNRIs, which suppress SNS activity less than SSRIs, are associated with lower rates of genital arousal problems than are SSRIs. Though there may be other mechanisms that contribute to the association between SSRIs and negative sexual side effects, SNS activity seems to play a strong role and may therefore be an important intervention target for this population. In addition, interventions that facilitate increased SNS activation affect the peripheral nervous system, so they are less likely to interfere with the central nervous system mechanisms that are presumably responsible for the antidepressants' beneficial therapeutic effects.

There are few treatment options for women who experience antidepressant-induced sexual dysfunction. Options including adding a drug to try to counteract the side effect, have the patient switch antidepressants in the hopes that a different antidepressant will not have the same side effect, or encourage the patient to take a "drug holiday," a structured interruption in treatment for a period of time, typically a few days. However, with respect to depression, drug holidays make little pharmacological sense, as they risk withdrawal symptoms, and they may lead to illness relapse (Baldwin & Foong, 2013).

Given the lack of strong treatment options for women with antidepressant-induced sexual problems, acute exercise is a viable intervention. As described earlier, acute exercise activates the SNS, which has been shown to play a mechanistic role in the relationship between antidepressants and adverse sexual side effects (Serretti & Chiesa, 2009). Recently, Lorenz and Meston (2012) examined the effect of acute exercise on genital arousal in women taking either SSRIs or SNRIs. The women participated in three counterbalanced experimental sessions, where they watched an erotic film while their genital sexual arousal (VPA) and their SNS activity was measured. During two of the three sessions, participants exercised for 20 min and viewed the nonsexual and erotic film sequence at either 5 min post-exercise or 15 min post-exercise. One session acted as a control, as women were simply asked to watch the film sequence without exercising. The authors hypothesized that the women who were on SSRIs were more likely to have increased SNS tone compared to their counterparts on SNRIs; therefore, their genital arousal would be greater 5 min post-exercise compared to 15 min post-exercise. Similarly, they expected that the women who were taking SNRIs would experience some of the benefits of the exercise intervention with respect to genital arousal, but to a lesser extent than those taking SSRIs. They also suggested that women who reported higher levels of impairment in genital arousal would experience the largest gains from the exercise intervention. The results showed that, as the authors hypothesized, SSRIs decrease SNS activity and genital arousal more so than SNRIs. That is, during the no-exercise control session, women taking SSRIs had lower genital arousal and SNS response to sexual stimuli than those taking SNRIs. More importantly, the authors found that, as anticipated, exercise-induced increases in genital arousal were greatest for those women reporting the lowest sexual arousal functioning.

Building upon these findings, a follow up study compared the effects of acute exercise immediately before sexual activity to exercise separate from sexual activity (Lorenz & Meston, 2014). Given that laboratory-based psychophysiological measures of female sexual arousal may not directly map on to reports of sexual function outside of the laboratory, Lorenz and Meston (2014) sought to examine potential differences between the effects of SNS activation on sexual responding (e.g., increased genital blood flow following acute exercise) and the general benefits of exercise on sexuality. Women who were experiencing antidepressant-induced sexual problems ($N=52$) were entered into a 9-week trial. Thirty-eight women out of the total sample met criteria for clinically relevant sexual dysfunction based on the Female Sexual Function Index (FSFI; Rosen et al., 2000), which has been shown to reliably differentiate between women with and without sexual dysfunction (Meston, 2003; Rosen et al., 2000). For the first 3 weeks, baseline levels of sexual activity were recorded. Participants were then randomized to either 3 weeks of exercise, three times a week, immediately prior to sexual activity or 3 weeks of exercise, also three times a week, at a time unrelated to sexual activity (at least 6 h between exercise and sexual activity). The women in this study were provided with a 30-min strength and cardio exercise video as well as a set of resistance bands in order to standardize the type of exercise across all participants. At the end of 3 weeks, participants crossed over to the other exercise condition.

Results revealed that, overall, exercise improved sexual desire, and for women who were experiencing clinically relevant sexual dysfunction at baseline, exercise improved overall sexual function. There was some evidence to suggest that exercise immediately before sexual activity was more beneficial than exercise in general. Overall, the results of this study indicate that exercise improves sexual function in women who report sexual problems due to antidepressant medication use, and there may be an additional benefit to exercising immediately prior to sexual activity.

Summary and Conclusions

The studies presented in this chapter strongly suggest that acute exercise increases physiological sexual arousal in women with normal or low levels of resting SNS activity. The most likely mechanism of action associated with the facilitatory effect of exercise on sexual arousal is SNS activation, although the roles of hormonal and other potential changes that occur with exercise cannot be ruled out. There appears to be an optimal level of SNS activation for the enhancement of genital arousal in women. Specifically, moderate increases in SNS activity have been associated with high physiological sexual arousal responses, while both very low and very high SNS activation are associated with lower physiological sexual arousal.

These findings have important clinical implications. For women who have normal baseline SNS levels and who are having problems becoming sexually aroused, as little as 20 min of acute exercise at a constant 70% of one's estimated maximum volume of oxygen uptake before sexual activity could help improve genital arousal. Acute exercise may also facilitate increased genital arousal in women who may have suppressed sympathetic activation due to hysterectomy, or antidepressant medication use, particularly SSRIs. As most of the treatment options for women with antidepressant-induced sexual dysfunction are pharmacologic in nature, acute exercise may be a valuable alternative for women seeking to increase their physiological sexual arousal without taking medication.

Drawing on the finding that high levels of SNS activation inhibited blood flow to the genitals, acute exercise prior to sexual activity may not be beneficial for women with high baseline SNS arousal. High SNS arousal is typical of women with high sexual anxiety, posttraumatic stress disorder, and childhood sexual abuse. For these women, treatments that decrease baseline SNS activity and SNS activity during sexual activity may prove more beneficial. In fact, chronic exercise training has been associated with lower SNS responses to acute exercise (Hackney, 2006). Level of chronic exposure to exercise is one of the most potent factors influencing the neuroendocrine stress response to a session of acute exercise. Women with elevated SNS arousal may benefit from regular exercise to reduce their basal SNS activity, which may, in turn, improve their sexual function.

Sexual arousal in women consists of both a genital (i.e., physiological) and psychological (i.e., the experience of being mentally "turned on") component, and both are important to a woman's overall sexual experience. This review focuses exclusively on genital sexual arousal because the studies presented were almost all conducted within a laboratory setting and the accurate measurement of psychological arousal is difficult to obtain in a contrived laboratory setting. Although laboratory studies often show a low concordance between physiological and psychological sexual arousal in women (for a review, see Chivers, Seto, Lalumière, Laan, & Grimbos, 2010), we would expect that in a real-life sexual scenario feedback from increased genital arousal post-exercise would serve to also enhance the psychological experience of arousal for most women.

It should also be noted that this review focused exclusively on the effects of acute exercise on women's sexual arousal response. The long-term, chronic effects of exercise on a woman's sexuality are also noteworthy. It is widely accepted that constructs such as self-esteem, body image, and body satisfaction are related to women's sexuality and overall sexual well-being. Exercise has been associated with improvements in self-esteem in both adolescents (e.g., Ekeland, Heian, & Hagen, 2005) and adults (e.g., McAuley, Mihalko, & Bane, 1997). Among healthy individuals, increased exercise has beneficial effects on body image (e.g., Adame & Johnson, 1989), and in women, researchers have noted a significant negative relationship between amount of exercise and body satisfaction (Tiggemann & Williamson, 2000). Exercise has also been linked to increased energy and decreased fatigue (for a review, see Berger & Motl, 2001), which collectively also play an important role in women's sexuality.

References

Adame DD, Johnson TC. Physical fitness, body image, and locus of control in college freshman men and women. Percept Mot Skills. 1989;68:400–2.
Baldwin DS, Foong T. Antidepressant drugs and sexual dysfunction. Br J Psychiatry. 2013;202:396–7.
Barton DA et al. Sympathetic activity in major depressive disorder: identifying those at increased cardiac risk? J Hypertens. 2007;25(10):2117–24.
Berger B, Motl R. Physical activity and quality of life. In: Singer R, Hausenblas H, Janelle M, editors. Handbook of sport psychology. New York, NY: Wiley; 2001. p. 636–71.
Berman JR. Physiology of female sexual function and dysfunction. Int J Impot Res. 2005;17 Suppl 1:S44–51.
Butler-Manuel SA et al. Pelvic nerve plexus trauma at radical and simple hysterectomy: a quantitative study of nerve types in the uterine supporting ligaments. J Soc Gynecol Investig. 2002;9(1):47–56.
Chivers ML et al. Agreement of self-reported and genital measures of sexual arousal in men and women: a meta-analysis. Arch Sex Behav. 2010;39(1):5–56.
Christensen NJ, Galbo H. Sympathetic nervous activity during exercise. Annu Rev Physiol. 1983;45:139–53.
Clayton A, Keller A, McGarvey E. Burden of phase-specific sexual dysfunction with SSRIs. J Affect Disord. 2006;91:27–32.
Dennerstein L, Wood C, Burrows G. Sexula response following hysterectomy and oophorectomy. Obstet Gynecol. 1977;56:316–22.
Ekeland E, Heian F, Hagen KB. Can exercise improve self esteem in children and young people? A systematic review of randomised controlled trials. Br J Sports Med. 2005;39(11):792–8. discussion 792–798.
Engelman E et al. Effects of clonidine on anesthetic drug requirements and hemodynamic response durign aortic surgery. Anesthesiology. 1989;71(2):178–87.
Farquhar CM, Steiner CA. Hysterectomy rates in the United States 1990–1997. Obstet Gynecol. 2002;99(2):229–34.
Fox CA, Fox B. Blood pressure and respiratory patterns during human coitus. J Reprod Fertil. 1969;19:405–15.
Geer JH, Morokoff P, Greenwood P. Sexual arousal in women: the development of a measurement device for vaginal blood volume. Arch Sex Behav. 1974;3(6):559–64.

Giuliano F et al. Vaginal physiological changes in a model of sexual arousal in anesthetized rats. Am J Physiol Regul Integr Comp Physiol. 2001;281(1):R140–9.

Giuliano F, Rampin O, Allard J. Neurophysiology and pharmacology of female genital response. J Sex Marital Ther. 2002;28 Suppl 1 2013:101–21.

Gothert M et al. Presynaptic 5-HT auto- and heteroreceptors in the human central and peripheral nervous system. Behav Brain Res. 1995;73(1-2):89–92.

Hackney AC. The male reproductive system and endurance exercise. Med Sci Sports Exerc. 1996;28(2):180–9.

Hackney AC. Stress and the neuroendocrine system: the role of exercise as a stressor and modifier of stress. Expert Rev Endocrinol Metabol. 2006;1(6):783–92.

Hamilton LD, Meston CM. Chronic stress and sexual function in women. J Sex Med. 2013;10(10):2443–54.

Hamilton LD, Fogle EA, Meston CM. The roles of testosterone and alpha-amylase in exercise-induced sexual arousal in women. J Sex Med. 2008;5(4):845–53.

Hancock M, Peveto C. Preganglionicneurons in the sacral spinal cord of the rat: an HRP study. Neurosci Lett. 1979;11:1–5.

Harte, C. & Meston, C.M., 2007. Gender comparisons in the concordance between physiological and subjective sexual arousal. In Paper presented at the International Society for the Study of Women's Sexual Health, Orlando, FL.

Harte CB, Meston CM. The inhibitory effects of nicotine on physiological sexual arousal in non-smoking women: Results from a randomized, double-blind, placebo-controlled, cross-over trial. J Sex Med. 2008;5(5):1184–97.

Hatch JP. Vaginal photoplethysmography: methodological considerations. Arch Sex Behav. 1979;8(4):357–74.

Heard-Davison A, Heiman JR, Kuffel S. Genital and subjective measurement of the time course effects of an acute dose of testosterone vs. placebo in postmenopausal women. J Sex Med. 2007;4(1):209–17.

Hew-Butler T et al. Acute changes in endocrine and fluid balance markers during high-intensity, steady-state, and prolonged endurance running: unexpected increases in oxytocin and brain natriuretic peptide during exercise. Eur J Endocrinol. 2008;159(6):729–37.

Hill EE et al. Exercise and circulating cortisol levels: the intensity threshold effect. J Endocrinol Invest. 2008;31(7):587–91.

Hull EM, Muschamp JW, Sato S. Dopamine and serotonin: influences on male sexual behavior. Physiol Behav. 2004;83(2):291–307.

Jovanovic UJ. The recording of physiological evidence of genital arousal in human males and females. Arch Sex Behav. 1971;1(4):309–20.

Komisaruk BR, Gerdes CA, Whipple B. "Complete" spinal cord injury does not block perceptual responses to genital self-stimulation in women. Arch Neurol. 1997;54(12):1513–20.

Krantz K. Innervation of the human vulva and vagina: a microscopic study. Obstet Gynecol. 1958;12:382–96.

Levin RJ. The physiology of sexual function in women. Clin Obstet Gynaecol. 1980;7(2):213.

Levin RJ. The mechanisms of human female sexual arousal. Annu Rev Sex Res. 1992;3:1–48.

Levin RJ. The physiology of sexual arousal in the human female: a recreational and procreational synthesis. Arch Sex Behav. 2002;31(5):405–11.

Licht CMM, Penninx BWJH, De Geus EJC. Response to depression and blood pressure control: all antidepressants are not the same. Hypertension. 2009;54(1):133512.

Linnamo V et al. Acute hormonal responses to submaximal and maximal heavy resistance and explosive exercises in men and women. J Strength Cond Res. 2005;19(3):566–71.

Lorenz TA, Harte CB, Hamilton LD, Meston CM. Evidence for a curvilinear relationship between sympathetic nervous system activation and women's hysiological sexual arousal. Psychophysiology. 2012;49(1):111–7.

Lorenz TA, Meston CM. Acute exercise improves physical sexual arousal in women taking antidepressants. Ann Behav Med. 2012;43(3):352–61.

Lorenz TA, Meston CM. Exercise improves sexual function in women taking antidepressants: results from a randomized crossover trial. Depress Anxiety. 2014;31(3):188–95.

McAuley E, Mihalko SL, Bane SM. Exercise and self-esteem in middle-aged adults: multidimensional relationships and physical fitness and self-efficacy influences. J Behav Med. 1997;20(1):67–83.

Merrill RM. Hysterectomy surveillance in the United States, 1997 through 2005. Med Sci Monit. 2008;14:CR24–31.

Meston CM. The effects of hysterectomy on sexual arousal in women with a history of benign uterine fibroids. Arch Sex Behav. 2004;33(1):31–42.

Meston CM, Gorzalka BB. The effects of sympathetic activation on physiological and subjective sexual arousal in women. Behav Res Ther. 1995;33(6):651–64.

Meston CM, Gorzalka BB. The effects of immediate, delayed, and residual sympathetic activation on sexual arousal in women. Behav Res Ther. 1996;34(2):143–8.

Meston CM, Heiman JR. Ephedrine-activated physiological sexual arousal in women. Arch Gen Psychiatry. 1998;55(7):652–6.

Meston CM, Gorzalka BB, Wright JM. Inhibition of subjective and physiological sexual arousal in women by clonidine. Psychosom Med. 1997;59:339–407.

Millan MJ, Lejeune F, Gobert A. Reciprocal autoreceptor and heteroreceptor control of serotonergic, dopaminergic and noradrenergic transmission in the frontal cortex: relevance to the actions of antidepressant agents. J Psychopharmacol. 2000;14(2):114–38.

Montejo AL, Rico-Villademoros F. Psychometric properties of the Psychotropic-Related Sexual Dysfunction Questionnaire (PRSexDQ-SALSEX) in patients with schizophrenia and other psychotic disorders. J Sex Marital Ther. 2008;34(3):227–39.

Nadelhaft I, McKenna K. Sexual dimorphism in sympathetic preganglionic neurons of the rat hypogastric nerve. J Comput Neurol. 1987;256:308–15.

Neuhber W. The central projections of visceral primary afferent neurons of the inferior mesenteric plexus and hypogastric nerve and the localization of the related sensory and preganglionic sympathetic cell bodies in the rat. Anat Embryol. 1982;163:413–25.

Palace EM, Gorzalka BB. The enhancing effects of anxiety on arousal in sexually dysfunctional and functional women. J Abnorm Psychol. 1990;99(4):403–11.

Paulose-Ram R et al. Trends in psychotropic medication use among US adults. Pharmacoepidemiol Drug Saf. 2007;16:560–70.

Rellini AH, Meston CM. Psychophysiological sexual arousal in women with a history of child sexual abuse. J Sex Marital Ther. 2006;32(1):5–22.

Riley AJ. Alpha adrenoceptors and human sexual function. In: Bancroft J, editor. The pharmacology of sexual function and dysfunction. New York, NY: Elsevier; 1995. p. 307–25.

Rojas Vega S, Hollmann W, Strüder HK. Influences of exercise and training on the circulating concentration of prolactin in humans. J Neuroendocrinol. 2012;24(3):395–402.

Rosen R et al. The Female Sexual Function Index (FSFI): a multidimensional self-report instrument for the assessment of female sexual function. J Sex Martial Ther. 2000;26(2):191–208.

Salonia A et al. Menstrual cycle-related changes in plasma oxytocin are relevant to normal sexual function in healthy women. Horm Behav. 2005;47(2):164–9.

Serretti A, Chiesa A. Treatment-emergent sexual dysfunction related to antidepressants: a meta-analysis. J Clin Psychopharmacol. 2009;29(3):259–66.

Simon JA. Identifying and treating sexual dysfunction in postmenopausal women: The role of estrogen. J Women's Heal. 2011;20(10):1453–65.

Shores MM et al. Short-term sertraline treatment suppresses sympathetic nervous system activity in healthy human subjects. Psychoneuroendocrinology. 2001;26(4):433–9.

Sintchak G, Geer JH. A vaginal plethysmograph system. Psychophysiology. 1975;12(1):113–5.

Sipski ML, Alexander CJ, Rosen R. Sexual arousal and orgasm in women: effects of spinal cord injury. Ann Neurol. 2001;49(1):35–44.

Sipski ML et al. Sexual responsiveness in women with spinal cord injuries: differential effects of anxiety-eliciting stimulation. Arch Sex Behav. 2004;33(3):295–302.

Smith S. Effects of antipsychotics on sexual and endocrine function in women: implications for clinical practice. J Clin Psychopharmacol. 2003;23(3 Suppl 1):27–32.

Smith AJ et al. The effects of aerobic exercise on estrogen metabolism in healthy premenopausal women. Cancer Epidemiol Biomarkers Prev. 2013;22(5):756–64.

Stahl SM. Mechanism of action of serotonin selective reuptake inhibitors. J Affect Disord. 1998;51(3):215–35.

Stahl SM. The psychopharmacology of sex, part 1: neurotransmitters and the 3 phases of human sexual response. J Clin Psychiatry. 2001;62(2):1–47.

Thakar R et al. Bladder, bowel and sexual function after hysterectomy for benign conditions. Br J Obstet Gynaecol. 1997;104(9):983–7.

Thakar R et al. Outcomes after total versus subtotal abdominal hysterectomy. N Engl J Med. 2002;347(17):1318–25.

Thayer JF, Yamamoto SS, Brosschot JF. The relationship of autonomic imbalance, heart rate variability and cardiovascular disease risk factors. Int J Cardiol. 2010;141(2):122–31.

Thiels C et al. Gender differences in routine treatment of depressed outpatients with the selective serotonin reuptake inhibitor sertraline. Int Clin Psychopharmacol. 2005;20(1):1–7.

Tiggemann M, Williamson S. The effect of exercise on body satisfaction and self-esteem as a function of gender and age. Sex Roles. 2000;43(1):119–27.

Vingren JL. Effect of resistance exercise on muscle steroid receptor protein content in strength-trained men and women. Steroids. 2009;74(13-14):1033–9.

Vingren JL et al. Testosterone physiology in resistance exercise and training. Sports Med. 2012;40(12):1037–53.

Wiedeking C, Ziegler MG, Lake CR. Plasma noradrenaline and dopamine-beta-hydroxylase during human sexual activity. J Psychiatr Res. 1979;15:139–45.

Yehuda R. Risk and resilience in posttraumatic stress disorder. J Clin Psychiatry. 2003;65:29–36.

Chapter 14
Sex Hormones, Menstrual Cycle and Resistance Exercise

Yuki Nakamura and Katsuji Aizawa

Introduction

During a normal menstrual cycle, women are exposed to a continuously changing profile of female sex steroid hormones. Estrogen starts to increase halfway through the follicular phase, and peaks just prior to ovulation. Estrogen and progesterone are both elevated during the middle of the luteal phase (Table 14.1) and have profound physiological effects (see earlier chapters in this book). To better understand the relationship between the menstrual cycle and resistance exercise in women, it is important to consider the hormonal fluctuations that occur throughout the menstrual cycle. This chapter attempts to address these points.

Estrogen receptors have been localized to skeletal muscle tissue as well as tendons and ligaments. Through these receptors estrogen is thought to influence the turnover of skeletal muscle and connective tissue proteins at rest in the postabsorptive phase and enhance sensitivity to anabolic stimuli (Hansen and Kjaer 2014). In women, estradiol (the principal estrogen, see Chap. 1) functions as an antioxidant and membrane stabilizer during exercise, particularly exercise that induces high levels of oxidative stress, such as intense aerobic and resistance exercise. The protective role of estradiol appears to be a primary factor in mitigating muscle damage due to exercise stress and is evidenced by the smaller inflammatory response found in women (Fleck and Kraemer 2014; Enns and Tiidus 2010).

Interesting, women experience a rapid decline in muscle mass and strength around menopause when estrogen levels decline dramatically. These changes may

---

Y. Nakamura, Ph.D. (✉)
St. Margaret's Junior College, 4-29-23 Kugayama,
Suginami, Tokyo 168-8626, Japan
e-mail: yuki.jp7@gmail.com

K. Aizawa, Ph.D.
Senshu University, 2-1-1 Higashimita, Tama-ku, Kanagawa, 214-8580, Japan

© Springer International Publishing Switzerland 2017
A.C. Hackney (ed.), *Sex Hormones, Exercise and Women*,
DOI 10.1007/978-3-319-44558-8_14

Table 14.1 Menstrual cycle phase with corresponding variations in basal body temperature and fluctuations of ovarian female sex hormones

Menstrual cycle phase (days of menstrual cycle[a])		Basal body temperature (BBT)	Estrogen concentration	Progesterone concentration
Follicular (1–13)	Early follicular (2–7)	Lower temperature	Low	Low
Ovulation (14)	Late follicular (9–13)	Lower temperature	High	Low
Luteal (15–28)	Mid-luteal (18–24)	Higher temperature	High	High

[a]Based on a 28-day cycle with ovulation occurring on day 14 (Janse de Jonge 2003)

at least partly be related to the hormonal changes during aging. The striking decline in muscle strength during perimenopause and after menopause can be reversed with hormone replacement therapy (Jabbour et al. 2006).

In contrast, there is a paucity of data on the effects of progesterone on skeletal muscle, although progesterone is purported to be catabolic (Oosthuyse and Bosch 2010). Another difficulty in interpreting menstrual cycle research stems from the interaction between estrogen and progesterone. During the early follicular phase, estrogen and progesterone levels are both low, but in the late follicular phase there are high estrogen concentrations and low progesterone concentrations. In the mid-luteal phase, levels of both estrogen and progesterone are high. To compare the increase in estrogen concentration relative to progesterone concentration, some studies have reported the estrogen/progesterone ratio in the luteal phase. This ratio may provide information about the opposing effects of estrogen and progesterone (Janse de Jonge 2003).

To understand the relationship between the menstrual cycle and exercise in women, researchers, athletes and coaches should take physical and mental symptoms related to menstruation into account, not only the effects of sex hormones on skeletal muscles. Furthermore, dysmenorrhea (painful menstruation) and premenstrual syndrome (PMS) which can involve mood swings, tender breasts, food cravings, fatigue, irritability, and depression, are commonly seen in eumenorrheic women. These symptoms in turn may affect performance and physical and mental conditions for training and performance during the menstrual cycle phases.

Muscle Strength During the Menstrual Cycle

Several review articles on muscle strength during the menstrual cycle (Constantini et al. 2005; Janse de Jonge 2003; Lebrun 1994) have reported that some studies found greater strength in the follicular phase or in the ovulatory phase than in the luteal phase, whereas other studies have reported that strength was greater in the mid-luteal phase. A majority of studies could not find any changes in muscle strength over the menstrual cycle. In particular, recent studies measuring estrogen and progesterone concentration in order to verify menstrual cycle phase have reported no changes over the menstrual cycle in isokinetic peak torque of knee extensors and flexors and maximum isometric strength of knee extensors (Bambaeichi et al. 2004), maximum voluntary isometric force of the first dorsal interosseous muscle (Elliott et al. 2003), or handgrip strength and isokinetic muscle strength of knee extensors (peak torque), muscle endurance, and one leg hop test (Fridén et al. 2003). Based on these results, from a very limited number of studies, it can be concluded there is little or no difference in muscle strength at various times during the menstrual cycle. However, since there are many factors that can potentially influence exercise performance such as self-expectations, negative attitudes toward menstruation, and weight gain, the effect of the menstrual cycle on performance is probably very individual-specific and much more research is needed.

Anabolic Hormones and Resistance Exercise in Women

Resistance exercise provides a potent stimulus for muscular adaptation. This process is mediated, at least in part, by acute and chronic hormonal responses to resistance training, including changes in testosterone, growth hormone (GH), dehydroepiandrosterone sulfate (DHEA-S), and insulin-like growth factor I (IGF-I) (Consitt et al. 2002; Fleck and Kraemer 2014; Kahn et al. 2002; Kraemer and Ratamess 2005). This is true for both sexes. However, the resistance exercise-induced anabolic hormone changes are considerably different in men and women.

Testosterone, a major androgenic-anabolic hormone, exerts a significant influence on anabolic functions in the human body, especially in males. Serum testosterone concentration is acutely elevated immediately following heavy resistance exercise in men, although several factors such as muscle mass, exercise intensity and volume, nutrition intake, and training experience play a role (Fleck and Kraemer 2014). At rest women have a 10- to 40-fold lower blood concentrations of testosterone than men (Kraemer et al. 1991; Vingren et al. 2010). Previous studies have reported that concentrations of testosterone do not change acutely after resistance exercise in women (Kraemer et al. 1991, 1993; Staron et al. 1994; Häkkinen and Pakarinen 1995) (Fig. 14.1), but some other data challenges this construct in relation to other exercise forms (Lane et al. 2015).

GH appears to be involved in the growth of skeletal muscle and many other tissues in the body. It also appears to play a vital role in the body's adaptation to the stimulus of resistance training (Fleck and Kraemer 2014). The GH response to resistance training is quite similar between the sexes. A high-intensity and high-volume resistance exercise program with short rest periods has been shown to induce a post-exercise increase in GH in both men and women (Kraemer et al. 1991; Häkkinen and Pakarinen 1995) (Fig. 14.2).

IGF-I is a salient biomarker for monitoring health, fitness, and training status. It also reflects nutritional status as well (Fleck and Kraemer 2014). The acute response

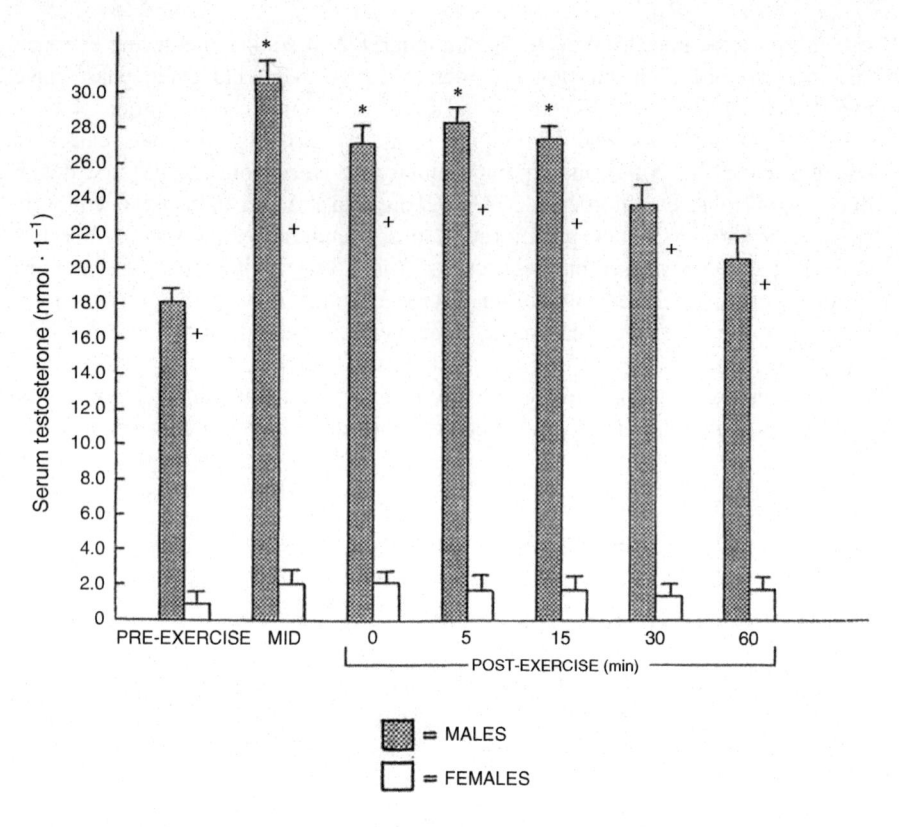

Fig. 14.1 Serum testosterone concentrations in men and women after the same resistance training session consisting of three sets of eight exercises at 10RM (ten repetition maximum) with 1 min of rest between sets and exercises (Kraemer et al. 1991). *Significantly different from pre-exercise value in the same sex; +significantly different from females at the same time point

of IGF-I to resistance exercise remains unclear. Most studies have shown no change in IGF-I during or immediately following an acute bout of resistance exercise (Kraemer et al. 1993; Consitt et al. 2001), whereas a few studies have shown acute elevations during and following resistance exercise (Kraemer et al. 1991; Kraemer and Ratamess 2005). However, long-term studies in women have shown elevations in resting IGF-I, particularly during high-volume training (Marx et al. 2001; Koziris et al. 1999). Interestingly, researches showed that GH and IGF-I appear to compensate for the attenuated testosterone response to signal muscle tissue growth in women and therefore may play a more central role in muscle hypertrophy than they do in men (Fleck and Kraemer 2014).

In women, about 90 % of circulating testosterone is derived from the metabolism of peripheral precursors, in particular from DHEA-S (Baulieu 1996; Labrie et al. 1997). DHEA-S is actually the predominant adrenal steroid hormone in both sexes. Regrettably, there is little information available on acute responses of DHEA-S to

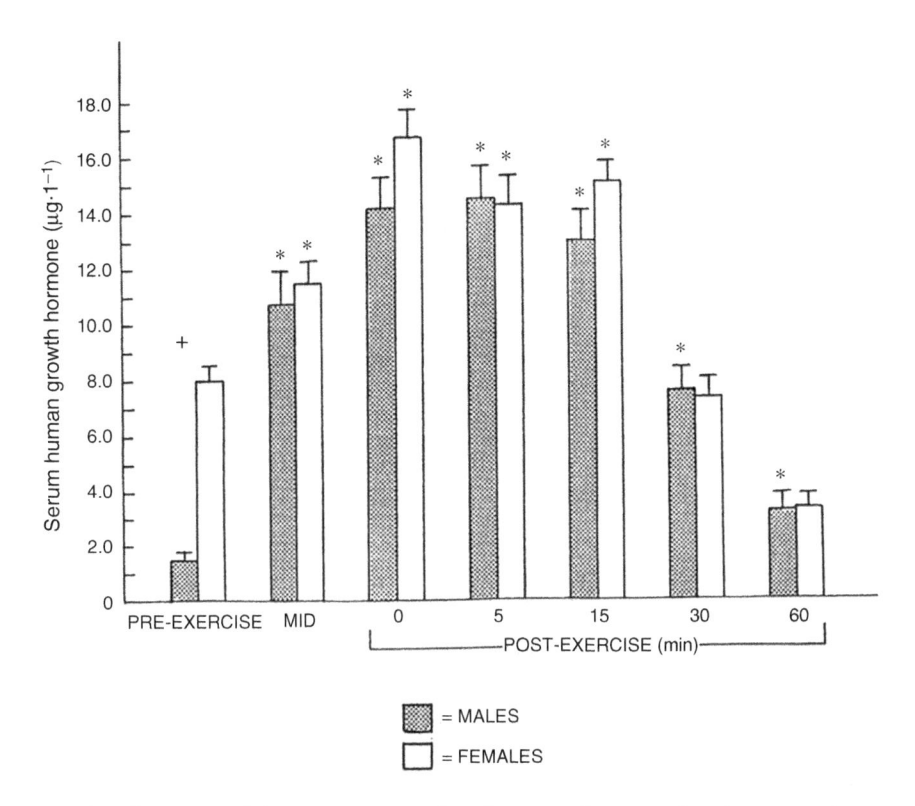

Fig. 14.2 Serum growth hormone concentrations in men and women after the same resistance training session consisting of three sets of eight exercises at 10RM with 1 min of rest between sets and exercises (Kraemer et al. 1991). *Significantly different from pre-exercise value in the same sex; +significantly different from females at the same time point

resistance exercise in women (Enea et al. 2011). Riechman et al. (2004) reported that acute resistance exercise increases blood DHEA-S levels in both men and women. Aizawa et al. (2003) have reported a dramatic increase in resting serum DHEA-concentrations after 8 weeks of resistance training. Furthermore, Aizawa et al. (2006) demonstrated that serum DHEA-S levels are positively correlated with leg extensor power in female athletes, but not in male athletes (Fig. 14.3). These findings suggest that blood DHEA-S levels in female athletes may reflect training-induced adaptation and plays an important role in muscular strength development. DHEA-S may also play a major biological role in women through its transformation into active androgens and estrogens (McMurray and Hackney 2000).

Thus, it is clear there are sex (gender) differences in basal anabolic hormone levels and responses to exercise. Nevertheless, women and men display similar relative changes in hypertrophy with resistance exercise. Although not discussed here, other hormones or mechanisms may also be responsive to resistance training and thus affect long-term adaptations to resistance training in women (see McMurray and Hackney 2000).

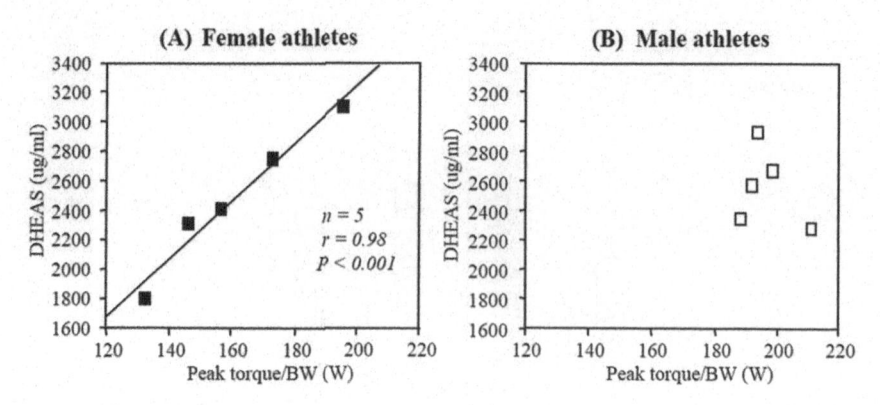

Fig. 14.3 Serum DHEA-S levels were positively correlated with leg extensor power (peak torque/body weight) in female athletes but not in males athletes (Aizawa et al. 2006)

Hormonal Responses to Resistance Exercise During Different Menstrual Cycle Phases

It has been suggested that many factors (e.g., sex, age, fitness level, nutritional status, exercise variables) influence hormonal responses to resistance exercise (Consitt et al. 2002; Kraemer and Ratamess 2005). When interpreting a woman's hormonal response to training, the potential effects of the menstrual cycle must be considered, because the hormonal responses to exercise are modified by the ovarian systems in women. Logically then understanding the potential effects of the menstrual cycle is vital for female athletes and their coaches.

Previous studies have reported that GH concentrations are higher in the periovulatory phase than in the early follicular phase (Faria et al. 1992; Ovesen et al. 1998). Kraemer et al. (1995) demonstrated that low-volume resistance exercise induces larger increases in estradiol, GH, and androstenedione in the mid-luteal phase than in the early follicular phase, although they did not compare the responses within the same individuals. Nakamura et al. (2011) have investigated the effect of the menstrual cycle on ovarian and anabolic hormonal responses to acute resistance exercise in young women. Specifically in this work eight eumenorrheic women and eight women with menstrual disorders including oligomenorrhea and amenorrhea were enrolled in the study. All subjects were recreationally active young women (18–30 years of age) and were not using oral contraceptives. The eumenorrheic women participated in two series of exercise sessions, one in the early follicular phase (days 4–7 of the menstrual cycle) and one in the mid-luteal phase (7–10 days after ovulation). The women with menstrual disorders participated in a series of exercise session on an arbitrary day. All subjects performed three sets each of resistance exercises (lat pull-downs, leg curls, bench presses, leg extensions, and squats) at 75–80 % of the one-repetition maximum with 1 min of rest between sets. Blood samples were obtained before exercise and immediately, 30 min, and 60 min after exercise. The effects of the menstrual cycle phase in eumenorrheic women are described in this section of the chapter, and the effects of menstrual status in women with menstrual disorders are described in the next section.

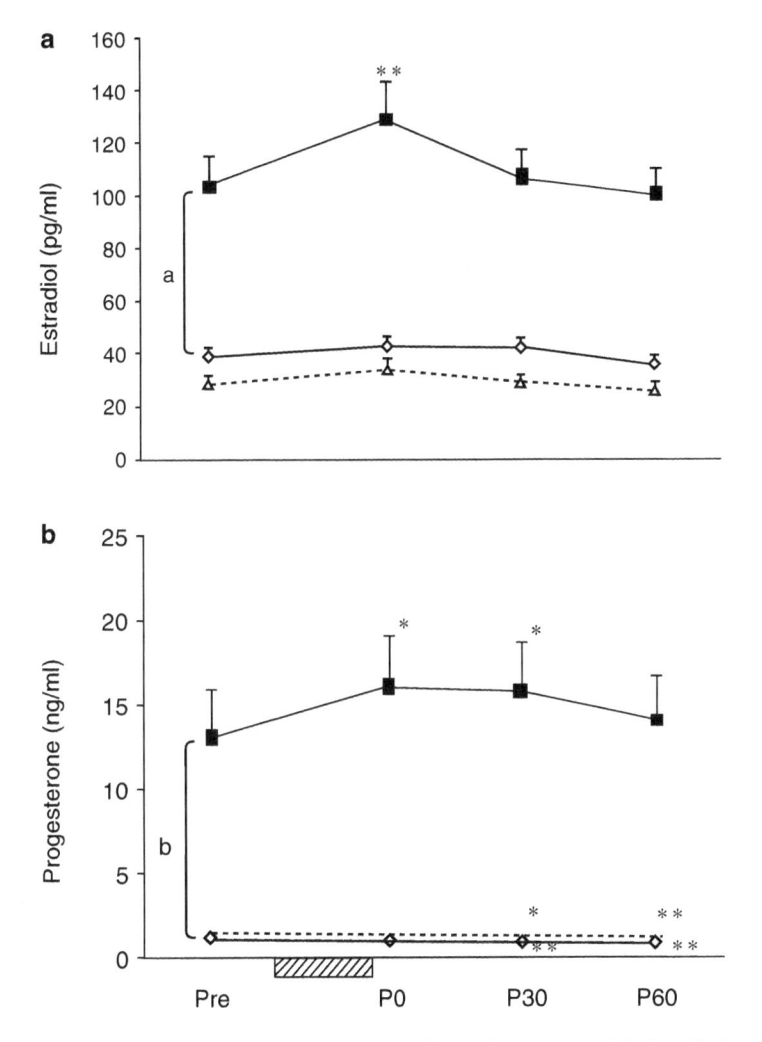

Fig. 14.4 Concentrations of ovarian hormones (estradiol and progesterone) before (Pre) and after resistance exercise: immediately after the end of the resistance exercise: (P0), 30 min after exercise. (P30) and 60 min after exercise (P60). In the mid-luteal phase, these hormones increased after exercise but they did not change in the early follicular phase and in women with menstrual disorders. Early follicular phase: *diamond*, mid-luteal phase: *filled square*, women with menstrual disturbance: *triangle*. Data are expressed as means ± SEM. *$P<0.05$, **$P<0.01$ versus Pre. ª$P<0.001$, ᵇ$P<0.01$ between Pre in the early follicular phase and Pre in the mid-luteal phase. The *hatched box* represents resistance exercise (Nakamura et al. 2011)

In the mid-luteal phase, serum estradiol and progesterone increased after exercise but they did not change after exercise in the early follicular phase (Fig. 14.4). Serum GH increased after exercise in both the early follicular and mid-luteal phases. On the other hand, total secretion (area under the curve) of GH was increased significantly after exercise in the mid-luteal phase, but not in the follicular phase (Fig. 14.5).

Hornum et al. (1997) also demonstrated that total secretion of GH after a high-intensity cycling exercise was greater in the periovulatory phase (estradiol levels were high) than in the follicular phase (estradiol levels were low). These findings indicate that menstrual cycle variations in circulating estradiol levels may affect exercise-induced GH secretion. Testosterone and IGF-I concentrations showed no significant increase in response to the resistance exercise protocols during either menstrual cycle phases (Fig. 14.5). These findings are consistent with previous studies (Consitt et al. 2001; Copeland et al. 2002; Häkkinen and Pakarinen 1995; Häkkinen et al. 2000; Kraemer et al. 1993). DHEA-S concentrations showed no significant increase immediately after resistance exercise in either menstrual cycle phases; however, there was a significant increase in DHEA-S 60 min after exercise in the early follicular phase. Cortisol, a catabolic hormone, also did not increase after resistance exercise in either menstrual cycle phases (Fig. 14.5). Likewise, Häkkinen and Pakarinen (1995) reported no changes in cortisol levels after acute resistance exercise in women. Kraemer et al. (1998), however, found significant elevations in cortisol after acute resistance exercise in men and women. It is possible that these differences in the response of cortisol to exercise are affected by the training status of the subjects (Kraemer et al. 1998), daily hormonal fluctuation, or both factors interacting (Hackney and Viru 2008).

The findings from these studies suggest that anabolic hormone responses to resistance exercise (e.g., levels of ovarian hormones, GH) may be influenced by menstrual cycle phase and the hormonal changes associated with the phases.

Hormonal Responses to Resistance Exercise with Different Menstrual Cycle Status

Menstrual disorders such as oligomenorrhea and amenorrhea are functional disorders characterized by altered gonadotropin-releasing hormone pulsatility, loss of pulsatile gonadotropin secretion (FSH and LH), and, in turn, altered ovarian steroidogenesis (Meczekalski et al. 2000). These reproductive hormonal changes have the potential to impact of a variety of other hormones (McMurray and Hackney 2000). For example, Waters et al. (2001) reported that amenorrheic athletes had significantly lower (four- to five-fold) GH responses to 50 min of submaximal exercise (70 % maximal oxygen consumption$_{2max}$) compared with eumenorrheic athletes. Yahiro et al. (1987) reported that serum testosterone levels increased in eumenorrheic runners, but not in amenorrheic runners, after acute treadmill exercise.

As mentioned in the preceding section, Nakamura et al. (2011) investigated changes in ovarian and anabolic hormones after acute resistance exercise in women with menstrual disorders including oligomenorrhea and amenorrhea. Serum estradiol and progesterone concentrations in these women with menstrual disorders did not increase after exercise (Fig. 14.4). Immediately after the end of resistance exercise, GH concentrations in eumenorrheic women increased significantly from pre-exercise levels, but this difference was not observed in women with menstrual disorders. However, a small, but statistically significantly higher increase in IGF-I in response to resistance exercise

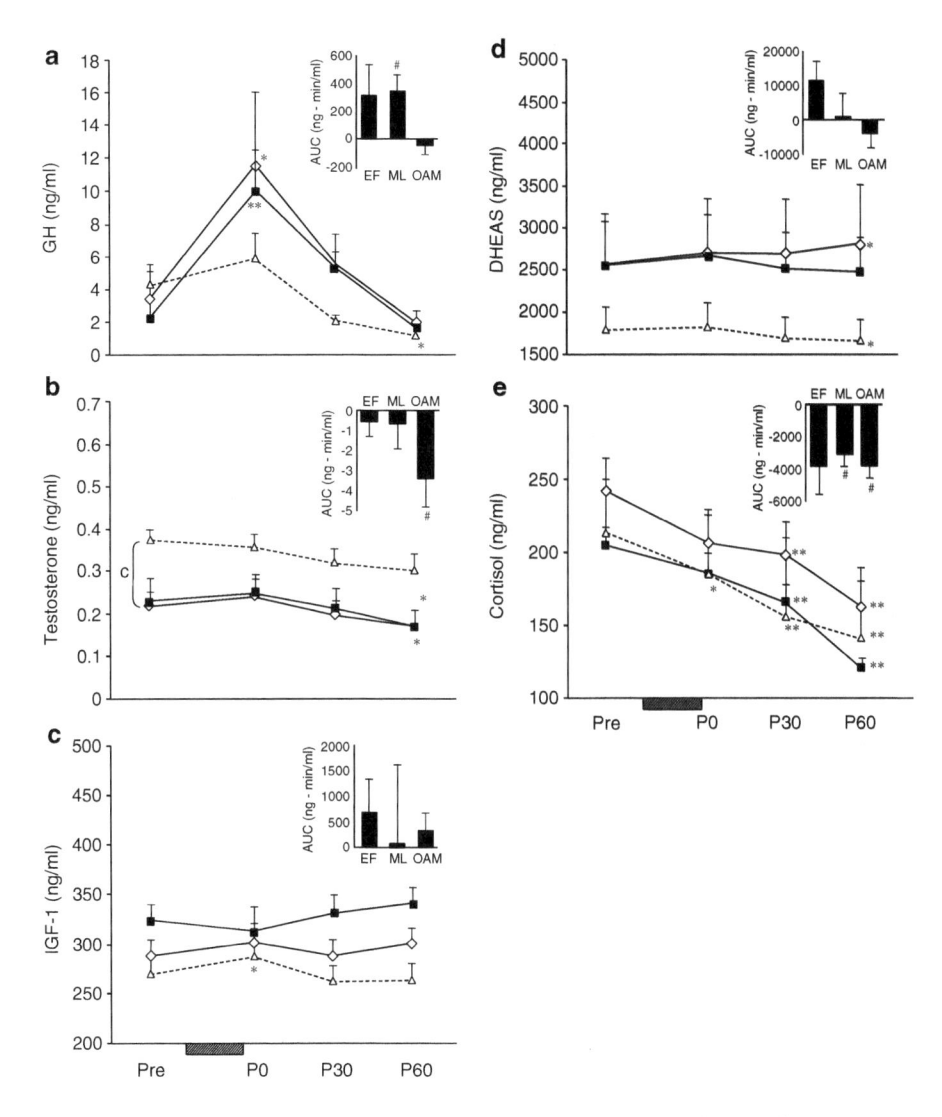

Fig. 14.5 Concentrations of anabolic hormones (GH, IGF-I, testosterone, and DHEA-S) and cortisol before (Pre) and after resistance exercise (immediately after the end of the resistance exercise (P0), 30 min after exercise (P30), and 60 min after exercise (P60). Early follicular phase: *diamond*, mid-luteal phase: *filled square*, women with menstrual disturbance: *triangle*. Data in the *small upper panels* represent the area under the curve (AUC). Data are expressed as means±SEM. *$P<0.05$, **$P<0.01$ versus Pre. $^c P<0.01$ between Pre in the early follicular (EF) phase and Pre in women with menstrual disorders (MD). The *hatched box* represents resistance exercise. #$P<0.05$ compared with zero (Nakamura et al. 2011)

was observed immediately after exercise in women with menstrual disorders. Testosterone and DHEA-S concentrations showed no significant increase in response to the resistance exercise protocols either, regardless of menstrual cycle status. However, total secretion (area under the curve) of testosterone was significantly lower in women with menstrual disorders. In addition, DHEA-S increased significantly 60 min after exercise in the early follicular phase in eumenorrheic women, but there was decreased significantly in women with menstrual disorders. And finally no significant differences in cortisol levels were found within any menstrual cycle status (Fig. 14.5).

The neuroendocrine mechanisms of exercise-induced GH release are not fully understood; however, GH secretion is controlled by hypothalamic hormones. These hormones include GH-releasing hormone, which exerts positive feedback, and somatostatin, which exerts negative feedback, on GH secretion (Giustina and Veldhuis 1998; Jenkins 1999). It is possible that the attenuated GH secretion of these women in response to acute resistance exercise is related to a disturbance in hypothalamic–pituitary function, but the mechanism of these events is not well understood at this time.

Findings from previous studies have suggested that estradiol stimulates GH secretion because estrogen replacement therapy increases GH secretion in postmenopausal women and prepubertal girls with Turner syndrome (Kanaley et al. 2005; Mauras et al. 1990). In addition, Kraemer et al. (1998) and Kanaley et al. (2005) demonstrated that GH responses to endurance exercise are higher in postmenopausal women receiving hormone replacement therapy than those who were not. This effect of estrogen may be due to a combination of withdrawal of somatostatin's (also known as growth hormone-inhibiting hormone [GHIH]) inhibitory tone, amplification of endogenous GH-releasing hormone release or its pituitary actions, and recruitment of other mechanisms that stimulate GH release (Giustina and Veldhuis 1998).

Specific endocrine differences between eumenorrheic women and women with menstrual disorders include cyclic fluctuations of estrogen and progesterone which are controlled by the hypothalamic–pituitary–gonadal axis (see Chap. 1). Women with menstrual disorders can be estrogen deficient on a long-term basis. Insufficient estrogen and progesterone feedback disturbs hypothalamic–pituitary axis responses (De Crée 1998). Thus, differences in ovarian hormone secretion status, that is, differences in hypothalamic–pituitary function between women with menstrual disorders and eumenorrheic women, may influence the GH response to acute resistance exercise. However, there appears to be no available information on anabolic hormonal responses to resistance exercise in women with menstrual disorders. There is also little information available on acute responses of DHEA-S to resistance exercise in such women. Riechman et al. (2004) reported that acute resistance exercise increases blood DHEA-S levels. Exercise-induced increases in DHEA-S concentrations have been attributed to an increased rate of secretion from the adrenal cortex in response to ACTH stimulation (Johnson et al. 1997). Meczekalski et al. (2000) investigated the hypothalamic–pituitary–adrenal axis in women with hypothalamic amenorrhea and reported that the ACTH response to corticotrophin-releasing hormone was significantly lower in amenorrheic women compared with healthy control women. Nakamura et al. (2011) reported DHEA-S levels were not significantly higher immediately after acute resistance exercise regardless of menstrual cycle status. Enea et al. (2009) reported short-term exercise does not induce increased adrenal steroid production in response to ACTH secretion. It is possible that a higher-volume resistance exercise program for a longer period could induce an increase in DHEA-S.

In summary, women with a menstrual disorder associated with low estradiol and progesterone levels have an attenuated anabolic hormonal response to acute resistance exercise. However, there is extremely limited evidence on this topic and more research is needed.

Menstrual Cycle Effects on Strength and Weight Training

The responses of sex hormones and anabolic hormones to acute resistance exercise varied by menstrual cycle status, suggesting that menstrual cycle status may influence exercise training-induced skeletal muscular adaptation. Thus, it would be possible that training programs for eumenorrheic women could be timed in accordance with the menstrual cycle to maximize anabolic effects. However, it is important to recognize that there are issues with the practicality of such an application to training. On the other hand, women with menstrual disorders associated with low serum estradiol and progesterone levels have an attenuated anabolic hormone response to acute resistance exercise, thus the long-term adaptations to resistance training may be different from that of eumenorrheic women.

Recent studies have begun investigating the trainability of muscle strength with menstrual cycle-triggered training. Sung et al. (2014) compared the effects of two different menstrual cycle-based leg strength training programs (follicular phase-based training versus luteal phase-based training) on muscle volume and microscopic morphological parameters. The increase in maximum isometric force with follicular phase-based training was higher than with luteal phase-based training, which was consistent with earlier findings of Reis et al. (1995). Follicular phase-based training was also associated with a higher increase in muscle diameter than luteal phase-based training. Moreover, they found significant increases in fiber type II diameter and cell nuclei-to-fiber ratio after follicular phase-based training but not luteal phase-based training. They recommend that eumenorrheic females should base the periodization of their strength training on their menstrual cycle.

In contrast, Sakamaki-Sunaga et al. (2015) reported no major differences among different training frequencies for arm curls during menstrual cycle phases with regards to muscle hypertrophy and strength. These investigators suggested that changes in female hormones caused by the menstrual cycle do not strongly affect muscle hypertrophy induced by resistance training.

It is notable that women with menstrual disorders characterized by low estradiol and progesterone serum concentrations show an attenuated GH response to acute resistance exercise (Nakamura et al. 2011). This could affect long-term adaptations to resistance training, but at this time there is no data available to clearly demonstrate this. Further studies are needed to demonstrate the short-term and long-term effects of changes in hormonal responses to resistance exercise on skeletal muscle by menstrual cycle status.

Conclusion

The fluctuations of sex steroid hormones have the potential influence muscle strength performance and hormonal response to resistance exercise in women. However, based on a number of studies investigated the effects of the menstrual cycle on muscle strength performance, it can be concluded there is little or perhaps no difference in muscle strength at various times during the menstrual cycle. On the other hand, though, there is very limited data about the hormonal response to resistance exercise in women as related to their sex hormone levels. A few studies do indicate that menstrual cycle state and status variations affect exercise-induced secretion of some hormones, and that there is a possibility of an effect on trainability of muscle strength to resistance training programs. But much more research work is needed on these topics. In addition, exercise performance and physiological response to exercise, resistance and otherwise, are probably very individual-specific and influenced by many factors and more research is also needed taking into account these individual-specific factors.

References

Aizawa K, Akimoto T, Inoue H, et al. Resting serum DHEAS level increases after 8-week resistance training among young. Eur J Appl Physiol. 2003;90:575–80.

Aizawa K, Hayashi K, Mesaki N. Relationship of muscle strength with dehydroepiandrosterone sulfate (DHEAS), testosterone and insulin-like growth factor-I in male and female athletes. Adv Exerc Sports Physiol. 2006;12:29–34.

Bambaeichi E, Reilly T, Cable NT, et al. The isolated and combined effects of menstrual cycle phase and time-of-day on muscle strength of eumenorrheic females. Chronobiol Int. 2004;21:645–60.

Baulieu EE. Dehydroepiandrosterone (DHEA): a fountain of youth? J Clin Endocrinol Metab. 1996;81:3147–51.

Consitt LA, Copeland JL, Tremblay MS. Hormone responses to resistance vs. endurance exercise in premenopausal females. Can J Appl Physiol. 2001;26:574–87.

Consitt LA, Copeland JL, Tremblay MS. Endogenous anabolic hormone responses to endurance versus resistance exercise and training in women. Sports Med. 2002;32:1–22.

Constantini NW, Dubnov G, Lebrun CM. The menstrual cycle and sport performance. Clin Sports Med. 2005;24:e51–82.

Copeland JL, Consitt LA, Tremblay MS. Hormonal responses to endurance and resistance exercise in females aged 19–69 years. J Gerontol A Biol Sci Med Sci. 2002;57:B158–65.

De Crée C. Sex steroid metabolism and menstrual irregularities in the exercising female. A review. Sports Med. 1998;25:369–406.

Elliott KJ, Cable NT, Reilly T, et al. Effect of menstrual cycle phase on the concentration of bioavailable 17-beta oestradiol and testosterone and muscle strength. Clin Sci (Lond). 2003;105:663–9.

Enea C, Boisseau N, Ottavy M, et al. Effects of menstrual cycle, oral contraception, and training on exercise-induced changes in circulating DHEA-sulphate and testosterone in young women. Eur J Appl Physiol. 2009;106:365–73. doi:10.1007/s00421-009-1017-6.

Enea C, Boisseau N, Fargeas-Gluck MA. Circulating androgens in women: exercise-induced changes. Sports Med. 2011;41:1–15. doi:10.2165/11536920-000000000-00000.

Enns DL, Tiidus PM. The influence of estrogen on skeletal muscle: sex matters. Sports Med. 2010;40:41–58. doi:10.2165/11319760-000000000-00000.
Faria AC, Bekenstein LW, Booth Jr RA, et al. Pulsatile growth hormone release in normal women during the menstrual cycle. Clin Endocrinol (Oxf). 1992;36:591–6.
Fleck SJ, Kraemer WJ. Designing resistance training programs. 4th ed. Champaign, IL: Human Kinetics; 2014.
Fridén C, Hirschberg AL, Saartok T. Muscle strength and endurance do not significantly vary across 3 phases of the menstrual cycle in moderately active premenopausal women. Clin J Sport Med. 2003;13:238–41.
Giustina A, Veldhuis JD. Pathophysiology of the neuroregulation of growth hormone secretion in experimental animals and the human. Endocr Rev. 1998;19:717–97.
Hackney AC, Viru A. Research methodology: endocrinologic measurements in exercise science and sports medicine. J Athl Train. 2008;43:631–9.
Häkkinen K, Pakarinen A. Acute hormonal responses to heavy resistance exercise in men and women at different ages. Int J Sports Med. 1995;16:507–13.
Häkkinen K, Pakarinen A, Kraemer WJ, et al. Basal concentrations and acute responses of serum hormones and strength development during heavy resistance training in middle-aged and elderly men and women. J Gerontol A Biol Sci Med Sci. 2000;55:B95–105.
Hansen M, Kjaer M. Influence of sex and estrogen on musculotendinous protein turnover at rest and after exercise. Exerc Sport Sci Rev. 2014;42:183–92. doi:10.1249/JES.0000000000000026.
Hornum M, Cooper DM, Brasel JA, et al. Exercise-induced changes in circulating growth factors with cyclic variation in plasma estradiol in women. J Appl Physiol. 1997;82:1946–51.
Jabbour HN, Kelly RW, Fraser HM, et al. Endocrine regulation of menstruation. Endocr Rev. 2006;27:17–46.
Janse de Jonge XA. Effects of the menstrual cycle on exercise performance. Sports Med. 2003;33:833–51.
Jenkins PJ. Growth hormone and exercise. Clin Endocrinol (Oxf). 1999;50:683–9.
Johnson LG, Kraemer RR, Haltom R, et al. Effects of estrogen replacement therapy on dehydroepiandrosterone, dehydroepiandrosterone sulfate, and cortisol responses to exercise in postmenopausal women. Fertil Steril. 1997;68:836–43.
Kahn SM, Hryb DJ, Nakhla AM, et al. Sex hormone-binding globulin is synthesized in target cells. J Endocrinol. 2002;175:113–20.
Kanaley JA, Giannopoulou I, Collier S, et al. Hormone-replacement therapy use, but not race, impacts the resting and exercise-induced GH response in postmenopausal women. Eur J Endocrinol. 2005;153:527–33.
Koziris LP, Hickson RC, Chatterton Jr RT, et al. Serum levels of total and free IGF-I and IGFBP-3 are increased and maintained in long-term training. J Appl Physiol. 1999;86:1436–42.
Kraemer WJ, Ratamess NA. Hormonal responses and adaptations to resistance exercise and training. Sports Med. 2005;35:339–61.
Kraemer WJ, Gordon SE, Fleck SJ, et al. Endogenous anabolic hormonal and growth factor responses to heavy resistance exercise in males and females. Int J Sports Med. 1991;12:228–35.
Kraemer WJ, Fleck SJ, Dziados JE, et al. Changes in hormonal concentrations after different heavy-resistance exercise protocols in women. J Appl Physiol. 1993;75:594–604.
Kraemer RR, Heleniak RJ, Tryniecki JL, et al. Follicular and luteal phase hormonal responses to low-volume resistive exercise. Med Sci Sports Exerc. 1995;27:809–17.
Kraemer RR, Johnson LG, Haltom R, et al. Effects of hormone replacement on growth hormone and prolactin exercise responses in postmenopausal women. J Appl Physiol. 1998;84:703–8.
Labrie F, Belanger A, Cusan L, et al. Marked decline in serum concentrations of adrenal C19 sex steroid precursors and conjugated androgen metabolites during aging. J Clin Endocrinol Metab. 1997;82:2396–402.
Lane AR, O'Leary CB, Hackney AC. Menstrual cycle phase effects free testosterone responses to prolonged aerobic exercise. Acta Physiol Hung. 2015;102(3):336–41.

Lebrun CM. The effect of the phase of the menstrual cycle and the birth control pill on athletic performance. Clin Sports Med. 1994;13:419–41.

Marx JO, Ratamess NA, Nindl BC, et al. Low-volume circuit versus high-volume periodized resistance training in women. Med Sci Sports Exerc. 2001;33:635–43.

Mauras N, Rogol AD, Veldhuis JD. Increased hGH production rate after low-dose estrogen therapy in prepubertal girls with Turner's syndrome. Pediatr Res. 1990;28:626–30.

McMurray RG, Hackney AC. Endocrine responses to exercise and training. In: Garrett W, Kirkendall DT, editors. Exercise and sport science. Philadelphia, PA: Lippincott, Williams & Wilkins; 2000. p. 135–61.

Meczekalski B, Tonetti A, Monteleone P, et al. Hypothalamic amenorrhea with normal body weight: ACTH, allopregnanolone and cortisol responses to corticotropin-releasing hormone test. Eur J Endocrinol. 2000;142:280–5.

Nakamura Y, Aizawa K, Imai T, et al. Hormonal responses to resistance exercise during different menstrual cycle states. Med Sci Sports Exerc. 2011;43:967–73. doi:10.1249/MSS.0b013 e3182019774.

Oosthuyse T, Bosch AN. The effect of the menstrual cycle on exercise metabolism: implications forexerciseperformanceineumenorrhoeicwomen.SportsMed.2010;40:207–27.doi:10.2165/11317090-000000000-00000.

Ovesen P, Vahl N, Fisker S, et al. Increased pulsatile, but not basal, growth hormone secretion rates and plasma insulin-like growth factor I levels during the periovulatory interval in normal women. J Clin Endocrinol Metab. 1998;83:1662–7.

Reis E, Frick U, Schmidtbleicher D. Frequency variations of strength training sessions triggered by the phases of the menstrual cycle. Int J Sports Med. 1995;16:545–50.

Riechman SE, Fabian TJ, Kroboth PD, et al. Steroid sulfatase gene variation and DHEA responsiveness to resistance exercise in MERET. Physiol Genomics. 2004;17:300–6.

Sakamaki-Sunaga M, Min S, Kamemoto K, et al. Effects of menstrual phase-dependent resistance training frequency on muscular hypertrophy and strength. J Strength Cond Res. 2015;30(6):1727–34.

Staron RS, Karapondo DL, Kraemer WJ, et al. Skeletal muscle adaptations during early phase of heavy-resistance training in men and women. J Appl Physiol. 1994;76:1247–55.

Sung E, Han A, Hinrichs T, et al. Effects of follicular versus luteal phase-based strength training in young women. SpringerPlus. 2014;3:668. doi:10.1186/2193-1801-3-668.

Vingren JL, Kraemer WJ, Ratamess NA, et al. Testosterone physiology in resistance exercise and training: the up-stream regulatory elements. Sports Med. 2010;40:1037–53. doi:10.2165/11536910000000000-00000.

Waters DL, Qualls CR, Dorin R, et al. Increased pulsatility, process irregularity, and nocturnal trough concentrations of growth hormone in amenorrheic compared to eumenorrheic athletes. J Clin Endocrinol Metab. 2001;86:1013–9.

Yahiro J, Glass AR, Fears WB, et al. Exaggerated gonadotropin response to luteinizing hormone-releasing hormone in amenorrheic runners. Am J Obstet Gynecol. 1987;156:586–91.

Chapter 15
Effects of Sex Hormones and Exercise on Adipose Tissue

Victoria J. Vieira-Potter

Overview of Functions of Adipose Tissue

In the human body, adipose (i.e., fat) tissue makes up between five and upwards of 50 % of total body mass. In severe cases of obesity, adipose tissue can make up over 80 % of body mass. Whereas ~20 % of the mass of an average adult male constitutes adipose tissue, this percentage is much greater among age-matched females, who have an average body fat mass of ~28 % (Thompson et al. 2012). The major function of adipose tissue is energy storage in the form of lipid as triacylglycerol (TAG), which is the most efficiently stored source of energy. Indeed, total body adipose tissue supplies up to ~800,000 kcal of energy whereas energy stored as glycogen in skeletal muscle and liver combined supplies only a fraction of that amount of energy. If the amount if energy stored in adipose tissue was to be stored as glycogen, it would take up ~500 % more volume (Frayn et al. 2003). Thus, energy storage in adipose tissue allows for survival over relatively long periods of inadequate energy intake, and is therefore a key evolutionarily advantageous feature.

While it has long been thought that the total number of adipocytes over the course of a lifetime is constant, newer evidence suggests that cell turnover does occur, albeit not at the rate of some other human cell types. Estimates are that the half-life of an adipocyte is ~300–400 days (Strawford et al. 2004) but more studies are necessary to validate that estimate. What is evident is that turnover does occur, counter to previous belief. Because of the body's almost constant reliance on a shift between adipocyte storage and lipolysis, the adipocyte cell is one that is plastic throughout its life and has tremendous capacity to expand and shrink depending on the circumstance. This plasticity requires considerable remodeling to accommodate these cycles of expansion and shrinking. This remodeling is achieved with the help

---

V.J. Vieira-Potter, Ph.D. (✉)
Department of Nutrition and Exercise Physiology, University of Missouri,
204 Gwynn Hall, Columbia, MO 65211, USA
e-mail: vieirapotterv@missouri.edu

of resident and acquired immune cells, such as macrophages. This may help explain, teleologically, why adipose tissue is a major site of immune cell localization, a topic to be discussed in more detail later.

Aside from its important energy storage role, adipose tissue serves many other essential functions such as organ structural support and temperature regulation/ insulation. Moreover, it is now appreciated that the adipose tissue plays important roles in immune and endocrine function and serves as an important mediator of immunity and energy balance. These later more recently discovered functions of adipose tissue have led to its classification as an endocrine organ and a new field of study called "immunometabolism" which investigates these interactions between the immune and endocrine systems (Ferrante 2013). Exercise and female sex hormones, as well as a variety of other biological and behavioral factors, profoundly affect the endocrine functions of adipose tissue. While the implications of this are only beginning to be investigated, it is quite possible that the influence of various factors (e.g., exercise, aging, sex hormones) on systemic metabolic health may be driven by changes that occur in the adipose tissue. Moreover, the sex differences that exist in age-related metabolism and metabolic responses to exercise training may be at least partially explained by sex hormone-mediated differences in adipose tissue metabolism.

The adipose tissue is a heterogeneous organ that is broadly classified as either "white" (i.e., WAT), accounting for ~95–99 % of total body fat mass and serving the main functions of energy storage and lipid mobilization, or "brown" (i.e., BAT), accounting for only a fraction of total body fat mass and functioning mainly to regulate body temperature via adaptive thermogenesis (Peirce et al. 2014). Unlike WAT, the major role of BAT is not in energy storage, but rather, energy dissipation as heat. The distinguishing characteristic of BAT is that it is mitochondria-dense and contains a multilocular phenotype such that lipid is stored as tiny droplets throughout the cell rather than as the one large droplet which is characteristic of adipocytes from WAT. The mitochondria found in brown adipocytes are unique in that they contain a high concentration of uncoupling protein-1 (UCP-1), a protein that uncouples oxidative phosphorylation from energy (i.e., ATP) production. This allows the brown adipocyte to produce heat rather than trapping substrate energy in a utilizable form. However, intriguing new research suggests that there is a great deal of plasticity in the major adipose tissue depots, such that some resident cells in WAT have the ability to take on a phenotype reminiscent of adipocytes from BAT; these cells have been classified as "brite" or "beige" adipocytes. On the other hand, it is likely that cells with similar plasticity are present in BAT such that they may, under certain environmental conditions (e.g., chronic energy overload as in obesity), take on a phenotype more similar to adipoctyes from WAT. This process in BAT, whereby adipocytes store more lipid and take on characteristics more similar to white adipocytes, has been described as "whitening" (Shimizu et al. 2014). Notably, both exercise and female sex hormones are among the growing list of factors that may influence "beigeing" of WAT. On the other hand, physical inactivity, obesity, and estrogen loss may trigger "whitening" of BAT. This exciting area of research is in its infancy.

Effects of Exercise and Estrogen on Adipocyte Lipolysis

Given its primary role in lipid energy storage, WAT is particularly important during fasting and exercise, especially when glycogen becomes limited. It is during fasting and endurance exercise that the process of adipocyte lipolysis becomes highly activated. Lipolysis is the major process that occurs uniquely in adipose tissue whereby the energy stored as lipid can be mobilized for use by other tissues. It is largely hormone-driven and is dependent upon the specific physiological condition (Fig. 15.1). During the fed state, the hormone insulin potently suppresses adipose tissue lipolysis whereas during the fasted state, when insulin levels are low and glucagon levels are high, lipolysis occurs unabated, resulting in an increase in circulating non-esterified free fatty acids (NEFAs) which serve as an important fuel for

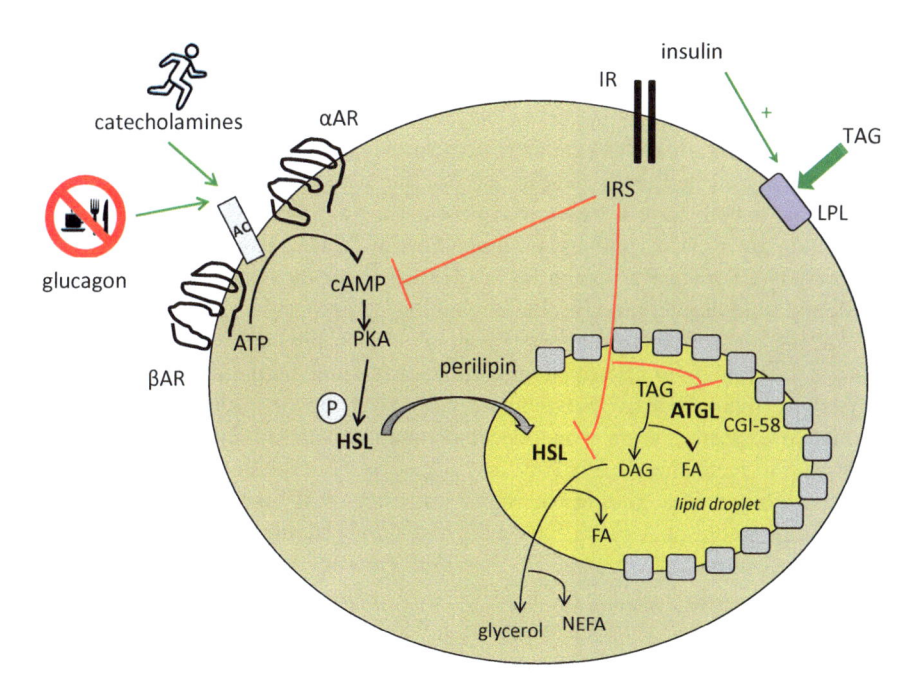

Fig. 15.1 Hormonal regulation of adipocyte lipolysis. Hormones released during exercise (i.e., catecholamines) and fasting (i.e., glucagon) bind to and activate membrane-bound ARs which trigger an AC-mediated increase in cAMP. cAMP activates PKA which phosphorylates and activates HSL to catalyze the hydrolysis of TAG stored in the lipid droplet; cAMP also activates perilipin allowing it to dissociate from the lipid droplet and thus facilitate lipolysis. During the fed state, insulin allows the adipocyte to take up fatty acids for storage via the activation of LPL and suppresses adipocyte lipolysis via activation of IRS, which leads to reduced cAMP/HSL activation. Insulin also inhibits ATGL which is another important lipase located in the lipid droplet which works closely with CGI-58. *AR* adrenergic receptor, *AC* adenylate cyclase, *cAMP* cyclic AMP, *PKA* protein kinase A, *HSL* hormone sensitive lipase, *IR* insulin receptor, *IRS* insulin receptor substrate, *TAG* triacylglycerol, *DAG* diacylglycerol, *FA* fatty acid, *NEFA* non-esterified fatty acid, *LPL* lipoprotein lipase

the energy-requiring skeletal and cardiac muscle cells. The mechanism of lipolysis involves increased activity of hormone sensitive lipase (HSL), an enzyme potently inhibited by insulin and activated by glucagon. On the other hand, during the fed state, insulin promotes fat storage in adipocytes by activating the enzyme lipoprotein lipase (LPL) (Wang and Eckel 2009) and inhibiting HSL. Not only does insulin increase TAG storage via LPL, but it also potentiates an increase in re-esterification of fatty acids in adipocytes for reasons that are not entirely clear (Frayn et al. 1994). In addition to being inhibited by insulin, adipocyte lipolysis is stimulated strongly by catecholamines (e.g., epinephrine and norepinephrine) which are released during exercise, and which result in beta-adrenergic-mediated mobilization of lipid (Hjemdahl and Linde 1983). Briefly, catecholamines bind to adipocyte cell surface adrenergic receptors, triggering intracellular signaling events culminating in the phosphorylation of HSL by protein kinase A (PKA); phosphorylated HSL mediates the hydrolysis of TAG molecules, resulting in the release of NEFAs and free glycerol from the adipocyte. Lipid droplet proteins such as perilipin are also important regulators of lipolysis and, when active, allow for the hydrolysis of lipid droplets within adipocytes. Other important players in the stimulation of lipolysis are adipose triglyceride lipase (ATGL) and comparative gene identification-58 (CG158). ATGL is a TAG hydrolase and the rate-limiting enzyme that promotes the catabolism of fat in both adipose and non-adipose tissues. Efficient ATGL activity requires activation by CG158, and upon stimulation of ATGL, release of fatty acids is increased. Alternatively, insulin, which decreases during exercise, deactivates both HSL and lipid droplet proteins, thereby inhibiting lipolysis.

During exercise, there is a strong positive relationship between adipocyte lipolysis and systemic fatty acid oxidation. In fact, net whole body fat oxidation is determined by many factors that regulate both WAT lipolysis and skeletal muscle oxidative capacity. With a net negative energy balance, fatty acid utilization increases to meet energy demands, and adipocytes shrink. As blood glucose levels become limited (e.g., during endurance exercise), WAT lipolysis increases as the body relies more heavily on fatty acid oxidation (Thompson et al. 2012). Thus, WAT lipolysis and skeletal muscle fatty acid oxidation are tightly linked such that WAT lipolysis increases the plasma NEFA concentration, and NEFAs are taken up by exercising muscles in a concentration-dependent manner. NEFA oxidation is dependent on both the intensity and the duration of the exercise. Given its near constant reliance on endocrine factors which regulate the flux between storage and lipolysis, and its primary role in secreting NEFAs into the circulation for transport throughout the body, it is not surprising that adipose tissue is among the most highly vascularized tissues in the human body. In fact, during resting conditions, blood perfusion is even greater in adipose tissue than in skeletal muscle (Thompson et al. 2012). During exercise, blood flow to both adipose tissue as well as skeletal muscle increases significantly. Undeniably, increased blood flow to adipose tissue during exercise is critical for neuro-endocrine control of lipid kinetics and NEFA mobilization to exercising skeletal muscle (Lambadiari et al. 2015).

Exercise training may also facilitate adaptations in adipose tissue lipolysis (Ogasawara et al. 2015) and fat oxidation to maximize fat utilization and preserve glycogen stores (Vicente-Salar et al. 2015). The importance of exercise-mediated regulation of adipocyte lipolysis is illustrated by evidence in rodents, which suggests that exercise training-induced cardiac tissue adaptations do not occur when adipose tissue lipolysis is prevented via genetic knock down of ATGL (Foryst-Ludwig et al. 2015). And, acute and chronic exercise may differentially affect lipolysis. For example, the cellular machinery associated with adipose tissue lipolysis undergoes significant and unique molecular changes with both acute and chronic exercise training (Ogasawara et al. 2015). There have been limited studies on how different types and intensities of exercise affect these changes. However, in one study of eumenorrheic women who were examined for substrate metabolism during a submaximal exercise bout at two different menstrual cycle phases (i.e., midfollicular characterized by higher estrogen levels and midluteal characterized by lower estrogen levels), significant differences in substrate utilization were noted. Specifically, carbohydrate oxidation was higher during the follicular compared to luteal phase. Correspondingly, lipid oxidation was higher during the luteal phase. Interestingly, at a greater exercise intensity, there were no longer significant differences in fuel utilization during menstrual phases suggesting that female sex hormones may affect fuel utilization during moderate but not intense exercise (Hackney et al. 1994).

Although sex differences have been appreciated, how estrogen affects adipose tissue-specific exercise training adaptations is completely unknown. While one study in humans failed to demonstrate significant sex differences between fatty acid and glycerol mobilization during rest or moderate-intensity exercise (Bulow et al. 2006), another study investigating the effects of short-term sub-maximal exercise on lipid mobilization showed that women have a more pronounced exercise-driven lipid mobilization response (Hellstrom et al. 1996). Although estrogen has been shown to enhance adipocyte lipolysis and fatty acid oxidation, postmenopausal women develop dyslipidemia, which may be related to an increase in basal lipolysis. Wohlers and Spangenburg, in mice, showed that loss of ovarian function results in increased ATGL protein content and decreased perilipin content; these differences compared to control, sham-operated animals associated with increased NEFA and glycerol levels, suggestive of increased basal lipolysis. Those differences were partially normalized with estrogen treatment, but not by exercise (Wohlers and Spangenburg 2010). In addition, premenopausal females have greater sensitivity to insulin's anti-lipolytic effect in adipose tissue causing them to be protected from adipose tissue loss (Luglio 2014). Interestingly, during endurance exercise, females may actually have a greater preference toward fat oxidation than males, which associates with greater glycogen preservation. Along those same lines, there is also some evidence that females have greater skeletal muscle intramyocellular lipid (IMCL) content and that a greater percentage of their IMCL stores associate directly with mitochondria following exercise, suggestive of a greater capacity to utilize those lipid stores (Devries 2016). The role of estrogen in this sex difference is not completely understood. In sum, definitive data on whether sex differences exist in exercise-mediated adipose tissue lipolysis are inconclusive and require further study.

Factors Affecting Adipose Tissue Distribution

WAT is classified broadly as subcutaneous and visceral depots. Visceral WAT describes that surrounding the internal organs whereas subcutaneous lies just beneath the skin throughout the body. Subcutaneous WAT is stored primarily around the hips and buttocks. The visceral intra-abdominal depot is most metabolically detrimental in that it associates strongly with insulin resistance and dyslipidemia. Estrogen appears to drive subcutaneous adipose tissue storage and estrogen-mediated adipose tissue distribution is thought to explain why females characteristically store fat in subcutaneous (e.g., hip, gluteal regions) whereas males tend to store fat viscerally. Other evidence that estrogen increases subcutaneous fat storage is that male-to-female transsexual individuals receiving estrogen therapy increase subcutaneous but not visceral fat deposition (Luglio 2014). This estrogen-dependent fat distribution pattern is considered metabolically protective and likely explains why premenopausal women are less likely to experience adverse obesity-associated metabolic outcomes compared to age-matched men (Lapid et al. 2014). Mechanistically, this might be due to the fact that subcutaneous fat is more insulin sensitive and thus serves an important blood glucose regulatory role. Equally important, this sex difference dissipates with age, when postmenopausal females begin to accumulate more visceral fat in the abdominal region concomitant with the natural cessation of ovarian hormones, including 17-β-estradiol (to be referred to simply as "estrogen" throughout this chapter). Also, in postmenopausal women who experience gains in adiposity with cessation of ovarian hormone production, estrogen replacement reduces visceral, but not subcutaneous fat storage (Mattiasson et al. 2002). Interestingly, despite increasing adipose tissue blood flow similarly in visceral and subcutaneous depots, catecholamine-driven lipolytic activation is greater in intra-abdominal compared to subcutaneous WAT (Enevoldsen et al. 2000). For this reason, exercise is particularly beneficial in reducing visceral fat and thus improving metabolic syndrome symptoms, such as dyslipidemia. The sex difference in adipose tissue distribution may also help explain why women compared to men are less responsive to exercise training in terms of body fat reduction.

As indicated above, the major sex difference in lipid metabolism and adipose tissue distribution is that lipid metabolism in females drives fat storage in subcutaneous WAT depots with the majority being deposited in lower body regions whereas males tend to favor central storage of lipid where it can be oxidized more readily (Varlamov et al. 2014). The earliest reports that ovarian hormones, particularly estrogen, can directly affect body fat levels via signaling specifically in adipocytes were from 1978 by Wade and Gray, who found that estrogen binds to a protein receptor in the cytosolic fraction of both white and brown adipose tissue depots (Wade and Gray 1978). It has also been appreciated since the 1980s that estrogen acts directly in the brain to augment food intake and stimulate voluntary exercise, and acts directly in adipocytes to decrease LPL activity and therefore limit excess lipid storage in adipose tissue (Wade et al. 1985). The aromatase knock-out mouse supports the notion that estrogen loss causes visceral WAT accumulation. In that rodent model in which endogenous estrogens cannot be synthesized, obesity is characterized by significant adipose accumulation in central (i.e., gonadal and intrarenal) depots (Endlich et al. 2013).

The sex difference in body fat content and distribution really begins to manifest during puberty, when increasing estrogen drives accretion of adipose tissue mass in females. Mechanistically, this may be due to an estrogen-mediated stimulation of preadipocyte differentiation in adipose tissue (Lapid et al. 2014). This effect of estrogen on adipose tissue development is not surprising since adipose tissue is essential for female reproductive capabilities. The increase in adipose tissue during pubertal development in females is a key factor which determines when reproductive maturity is reached. Notably, whereas a critical adiposity threshold needs to be reached in order for females to reach sexual maturity, this is not true for males. Leptin, a hormone produced and secreted by adipose tissue to be discussed in greater detail later, appears to be critical in this regard and is a powerful example of the importance of adipose tissue as an endocrine organ (Chehab et al. 1997). There is also sexual dimorphism in the effects of excess adipose tissue during development such that it potentiates early pubertal development in young females, whereas the opposite is true in young males where excess adiposity delays puberty (Crocker et al. 2014).

The important role of adipose tissue on female reproductive capabilities is also demonstrated by the fact that even moderate weight loss of 10–15 % of ideal body weight induces amenorrhea. Higher body fat percentage (26–28 %) in mature women has been thought to be necessary for regular ovulatory cycles and may influence reproductive ability in three major ways: (1) directly as adipose tissue is a source of estrogen via aromatization of androgen to estrogen by the aromatase enzyme present in adipose tissue; (2) shifting estrogen metabolism in such a way that influences its potency; (3) indirectly by changing the binding affinity of sex hormone binding globulin which binds estrogen, thus limiting its biological activity (Frisch 1991). It appears that ~22 % body fat is necessary to maintain a regular menstrual cycle; although some have reported regular cycles in athletes with <17 % body fat (Ramos and Warren 1995).

These sex differences in the relationship between adiposity and reproductive development are clearly related to differences in several endocrine factors, arguably the most important of which being estrogen. This is also illustrated by the enhancement of body fat gain in the subcutaneous region in early pregnancy (even in the absence of caloric increase), a period characterized by high levels of estrogen (O'Sullivan 2009). Estrogen's ability to enhance efficient fat storage in women is clearly metabolically beneficial in preparation for fertility, fetal development and lactation. Estrogen's ability to drive efficient fat storage may be due to its effect to suppress postprandial lipid oxidation (O'Sullivan et al. 2001). Taken together, estrogen promotes efficient fat storage, especially in subcutaneous depots, and potentiates lower rates of lipid oxidation, thus favoring energy retention in adipose tissue. Estrogen also appears to suppress visceral adipose tissue accumulation by suppressing de novo lipogenesis in this depot.

Role of Estrogen Receptors in Adipose Tissue Metabolism

The multitude of estrogen's effects on physiological and endocrine processes is virtually all mediated via its specific receptors. The best characterized receptors are the alpha and beta forms which are both classical nuclear receptors; it is estrogen receptor alpha (ERα) that is most heavily expressed in adipose tissue and likely modulates estrogen's metabolic effects on this tissue. But ERs α and β are expressed throughout the body and brain and ERα is thought to drive many global effects of estrogen, including adipose tissue deposition and fuel partitioning (Rettberg et al. 2014). Although the classical (i.e., genomic) pathway is thought to mediate most of estrogen's actions in the body, it is now known that non-genomic signaling also occurs. Via activation of membrane-bound ERs, estrogen (and possibly other ER ligands) can trigger a signaling cascade including PKA and mitogen-activated protein kinase (MAPK) cascades, which may facilitate cellular nitric oxide production and/or increase glucose transporter (i.e., GLUT4) translocation, thus improving insulin signaling (Wehling et al. 2006). The important role of adipose tissue ERα in mediating effects of estrogen is illustrated by rodent studies involving mice null for this receptor, which experience significant adiposity gains and disturbances in metabolic health. Studies of mutant mice will ERα selectively knocked out of adipose tissue recapitulates the adverse metabolic phenotype induced by removing ovarian estrogen production (e.g., insulin resistance), suggesting that many of the adipose tissue-specific adverse effects of estrogen loss are mediated through loss of signaling through this receptor. Together, these studies demonstrate the metabolically protective role of estrogen, signaling through ERα, in adipose tissue. The well known sex difference in systemic insulin sensitivity, where premenopausal women have significantly greater sensitivity than age-matched men, is likely driven by enhanced insulin sensitivity of adipose tissue in females; and this is likely mediated, at least in part, by ERα (Davis et al. 2013). Indeed, isolated adipocytes from the intra-abdominal region of females have been shown to have greater sensitivity to insulin compared to those from the same region in males (Kim et al. 2014).

It is well established that exercise training is among the most effective strategies to improve systemic insulin sensitivity. Given the role of ERα in enhancing insulin sensitivity, one study investigated the effect of exercise training on ERα expression in skeletal muscle. Interestingly, that study showed that exercise increased muscle ERα expression, but only in female rats; later work showed this effect to be muscle cell type-specific with increases being most evident in gastrocnemius muscle (Lemoine et al. 2002). Interestingly, even in adult men, exercise has been shown to increase skeletal muscle ERα (Wiik et al. 2005). Whether exercise-mediated changes in ERα are related to its insulin sensitizing effects has not been addressed but is an intriguing idea. While exercise is thought to mostly improve skeletal muscle insulin sensitivity, data also suggests that exercise enhances adipocyte insulin sensitivity. Studies are necessary to determine if exercise can increase adipocyte ERα expression and if this explains part of the mechanism by which exercise improves adipose tissue insulin sensitivity. Only one published study to date has addressed that question of whether exercise increases adipose tissue ERα, but that study was performed on male rodents only; nonetheless, those authors did not report an increase in adipose tissue ERα (Metz et al. 2016). While the influence of ERα and estrogen on the insulin-sensitizing role of exercise training on adipose tissue insulin sensitivity remains largely unknown, there is evidence in female rodents that aerobic fitness improves adipose tissue sensitivity across WAT and BAT depots. Remarkably, the adipose tissue insulin sensitivity difference between high and low-aerobically fit rats in that study was even more robust than that observed in skeletal muscle (Park et al. 2016).

Effects of Exercise and Estrogen on Brown Adipose Tissue (BAT)

While the vast majority of adipose tissue in the human body is WAT, as mentioned earlier, BAT also exists and has received significant attention recently. Until around 2007, it was thought that adult humans did not have physiologically relevant amounts of BAT. However, with new technologies allowing for BAT metabolic detection, now it is known that we do harbor some BAT. Further, although making up only a fraction of total adipose tissue mass, it appears to be very relevant from a metabolic standpoint. Due to its reliance on mitochondrial fatty acid oxidation that occurs in its specialized adipocytes to produce heat, BAT contributes to energy expenditure. In addition, studies have demonstrated that BAT activity also improves glucose homeostasis. While the major stimulus for BAT activity is cold, since the realization that functional BAT exists in adult humans, a growing body of research has investigated alternative mechanisms to activate BAT. This new research emphasis has been partially driven by the possibility of targeting BAT as an obesity-mitigating therapeutic. The mechanism behind the classic BAT stimulus, cold exposure, involves activation of the sympathetic nervous system (SNS). Upon SNS activation, norepinephrine (NE) is released into the circulation and binds to β-adrenergic receptors on the surface of brown adipocytes. This binding triggers an activation cascade involving G-proteins and adenylate cyclase activation, which ultimately results in lipolysis; the fatty acids released activate UCP-1, which then uncouples oxidative phosphorylation, and produces heat. Simultaneously, NE stimulates BAT glucose uptake; it is the stimulation of glucose uptake that allows positron emission tomography/computed tomography (PET/CT) scan technology to detect BAT activity and it is this technology that allowed for the discovery that human adults have functional BAT.

Falling under the physiological adaptation principle of hormesis, low levels of reactive oxygen species (ROS) have been shown to be, not only not detrimental, but *necessary* for the proper thermogenic functioning of BAT (Ro et al. 2015). When chemical antioxidants are over-expressed in BAT adipocytes, UCP-1 expression, and the associated thermogenesis, is suppressed. On the other hand, excessive ROS caused by dysfunctional mitochondria lead to oxidative damage, which impairs proper BAT function. Exercise may act to enhance "mitohormesis." Mitohormesis applies the definition of hormesis (i.e., *the process by which exposure to a low dose of a mild stressor promotes adaptive changes which enhance the capacity to tolerate subsequent stressors*) specifically to the mitochondria, suggesting that mitochondrial stress leads to healthy adaptations allowing the mitochondria to maintain cellular homeostasis upon subsequent stress (Merry and Ristow 2015). Exercise may promote this process by inducing low levels of ROS that then enhance oxidative metabolism. Since exercise stimulates the SNS and catecholamine release (i.e., NE and epinephrine), it has been hypothesized that exercise may activate BAT. That hypothesis was tested in a few rodent studies. In one such study, mitochondria were harvested from BAT of trained and untrained rats both before and after an exhaustive exercise bout (Gohil et al. 1984). What was found was that exercise actually reduced the oxidative capacity of BAT. However, early animal studies revealed that exercise trained rats have greater capacity for NE-stimulated BAT thermogenesis (Hirata 1982a, b); that is, those findings suggested that exercise may not activate BAT per se, but may increase its sensitivity to stimulated activity. However, this line of research has produced conflicting results. In fact, several studies using a variety of exercise modalities have reported that exercise training reduces the SNS response in BAT (Richard et al. 1992; Nozu et al. 1992; Yamashita et al. 1993; Larue-Achagiotis et al. 1995). This is quite the opposite of what happens with exercise training in skeletal muscle (Joseph et al. 2006). While some investigators who have reported that BAT thermogenic activity increases following exercise training in mice (Oh-ishi et al. 1996), others have reported an exercise-mediated reduction in BAT thermogenesis (Leblanc et al. 1982). This latter finding perhaps makes more physiological sense, as the authors speculate that an exercise-mediated reduction in thermogenesis would prevent energy wasting. Recent studies have confirmed that latter theory, that exercise is more likely to reduce than activate BAT activity. While there is a noticeable gap in the animal literature on the metabolic effects of BAT between ~1990 and 2007, there has been a resurgence of basic animal studies on BAT activity following the discoveries between the years 2007 and 2009 that human adults indeed harbor thermogenically active BAT (Sanchez-Delgado et al. 2015). It has since been discovered that BAT activity decreases with age, correlates inversely with BMI and obesity and is greater among premenopausal women compared to age-matched men (Sanchez-Delgado et al. 2015). In a cross-sectional study of adult males, cold-induced BAT activation was significantly lower among exercise-trained compared to weight and sex-matched sedentary controls (Vosselman et al. 2015). A renewed interest in the potential effect of exercise to increase non-exercise thermogenesis came about after a comprehensive study led by Speigelman and colleagues in 2012, in which it was found that exercise induced skeletal muscle secretion of a hormone (irisin) that was shown to increase UCP-1 expression in WAT in humans and animals (Bostrom et al. 2012).

A very interesting observation was made recently that adipocytes from BAT express ERα and that this receptor is essential for brown adipogenesis. A study of human fetal BAT demonstrated that it expresses both ERα and β, with ERα being the predominant form. This not only suggests that, like WAT, BAT is regulated by estrogens but also implicates estrogen as playing a role in BAT development (Velickovic et al. 2014). Thus, it is perhaps not surprising that females have more BAT than males and that estrogen regulates BAT thermogenesis (Martinez de Morentin et al. 2014). It also appears that there is sexual dimorphism in mitochondrial function of BAT such that female BAT has greater mitochondrial content and is less susceptible to oxidative stress (Nadal-Casellas et al. 2012); these protective characteristics are lost with ovariectomy in rodents and only partially restored with estrogen replacement, suggesting estrogen as well as other ovarian hormones may protect BAT mitochondrial function (Nadal-Casellas et al. 2011). It has been hypothesized that post-ovariectomy weight gain in rodents, and possibly, weight gain post-menopause in humans, is due in part to reduced BAT activity. Interestingly, early evidence cited that estrogen may increase energy expenditure independent of increased physical activity by increasing adaptive thermogenesis in BAT. While not all preclinical studies have supported this hypothesis (Nigro et al. 2014), it is possible that estrogens regulate BAT thermogenesis and that loss of estrogen signaling affects energy homeostasis in part by reducing non-activity energy expenditure via BAT activity (Martinez de Morentin et al. 2014). It is also important to note that estrogen is an antioxidant and increases gene expression of natural antioxidant molecules which may protect adipocytes from mitochondrial oxidative stress. This point will be discussed further in the section to follow.

Mitochondrial Function and Browning of WAT (*Can Exercise and Estrogen Make Fat Cells Fit?*)

While BAT is characteristically the mitochondria-dense depot, all adipocytes contain mitochondria. In fact, mitochondria are essential for many adipocyte functions including lipolysis, triglyceride re-esterification and storage, and adipokine production. And it has been appreciated since the early 1990s that exercise training induces mitochondrial adaptations in WAT that are similar to those that occur in skeletal muscle (Stallknecht et al. 1991). It appears that the exercise-mediated increase in mitochondrial biogenesis in adipose is driven by catecholaminergic mechanisms. Moreover, 'healthy' adipoctyes are known to have highly functional mitochondria whereas 'unhealthy' adipocytes are characterized by a profile of high inflammatory/oxidative stress associated with dysfunctional mitochondria (Vieira-Potter et al. 2015). Thus, it is possible that exercise training enhances adipocyte function in part via its positive effects on adipocyte mitochondria. This may help explain the evidence that exercise training mitigates metabolic dysfunction by enhancing adipocyte differentiation in BAT and/or increasing WAT browning (Xu et al. 2011). A recent elegant study showed that the transplantation of subcutaneous WAT from exercise-trained rodents into sedentary, insulin resistant rodents led to remarkable improvements in insulin sensitivity in the recipient rodents (Stanford et al. 2013). Moreover, that study showed the increased insulin-stimulated glucose disposal in the recipient mice was not due to increased glucose uptake into the transplanted fat; rather, those mice experienced increased glucose uptake into skeletal muscle and BAT, strongly suggesting an exercise-induced endocrine effect of the WAT. This suggests that exercise may affect the endocrine function of brown and WAT to facilitate systemic metabolic enhancements.

It is well established that exercise upregulates skeletal muscle peroxisome proliferator-activated receptor gamma coactivator 1 alpha (PGC1-α), which is linked to mitochondrial biogenesis, angiogenesis, and fiber-type switching. Moreover, in individuals with type 2 diabetes, skeletal muscle PGC-1α mRNA levels are reduced (Patti et al. 2003) whereas the attenuated levels are restored by various types of exercise ranging from acute to chronic endurance (Summermatter and Handschin 2012). In one study, mice with upregulated PGC-1α were not only resistant to obesity and diabetes but also had a prolonged life span (Bostrom et al. 2012). Human white adipocytes transfected with PGC-1α present increased levels of UCP-1, suggesting PGC-1α can remodel WAT into BAT (i.e., browning of WAT) (Tiraby et al. 2003). Importantly, exercise may also increase adipose tissue PGC-1α. One study (Sutherland et al. 2009) demonstrated that 2 h of daily swimming exercise training for a month led to increases in markers of WAT mitochondrial biogenesis such as cytochrome-C oxidase (COXIV) and Core1 expressions and citrate synthase activity, which are all driven by increased PGC-1α and mitochondrial transcription factor A (Tfam). Recently, the newly identified "exercise hormone," irisin has received much attention due to its potential browning effect on WAT. The Fndc5 gene stimulated by PGC-1α in exercising muscle forms irisin, which is secreted into circulation, and stimulates a biological program making WAT more like BAT via upregulated PGC-1α and UCP-1 expression. Spiegelman and Bostrom (Bostrom et al. 2012) demonstrated that exercise (i.e., voluntary wheel running and swimming) in mice drives the subcutaneous and visceral fat pads into a thermogenic gene program (e.g., enhanced mitochondrial content and increased levels of UCP-1 gene expression) via triggering an increase in circulating irisin. Exercise-mediated adaptations in adipose tissue mitochondria appear to require nitric oxide (NO) signaling via an endothelial NO synthase (eNOS)-dependent mechanism. Moreover, it has been suggested that an exercise-mediated increase in eNOS activity may explain its protective effects on adipose tissue immunometabolism (i.e., reduced inflammation, enhanced mitochondrial function, increased sensitivity to anti-lipolytic effect of insulin), although eliminating eNOS per se does not increase adipose tissue inflammation under sedentary conditions (Jurrissen et al. 2016).

Interestingly, estrogen may have similar effects on adipocyte mitochondria as those induced by exercise and a common mechanism may involve eNOS. ERα plays an important role in eNOS regulation (Sun et al. 2016) and may explain estrogen's role in increasing mitochondrial biogenesis and protecting against mitochondrial stress (Duckles and Krause 2011). The relationships between estrogen availability and adaptations to exercise in adipose tissue, and how such relationships may affect sex-specific effects of exercise on adipose tissue health, is an area of investigation that certainly required further exploration.

Roles Played by Exercise and Estrogen in Adiposity Reduction

The importance of exercise and total physical activity on adiposity reduction in states of energy surplus (e.g., obesity) is controversial. Although epidemiological data from the National Weight Control Registry demonstrate that exercise at the quantity of at least 1 h per day is a strong predictor of successful long-term weight loss, some researchers argue that calorie reduction is more effective in inducing an energy deficit resulting in weight loss. Some researchers suggest that exercise in the absence of dietary restriction results in compensatory dietary intake, thereby mitigating exercise-mediated weight loss (Thomas et al. 2012). From an energy-balance standpoint, any net energy deficit (i.e., due to dietary or exercise-mediated deficit) will result in a reduction in adipose (and lean) mass. Accordingly, in order for exercise to reduce total adiposity, it must induce an energy deficit that is not replaced by dietary energy. The direct versus indirect effects of exercise on adiposity are difficult to separate. That is, it is possible that exercise affects adipose tissue both by inducing an energy deficit that triggers mobilization to satisfy that need, and by more directly affecting adipocyte metabolism. It does appear that adipocyte lipolysis and skeletal muscle fat oxidation are higher, even during the resting state, following endurance exercise and that protein degradation is downregulated (Vicente-Salar et al. 2015). This suggests that training adaptations may occur in adipose tissue that are unique from the energy deficit effects of exercise. The mitochondrial adaptations in adipose tissue, and enhanced sensitivity to hormone-regulated lipolysis, described in the above sections, would certainly serve as examples of these exercise-specific effects.

In general, exercise training significantly reduces mean adipocyte size and adipocyte lipid content, as well as increases WAT gene expression of important metabolically protective proteins such as GLUT4 and PGC1-α, suggesting that exercise may facilitate exercise-mediated fat mobilization which is necessary for fat loss. On the other hand, in many cases, adipocyte molecular changes that occur with exercise training are independent of any exercise-mediated weight loss (Stanford et al. 2015). One study even showed that exercise training led to significantly greater gene expression changes in subcutaneous WAT compared to exercise-induced changes in skeletal muscle (Stanford et al. 2013). Thus, an important consideration in evaluating the literature on the role of exercise in weight loss is that exercise affects the 'quality' of adipose tissue even in instances when exercise training does not lead to total adipose tissue reduction. In this next section, the idea that adipose tissue is an endocrine organ will be discussed in greater detail to allow for a more in-depth investigation of how exercise might affect the 'quality' (e.g., regulatory function, insulin sensitivity, inflammation, endocrine role, etc.) of adipose tissue. Further, the idea that sex differences may exist in these attributes of adipose tissue will be discussed, along with a discussion of how the effects of exercise may differ depending on sex and other factors.

Adipose Tissue as an Endocrine Organ Susceptible to Inflammation

Research over the past two decades has revealed the adipose tissue as an immune site harboring a unique collection of cells (Giordano et al. 2014). In fact, mature adipocytes make up only ~50 % of WAT and that the remaining ~50 % comprises the stromal vascular cell (SVC) fraction which includes preadipocytes, fibroblasts, immune cells, endothelial cells, and smooth muscle cells (van Harmelen et al. 2005; Gesta et al. 2007) allowing WAT to serve functions to maintain vascular, metabolic, endocrine, and immunological homeostasis, in addition to energy storage and mobilization. The idea that WAT is little more than a storage depot was challenged in 1994 with the ground-breaking discovery of the hormone leptin (Halaas et al. 1995). Leptin is produced and secreted by adipocytes and its major role is in regulating whole body energy balance through its interaction with receptors in the ventral medial region of the hypothalamus (Campfield et al. 1996). While the major role of leptin is to act as a lipostat both suppressing appetite and increasing thermogenesis, it also has a multitude of other effects that span many physiological processes. Importantly, leptin is also at the interface between the body's energy reserves and reproduction, highlighting the vital role that adipose tissue plays in female reproduction (Thong et al. 2000). The first indication of the importance of adipose-derived leptin in reproduction came with the discovery that the few humans born with a genetic defect preventing them from producing leptin are not only obese due to disturbed energy balance regulation, but do not reach sexual maturity. It is now known that leptin receptors are expressed not only in brain but also in human ovaries (Thong et al. 2000) and other tissues. There is also a sexual dimorphism in circulating leptin such that women have greater levels than men, even when the greater total adiposity in women is accounted for. In healthy women, leptin increases during the luteal phase of the menstrual cycle (Thong et al. 2000). Moreover, this rise in leptin parallels ovarian hormones, suggesting a relationship between sex hormones and leptin production, although mechanisms remain unknown. Interestingly, exercise-induced amenorrhea, which is very common among reproductive-aged females undergoing intense training, associates with an absence of diurnal leptin rhythm (Thong et al. 2000) which is accompanied by reduced basal metabolic rate. In amenorrheic athletes, it has been hypothesized that their significantly lower circulating leptin levels are attributed to their low body fat content; however, studies have demonstrated that he lower leptin levels during amenorrhea are not fully accounted for my lower percent body fat, suggesting that another factor is responsible for leptin suppression in these individuals. Other factors that may play a role are low total energy intake and low circulating insulin (which has been shown to increase adipose tissue leptin gene expression). Importantly, exogenous leptin administration alone is not effective in restoring reproductive function in amenorrheic women unless sufficient glucose is available. Clearly, the relationships between reproductive capabilities, metabolism, and leptin are complex and not fully understood.

While low leptin levels associate with amenorrhea, obesity results in high leptin levels which has been shown to be a causative feature of obesity-related breast cancer (Schmidt et al. 2015). Since aromatase enzyme is present in adipose tissue, adipose tissue produces estrogen, which is produced from an androgen precursor. For this reason, adipose tissue is the major tissue responsible for estrogen production post-menopause. Moreover, excess local estrogen production in mammary tissue of obese women is thought to contribute to the increased risk of breast cancer among obese women (Howe et al. 2013).

In addition to leptin, many adipose tissue-derived hormones, cytokines, and chemokines have been discovered and are collectively called "adipokines." The immunometabolic processes which occur in adipose tissue directly affect somatic metabolic function (Ferrante 2013). Because of this rich immune cell composition which includes adaptive (e.g., B and T lymphocytes) as well as innate immune cells (e.g., macrophages, dendritic cells, mast cells, eosinophils), adipose tissue is now classified as an immune organ, the latest organ to be classified as such (Bloor and Symonds 2014). Modulating adipose tissue inflammation can independently affect whole body metabolic function (Xu et al. 2013; Ko et al. 2014; Miao et al. 2014).

Chronic inflammation in WAT links obesity with insulin resistance and obesity-related metabolic disease (Osborn and Olefsky 2012). This relationship was first recognized with the discovery that WAT produces and secretes the pro-inflammatory cytokine, tumor necrosis factor (TNF)-α in rodent models of obesity (Hotamisligil et al. 1993). Although, there is evidence of immune cells in WAT as far back as the 1950s (Laqueur and Harrison 1951), with the adipose-derived TNF-α discovery, it was learned that inflammation actually causes insulin resistance in adipose tissue through a mechanism involving inhibition of serine/threonine phosphorylation of the docking protein, insulin receptor substrate (IRS)-1 (Hotamisligil et al. 1993). Other immune cells arising from the WAT including interleukin (IL)-6 (Kern et al. 2001), resistin (Cherneva et al. 2013), IL-1β (Gao et al. 2014), and interferon (IFN)-γ (O'Rourke et al. 2012) also directly modulate insulin sensitivity locally and systemically. Also noteworthy is that adipose tissue secretes not only inflammatory cytokines but also anti-inflammatory and insulin-sensitizing proteins such as adiponectin (Yamauchi et al. 2001) and IL-10 (Speaker et al. 2014). These secretions arise from the adipocytes themselves (e.g., adiponectin, leptin, resistin, visfatin), as well as from other infiltrating and resident immune cells including adipose tissue macrophages (e.g., IL-10, TNF-α) and T-lymphocytes (e.g., IFN-γ). It is thought that macrophages, mostly recruited from blood monocytes, are mostly responsible for the inflammatory cytokines present in obese WAT (Weisberg et al. 2003). Research in this area of adipose tissue immune cell production and release has been reviewed extensively (Fain 2006) and it can be concluded that a diverse array of immune cell interactions occur in WAT that are orchestrated by a growing list of adipose mediated secretions. One of the major conclusions from that body of work is that adipose tissue macrophage phenotype is a key determinant of the inflammatory status of the tissue. Thus, it is important to briefly summarize the concept of macrophage phenotype.

Macrophages have been classically classified into two broad classes based on their secretion profile and surface markers: M1 or "classical" and M2 or "alternative." Newer findings suggest that there are actually many more subgroups (Natoli and Monticelli 2014). It is recognized that macrophages can readily change state based on the local tissue environment (Sorisky et al. 2013). Especially under nutrient dense conditions, inflammatory (i.e., M1) macrophages infiltrate WAT and, like the inflammatory cytokines they secrete, negatively affect insulin resistance. Macrophages and monocytes are present in obese as well as lean WAT (Feuerer et al. 2009), although the prevalence increases with WAT expansion (Weisberg et al. 2003). In fact, it is estimated that ~10% of the SVC fraction from lean WAT may be made up of macrophages whereas this number increases to ~40–50% in obese WAT (McNelis and Olefsky 2014). The M1 macrophage plays a central role in host defense against bacterial and viral infections (i.e., innate immunity) while the M2 macrophage is associated with anti-inflammatory reactions and plays roles in tissue remodeling, fibrosis, and tumor progression (Natoli and Monticelli 2014); these classical macrophage roles also dictate their function in WAT. While the majority of macrophages present in obese WAT are of the classical M1 phenotype, those present in lean WAT tend to M2 (Feuerer et al. 2009).

Effects of Exercise and Estrogen on Adipose Tissue Inflammation

Certainly, by way of reducing total WAT, exercise can serve to counter obesity-associated WAT inflammation (Tchernof and Despres 2013). However, the anti-inflammatory effects of exercise go beyond simply reducing total adiposity since weight loss-independent, exercise-mediated reductions in WAT inflammation have been documented in humans (Bruun et al. 2006) and rodents (Bradley et al. 2008; Vieira et al. 2009). One study investigated the effects of a 15-week exercise intervention (i.e., 2–3 h of moderate intensity walking, swimming, or aerobics, 5 days per week) on weight loss, insulin sensitivity, and inflammation (systemic, as well as gene expression in WAT and skeletal muscle biopsy samples) in severely obese subjects (Bruun et al. 2006). Those subjects experienced improvements in insulin sensitivity and reduced systemic inflammation (Bruun et al. 2006). Importantly, that study also found that WAT inflammation decreased with exercise, an effect that was not found in the skeletal muscle. In a similar study with animals, a reduction in WAT gene expression of CD68 and CD14 (macrophage markers) and TNF-α were observed in morbidly obese rats exposed to acute swimming exercise for 12 weeks (Oliveira et al. 2013). Similarly, in obese mice, moderate exercise training (6 or 12 weeks of treadmill running) lowered systemic and as well as WAT inflammation, anti-inflammatory effects that predicted improvements in insulin resistance and hepatic steatosis (Vieira et al. 2009). Another group showed that 6 weeks of voluntary wheel running exercise decreased WAT inflammation in obese mice, even in the presence of high fat diet (Bradley et al. 2008). Likewise, in genetically obese rats, endurance exercise training in combination with the drug, metformin positively altered WAT secretion and plasma concentrations of leptin and IL-10, shifting the WAT toward an anti-inflammatory phenotype (Jenkins et al. 2012). In another study using high fat diet-fed mice by Kawanishi et al., exercise training resulted in a marked reduction in WAT inflammation despite not weight-reducing effect of exercise (Kawanishi et al. 2010). Those authors went on to show that exercise was associated, not only with a reduction in total WAT macrophage content but with an M1 → M2 macrophage phenotype switch, which may help explain its anti-inflammatory effect (Kawanishi et al. 2010). Acute exercise has also been reported to have anti-inflammatory effects in WAT: a mild–moderate 3-h exercise bout reduced inflammation in the epididymal WAT (a major visceral fat depot) of rats as indicated by decreased mRNA levels of inflammatory cytokines including TNF-α and IL-1β. Similar to the study by Kawanishi et al., there was also a switch in macrophage phenotype from pro-inflammatory anti-inflammatory phenotype in that study, suggesting that the mechanism may involve the acute hormonal/physiological/immunological changes associated with exercise (Oliveira et al. 2013).

Exercise may also facilitate interactions between adipocytes and immune cells in adipose tissue, although more studies are necessary in this area. Adipocyte lipolysis was discussed in detail above and it well appreciated that exercise profoundly affects lipolysis, both acutely and perhaps induces chronic adaptations in this regard. Interestingly, macrophages also are capable of undergoing lipolysis, although they exhibit intracellular lipolysis mediated through lipophagy (Singh et al. 2009) unlike adipocytes, which exhibit extracellular lipolysis. These processes may work in concert to regulate lipid trafficking and metabolism (Xu et al. 2013). Mice lacking CGI-58, the lipid droplet-associated protein described above, have dysfunctional lipophagy in macrophages. And downregulation of this protein increased inflammation via inflammasome activation via a mechanism involving macrophage-produced ROS (Miao et al. 2014). Animals lacking CGI-58 also experience a suppression of PPARγ-dependent mitochondrial function, which leads to increased ROS release from mitochondria. That study by Miao et al. demonstrated a PPARγ-mitochondria-ROS-inflammation pathway in macrophages (Miao et al. 2014) and offers a good example of how adipocyte and macrophage function may be united via lipid metabolism pathways. Given the evidence cited above that exercise may improve mitochondrial function in adipose tissue, it is possible that exercise may improve adipose tissue function by limiting inflammation by improving the phenotype of both mitochondria and adipose resident immune cells.

In one study, Rahman and colleagues reported that suppression of the inflammasome NLRP3 was associated with an improved metabolic phenotype in addition to suppression of inflammation. An interesting and unexpected finding from that study was that lower inflammatory activation was also associated with improved adipocyte mitochondrial function. Indeed, mitochondrial dysfunction is emerging as an important trigger of inflammation and oxidative stress in many tissues including WAT. Hahn and coworkers used an adipocyte cell line, 3T3-L1, to elucidate mechanisms by which inflammatory cytokines may affect mitochondrial metabolism. Every pro-inflammatory cytokine investigated in that study, TNF-α, IL-6, and IL-1β, impaired adipocyte mitochondrial function as indicated by reduced gene expression of mitochondrial biogenesis indicators, PGC1α and eNOS. Inflammation also induced mitochondrial fragmentation and dysregulated mitochondrial fusion (Hahn et al. 2014). Since free fatty acids were shown to directly decrease CGI-58 expression in macrophages, via way of enhancing lipolytic regulation, exercise may also reduce the availability of potentially lipotoxic fatty acids which can cause inflammatory macrophage activation and insulin resistance.

Other research has demonstrated that the transcriptional regulator of fasting lipolysis, IRF4, both enhances adipocyte lipolysis and suppresses macrophage inflammation (Fabrizi et al. 2014); and mice with a myeloid-specific deletion of IRF4 are insulin resistant. Thus, IRF4 may serve as a communication link between adipocytes and macrophages that regulates lipid handling in adipocytes by promoting adipocyte lipolysis while also decreasing classical M1 macrophage activation (Fabrizi et al. 2014). The effects of exercise training on IRF4 remain unknown but this may serve as another potential mechanism by which exercise enhances lipolytic regulation and reduces inflammation. Saturated free fatty acids have been reported to activate DNA methyltransferase (DNAMT) enzymes (Yang et al. 2014) which may mechanistically link fatty acid exposure to inflammation. DNAMT3b was shown by those researchers to directly methylate PPARλ at its promoter region, thereby leading to M1 macrophage polarization. The trigger may be macrophage ROS production, as ROS lead to oxidative damage of phospholipids, protein, and DNA. Thus, cross talk exists between macrophage-derived cytokines and adipocytes, as well as between adipocyte mitochondria and macrophages themselves. This cycle of ROS production and inflammatory activation clearly potentiates inflammatory cascades. On the other hand, enhancing mitochondrial fatty acid oxidation may decrease inflammation. Activation of macrophage AMP-activated protein kinase (AMPK), an important cellular fuel gauge and regulator of lipid metabolism, can significantly abrogate inflammatory signaling events (Filippov et al. 2013). Interestingly estrogen is also known to activate AMPK (D'Eon et al. 2005) as well as reduce adipose tissue inflammation where exercise has strikingly similar effects (Higa et al. 2014).

Another possible mechanism by which exercise reduces WAT inflammation involves paracrine effects due to proteins secreted into the circulation by skeletal muscle cells (i.e., myokines) upon an exercise stimulus. Similar to adipokines, myokines have been shown to exhibit their effects both locally and peripherally. IL-6 is one such recently identified myokine that has shown potential in possessing a protective metabolic role. IL-6 may exert beneficial metabolic effects via enhancement of lipolysis and mitigation of the inflammatory response in WAT (Pedersen and Hojman 2012). Interestingly, IL-6 is commonly secreted by enlarged adipocytes and has been associated with reduced insulin action in WAT and systemically (Fried et al. 1998). However, Pedersen et al. (Petersen and Pedersen 2005) demonstrated that IL-6 may be a protective factor produced by exercising muscle cells and released into the circulation during and after exercise. Indeed, plasma IL-6 level increases exponentially with exercise and is related to exercise intensity, duration, mass muscle recruited, and endurance capacity of an individual. Produced by both type I and II muscle fibers, IL-6 acts to regulate glucose and lipid metabolism. In skeletal muscle, IL-6 activates AMPK and PI3 kinase to enhance glucose uptake and fat oxidation, and also exerts effects in a hormone-like fashion affecting other tissues such as liver (e.g., hepatic glucose production) and WAT (e.g., enhanced lipolysis). Notably, IL-6 lessens circulating TNF-α levels, implying an anti-inflammatory role. Starkie et al. (Starkie et al. 2003) used a model of low-grade inflammation established with a low dose of *E. coli* endotoxin administered to healthy individuals. The TNF-α response induced by endotoxin was totally blunted by a 3-h bout of cycling exercise or an infusion with recombinant human IL-6. Consistent with those multiple beneficial effects, mice with IL-6 deficiency develop obesity and insulin resistance, effects that are reversed with IL-6 administration (Wallenius et al. 2002). Thus, provocation of an increase in muscle IL-6 secretion may help explain some of the metabolic and anti-inflammatory effects of exercise.

Similar to anti-inflammatory effects of myokines during exercise, adipocyte-released adiponectin levels, which are inversely proportional to abdominal fat mass and insulin resistance, significantly increase with both acute and short-term aerobic exercise training (Saunders et al. 2012). Adiponectin inhibits nuclear factor kB (NFkB), an essential transcription factor for the expression of inflammatory and stress related proteins (Villarreal-Molina and Antuna-Puente 2012). What is counter-intuitive is that adiponectin has been shown to stimulate rapid TNF-α secretion in human and mouse macrophages. This, in turn, stimulates IL-10, an anti-inflammatory cytokine, thus creating tolerance to further LPS stimulation (Tsatsanis et al. 2005). Thus, regular exercise training may protect against chronic low-grade systemic inflammation as well as adipocyte inflammation via the increased secretion of immunomodulatory factors such as adiponectin from adipocytes, and IL-6 produced by skeletal muscle cells.

WAT browning, which was described above as being associated with improved insulin sensitivity, is also associated with reduced inflammation, offering yet another hypothetical mechanism by which exercise is anti-inflammatory. A possible mechanism between browning and suppressed inflammation may be that PGC-1α directly suppresses ROS in WAT (St-Pierre et al. 2006). ROS are often associated with obesity-associated diseases; they increase oxidative stress and trigger inflammatory cytokine production (St-Pierre et al. 2006). Anti-inflammatory effects of PGC-1α have been demonstrated in vitro using skeletal muscle cell lines. That is, enhanced expression of PGC-1α in C2C12 myotubes suppressed inflammatory cytokine production (Handschin et al. 2007). It is possible that, via upregulation of PGC-1 in WAT, exercise may reduce WAT inflammation, thus constituting another possible anti-inflammatory mechanism.

Quite similar to what happens to adipose tissue with obesity, ovarian estrogen deprivation via ovariectomy induces inflammation in adipose tissue (Vieira Potter et al. 2012), and this can be effectively mitigated with estrogen replacement (Bluher 2013). Exercise training is equally effective as estrogen replacement in preventing fat gain post-ovariectomy (Endlich et al. 2013) but whether exercise mitigates ovariectomy-induced adipose tissue inflammation does not appeared to have been investigated.

Role of Sex in Exercise-Mediated Adipose Tissue Responses

It is well appreciated that there are sex differences in metabolic responses to exercise. During exercise, women utilize proportionally more lipid and less carbohydrate than men, are better preservers of hepatic glycogen, and exhibit lower hepatic glucose production (Varlamov et al. 2014). Moreover, premenopausal women, when compared to age-matched men, have greater substrate flexibility exemplified by their ability to attenuate use of carbohydrate at high altitude (Braun et al. 2000). The mechanism is thought to involve estrogen-mediated enhancements of adipocyte lipolysis (Braun and Horton 2001). Estrogens have been shown to directly suppress triglyceride synthesis by both reducing lipogenesis in liver and increasing WAT lipolysis (Varlamov et al. 2014; Gao et al. 2006). Indeed, lipolysis rates are unequivocally greater in young women compared to age-matched men, with rates of FFA release being ~40% greater in women than men relative to energy needs and independent of differences in relative rats of fat oxidation (Santosa and Jensen 2015). The sex differential metabolic responses during exercise may be due to differences in sympathetic nerve activity or muscle fiber type distribution (Varlamov et al. 2014). For example, over 3000 genes are differentially expressed in male and female skeletal muscle. One skeletal muscle sex difference is that females tend to have more slower-twitch fibers; this is thought to be responsible for their increased endurance and greater oxidative capacity (Haizlip et al. 2015). Interestingly, estrogen loss impairs glucose uptake during exercise (Bostrom et al. 2012). In rodents, ovariectomy reduces key oxidative enzymes in skeletal muscle whereas estrogen replacement prevents this (Campbell and Febbraio 2001).

Aging in both sexes induces a change in body composition characterized by greater adiposity and less lean mass (Calles-Escandon and Poehlman 1997), and age-related physical activity reduction is at least partially responsible for these changes. Alterations in fat oxidation is also a contributing factor; clearly, it is difficult to differentiate cause and effect among the compilation of factors that occur with aging including less relative lean mass, physical inactivity, and hormone changes. Skeletal muscle-specific effects (i.e., age-related sarcopenia) also likely play an important role. Research suggests that female reproductive hormones are permissive to fatty acid oxidation, and their decline during menopause contributes to the reduction in fatty acid metabolism seen in this population. This may help explain the shift in body fat distribution toward an increase in visceral adiposity (Tchernof et al. 1998). Hormone replacement therapy has been shown to reduce visceral adipose tissue post-menopause (Sites et al. 2001). Not surprisingly, exercise training has been shown to be particularly therapeutic and preventative regarding this constellation of risk factors associated with aging in women. In rodents, ovariectomy increases adiposity across depots whereas both estrogen replacement and exercise prevent these effects (Shinoda et al. 2002).

Summary

The adipose tissue is an essential organ that not only serves as the body's main energy storage reservoir but also fulfills many other essential physiological roles including but not limited to organ protection, energy balance regulation, neuroendocrine control, immune homeostasis, and thermoregulation. Although the vast majority of adipose tissue in the human body is considered white (i.e., WAT), with its primary function being energy storage in a unified lipid droplet that makes up most of the cell, brown (i.e., BAT) is now known to exist in the adult human, albeit only representing a fraction of total body adipose tissue. BAT is different from WAT in that its main function is thermoregulation, which it carries out by producing heat via uncoupling of mitochondrial oxidative phosphorylation. To do this, adipocytes from BAT have a multilocular phenotype and contain many mitochondria which contain UCP-1; these specialized mitochondria oxidize fatty acids which are stored in close proximity in the numerous small lipid droplets which surround them. Important sex differences exist in BAT in that females tend to have more of it, and BAT from females tends to be more active than that from males. Interestingly estrogen receptors are expressed on adipocytes from both WAT and BAT and estrogen is thought to be an important signal required for preadipocyte differentiation in both types of fat. WAT is sub-classified into visceral and subcutaneous depots, with excess visceral being most metabolically detrimental. Subcutaneous, on the other hand, associates with a healthier overall metabolic phenotype and estrogen is the major driver of subcutaneous WAT deposition. This likely contributes to the overall mechanism explaining the significantly greater insulin sensitivity among females compared to males. Despite having greater body fat percentage compared to males, females are more insulin sensitive and this appears consistent across species. Females also tend to be protected against the increase in insulin resistance associated with high fat diet, which appears to be due to estrogen. Moreover, this sex difference is largely explained by estrogen. Postmenopausal women as well as ovariectomized experimental animals develop increased visceral adiposity and severe metabolic dysfunction, whereas premenopausal women characteristically exemplify a gynoid versus android body fat distribution profile.

Adipocyte lipolysis is the major physiological process that occurs in adipose tissue which allows its stored energy to be released for use by other tissues. It is largely driven by the hormonal milieu induced by either fasting or exercise, but estrogen is known to also be a powerful modulator of adipoctye lipolysis. Estrogen's ability to suppress adipocyte lipolysis may explain why it is more difficult for females to reduce total body adiposity with diet and exercise, and also why postmenopausal women experience dysregulated lipolysis which associates with the development of insulin resistance. Indeed, women are more sensitive in terms of insulin-mediated suppression of lipolysis (Varlamov et al. 2014).

Most of the established metabolic effects of estrogen on adipose tissue are mediated through its major receptors, ERα and ERβ. Via ERα, estrogen improves adipose tissue health by reducing inflammation, de novo lipogenesis, and insulin resistance. Intriguingly, exercise appears to have similar effects on adipose tissue and may therefore be particularly beneficial among postmenopausal women who experience the negative effects of loss of adipocyte estrogen signaling.

In conclusion, estrogen profoundly affects adipose tissue throughout the lifespan, from its very development in utero, to its function throughout adolescence, the reproductive stage, and aging. While estrogen replacement therapy remains controversial, most of the negative effects of menopause and/or estrogen loss via ovariectomy in rodents can be minimized or completely rescued with estrogen therapy. While the mechanisms by which exercise and/or estrogen reduce adipose tissue inflammation are not fully understood, one hypothesis is that both may directly affect macrophage phenotype by causing a shift from inflammatory to anti-inflammatory activation (Kawanishi et al. 2010; Toniolo et al. 2015).

References

Bloor ID, Symonds ME. Sexual dimorphism in white and brown adipose tissue with obesity and inflammation. Horm Behav. 2014;66(1):95–103.
Bluher M. Importance of estrogen receptors in adipose tissue function. Mol Metabol. 2013;2(3):130–2.
Bostrom P, Wu J, Jedrychowski MP, Korde A, Ye L, Lo JC, et al. A PGC1-alpha-dependent myokine that drives brown-fat-like development of white fat and thermogenesis. Nature. 2012;481(7382):463–8.
Bradley RL, Jeon JY, Liu FF, Maratos-Flier E. Voluntary exercise improves insulin sensitivity and adipose tissue inflammation in diet-induced obese mice. Am J Physiol Endocrinol Metab. 2008;295(3):E586–94.
Braun B, Horton T. Endocrine regulation of exercise substrate utilization in women compared to men. Exerc Sport Sci Rev. 2001;29(4):149–54.
Braun B, Mawson JT, Muza SR, Dominick SB, Brooks GA, Horning MA, et al. Women at altitude: carbohydrate utilization during exercise at 4,300 m. J Appl Physiol (1985). 2000;88(1): 246–56.
Bruun JM, Helge JW, Richelsen B, Stallknecht B. Diet and exercise reduce low-grade inflammation and macrophage infiltration in adipose tissue but not in skeletal muscle in severely obese subjects. Am J Physiol Endocrinol Metab. 2006;290(5):E961–7.
Bulow J, Gjeraa K, Enevoldsen LH, Simonsen L. Lipid mobilization from human abdominal, subcutaneous adipose tissue is independent of sex during steady-state exercise. Clin Physiol Funct Imaging. 2006;26(4):205–11.
Calles-Escandon J, Poehlman ET. Aging, fat oxidation and exercise. Aging. 1997;9(1-2):57–63.
Campbell SE, Febbraio MA. Effects of ovarian hormones on exercise metabolism. Curr Opin Clin Nutr Metab Care. 2001;4(6):515–20.
Campfield LA, Smith FJ, Guisez Y, Devos R, Burn P. OB protein: a peripheral signal linking adiposity and central neural networks. Appetite. 1996;26(3):302.
Chehab FF, Mounzih K, Lu R, Lim ME. Early onset of reproductive function in normal female mice treated with leptin. Science. 1997;275(5296):88–90.
Cherneva RV, Georgiev OB, Petrova DS, Mondeshki TL, Ruseva SR, Cakova AD, et al. Resistin – the link between adipose tissue dysfunction and insulin resistance in patients with obstructive sleep apnea. J Diabetes Metab Disord. 2013;12(1):5.
Crocker MK, Stern EA, Sedaka NM, Shomaker LB, Brady SM, Ali AH, et al. Sexual dimorphisms in the associations of BMI and body fat with indices of pubertal development in girls and boys. J Clin Endocrinol Metab. 2014;99(8):E1519–29.

Davis KE, Neinast MD, Sun K, Bills JD, Zehr JA, Zeve D, Hahne LD, et al. The sexually dimorphic role of adipose and adipocyte estrogen receptors in modulating adipose tissue expansion, inflammation, and fibrosis. Mol Metab. 2013;2(3):227–42.

D'Eon TM, Souza SC, Aronovitz M, Obin MS, Fried SK, Greenberg AS. Estrogen regulation of adiposity and fuel partitioning. Evidence of genomic and non-genomic regulation of lipogenic and oxidative pathways. J Biol Chem. 2005;280(43):35983–91.

Devries MC. Sex-based differences in endurance exercise muscle metabolism: impact on exercise and nutritional strategies to optimize health and performance in women. Exp Physiol. 2016;101(2):243–9.

Duckles SP, Krause DN. Mechanisms of cerebrovascular protection: oestrogen, inflammation and mitochondria. Acta Physiol (Oxf). 2011;203(1):149–54.

Endlich PW, Claudio ER, da Silva Goncalves WL, Gouvea SA, Moyses MR, de Abreu GR. Swimming training prevents fat deposition and decreases angiotensin II-induced coronary vasoconstriction in ovariectomized rats. Peptides. 2013;47:29–35.

Enevoldsen LH, Stallknecht B, Fluckey JD, Galbo H. Effect of exercise training on in vivo lipolysis in intra-abdominal adipose tissue in rats. Am J Physiol Endocrinol Metab. 2000;279(3):E585–92.

Fabrizi M, Marchetti V, Mavilio M, Marino A, Casagrande V, Cavalera M, et al. IL-21 is a major negative regulator of IRF4-dependent lipolysis affecting Tregs in adipose tissue and systemic insulin sensitivity. Diabetes. 2014.

Fain JN. Release of interleukins and other inflammatory cytokines by human adipose tissue is enhanced in obesity and primarily due to the nonfat cells. Vitam Horm. 2006;74:443–77.

Ferrante Jr AW. Macrophages, fat, and the emergence of immunometabolism. J Clin Invest. 2013;123(12):4992–3.

Feuerer M, Herrero L, Cipolletta D, Naaz A, Wong J, Nayer A, et al. Lean, but not obese, fat is enriched for a unique population of regulatory T cells that affect metabolic parameters. Nat Med. 2009;15(8):930–9.

Filippov S, Pinkosky SL, Lister RJ, Pawloski C, Hanselman JC, Cramer CT, et al. ETC-1002 regulates immune response, leukocyte homing, and adipose tissue inflammation via LKB1-dependent activation of macrophage AMPK. J Lipid Res. 2013;54(8):2095–108.

Foryst-Ludwig A, Kreissl MC, Benz V, Brix S, Smeir E, Ban Z, et al. Adipose tissue lipolysis promotes exercise-induced cardiac hypertrophy involving the lipokine C16:1n7-palmitoleate. J Biol Chem. 2015;290(39):23603–15.

Frayn KN, Shadid S, Hamlani R, Humphreys SM, Clark ML, Fielding BA, et al. Regulation of fatty acid movement in human adipose tissue in the postabsorptive-to-postprandial transition. Am J Physiol. 1994;266(3 Pt 1):E308–17.

Frayn KN, Karpe F, Fielding BA, Macdonald IA, Coppack SW. Integrative physiology of human adipose tissue. Int J Obes Relat Metab Disord. 2003;27(8):875–88.

Fried SK, Bunkin DA, Greenberg AS. Omental and subcutaneous adipose tissues of obese subjects release interleukin-6: depot difference and regulation by glucocorticoid. J Clin Endocrinol Metab. 1998;83(3):847–50.

Frisch RE. Body weight, body fat, and ovulation. Trends Endocrinol Metab. 1991;2(5):191–7.

Gao H, Bryzgalova G, Hedman E, Khan A, Efendic S, Gustafsson JA, et al. Long-term administration of estradiol decreases expression of hepatic lipogenic genes and improves insulin sensitivity in ob/ob mice: a possible mechanism is through direct regulation of signal transducer and activator of transcription 3. Mol Endocrinol. 2006;20(6):1287–99.

Gao D, Madi M, Ding C, Fok M, Steele T, Ford C, et al. Interleukin-1beta mediates macrophage-induced impairment of insulin signaling in human primary adipocytes. Am J Physiol Endocrinol Metab. 2014.

Gesta S, Tseng YH, Kahn CR. Developmental origin of fat: tracking obesity to its source. Cell. 2007;131(2):242–56.

Giordano A, Smorlesi A, Frontini A, Barbatelli G, Cinti S. White, brown and pink adipocytes: the extraordinary plasticity of the adipose organ. Eur J Endocrinol. 2014;170(5):R159–71.

Gohil K, Henderson S, Terblanche SE, Brooks GA, Packer L. Effects of training and exhaustive exercise on the mitochondrial oxidative capacity of brown adipose tissue. Biosci Rep. 1984;4(11):987–93.

Hackney AC, McCracken-Compton MA, Ainsworth B. Substrate responses to submaximal exercise in the midfollicular and midluteal phases of the menstrual cycle. Int J Sport Nutr. 1994;4(3):299–308.

Hahn WS, Kuzmicic J, Burrill JS, Donoghue MA, Foncea R, Jensen MD, et al. Proinflammatory cytokines differentially regulate adipocyte mitochondrial metabolism, oxidative stress, and dynamics. Am J Physiol Endocrinol Metab. 2014;306(9):E1033–45.

Haizlip KM, Harrison BC, Leinwand LA. Sex-based differences in skeletal muscle kinetics and fiber-type composition. Physiology. 2015;30(1):30–9.

Halaas JL, Gajiwala KS, Maffei M, Cohen SL, Chait BT, Rabinowitz D, et al. Weight-reducing effects of the plasma protein encoded by the obese gene. Science. 1995;269(5223):543–6.

Handschin C, Choi CS, Chin S, Kim S, Kawamori D, Kurpad AJ, et al. Abnormal glucose homeostasis in skeletal muscle-specific PGC-1alpha knockout mice reveals skeletal muscle-pancreatic beta cell crosstalk. J Clin Invest. 2007;117(11):3463–74.

Hellstrom L, Blaak E, Hagstrom-Toft E. Gender differences in adrenergic regulation of lipid mobilization during exercise. Int J Sports Med. 1996;17(6):439–47.

Higa TS, Spinola AV, Fonseca-Alaniz MH, Evangelista FS. Remodeling of white adipose tissue metabolism by physical training prevents insulin resistance. Life Sci. 2014;103(1):41–8.

Hirata K. Blood flow to brown adipose tissue and norepinephrine- induced calorigenesis in physically trained rats. Jpn J Physiol. 1982a;32(2):279–91.

Hirata K. Enhanced calorigenesis in brown adipose tissue in physically trained rats. Jpn J Physiol. 1982b;32(4):647–53.

Hjemdahl P, Linde B. Influence of circulating NE and Epi on adipose tissue vascular resistance and lipolysis in humans. Am J Physiol. 1983;245(3):H447–52.

Hotamisligil GS, Shargill NS, Spiegelman BM. Adipose expression of tumor necrosis factor-alpha: direct role in obesity-linked insulin resistance. Science. 1993;259(5091):87–91.

Howe LR, Subbaramaiah K, Hudis CA, Dannenberg AJ. Molecular pathways: adipose inflammation as a mediator of obesity-associated cancer. Clin Cancer Res. 2013;19(22):6074–83.

Jenkins NT, Padilla J, Arce-Esquivel AA, Bayless DS, Martin JS, Leidy HJ, et al. Effects of endurance exercise training, metformin, and their combination on adipose tissue leptin and IL-10 secretion in OLETF rats. J Appl Physiol. 2012;113(12):1873–83.

Joseph AM, Pilegaard H, Litvintsev A, Leick L, Hood DA. Control of gene expression and mitochondrial biogenesis in the muscular adaptation to endurance exercise. Essays Biochem. 2006;42:13–29.

Jurrissen TJ, Sheldon RD, Gastecki ML, Woodford ML, Zidon TM, Rector RS, et al. Ablation of eNOS does not promote adipose tissue inflammation. Am J Physiol Regul Integr Comp Physiol. 2016;310(8):744–51.

Kawanishi N, Yano H, Yokogawa Y, Suzuki K. Exercise training inhibits inflammation in adipose tissue via both suppression of macrophage infiltration and acceleration of phenotypic switching from M1 to M2 macrophages in high-fat-diet-induced obese mice. Exerc Immunol Rev. 2010;16:105–18.

Kern PA, Ranganathan S, Li C, Wood L, Ranganathan G. Adipose tissue tumor necrosis factor and interleukin-6 expression in human obesity and insulin resistance. Am J Physiol Endocrinol Metab. 2001;280(5):E745–51.

Kim JH, Cho HT, Kim YJ. The role of estrogen in adipose tissue metabolism: insights into glucose homeostasis regulation. Endocr J. 2014;61(11):1055–67.

Ko SH, Lee JK, Lee HJ, Ye SK, Kim HS, Chung MH. 8-Oxo-2'-deoxyguanosine ameliorates features of metabolic syndrome in obese mice. Biochem Biophys Res Commun. 2014;443(2):610–6.

Lambadiari V, Triantafyllou K, Dimitriadis GD. Insulin action in muscle and adipose tissue in type 2 diabetes: the significance of blood flow. World J Diabetes. 2015;6(4):626–33.

Lapid K, Lim A, Clegg DJ, Zeve D, Graff JM. Oestrogen signalling in white adipose progenitor cells inhibits differentiation into brown adipose and smooth muscle cells. Nat Commun. 2014;5:5196.

Laqueur GL, Harrison MB. Glandular adipose tissue associated with cytotoxic suprarenal contraction and diabetes mellitus. Am J Pathol. 1951;27(2):231–45.

Larue-Achagiotis C, Rieth N, Goubern M, Laury MC, Louis-Sylvestre J. Exercise-training reduces BAT thermogenesis in rats. Physiol Behav. 1995;57(5):1013–7.

Leblanc J, Dussault J, Lupien D, Richard D. Effect of diet and exercise on norepinephrine-induced thermogenesis in male and female rats. J Appl Physiol. 1982;52(3):556–61.

Lemoine S, Granier P, Tiffoche C, Berthon PM, Rannou-Bekono F, Thieulant ML, et al. Effect of endurance training on oestrogen receptor alpha transcripts in rat skeletal muscle. Acta Physiol Scand. 2002;174(3):283–9.

Luglio HF. Estrogen and body weight regulation in women: the role of estrogen receptor alpha (ER-alpha) on adipocyte lipolysis. Acta Med Indones. 2014;46(4):333–8.

Martinez de Morentin PB, Gonzalez-Garcia I, Martins L, Lage R, Fernandez-Mallo D, Martinez-Sanchez N, et al. Estradiol regulates brown adipose tissue thermogenesis via hypothalamic AMPK. Cell Metab. 2014;20(1):41–53.

Mattiasson I, Rendell M, Tornquist C, Jeppsson S, Hulthen UL. Effects of estrogen replacement therapy on abdominal fat compartments as related to glucose and lipid metabolism in early postmenopausal women. Horm Metab Res. 2002;34(10):583–8.

McNelis JC, Olefsky JM. Macrophages, immunity, and metabolic disease. Immunity. 2014;41(1):36–48.

Merry TL, Ristow M. Mitohormesis in exercise training. Free Radic Biol Med. 2015;pii:S0891-5849(15)01141-7.

Metz L, Gerbaix M, Masgrau A, Guillet C, Walrand S, Boisseau N, et al. Nutritional and exercise interventions variably affect estrogen receptor expression in the adipose tissue of male rats. Nutr Res. 2016;36(3):280–9.

Miao H, Ou J, Ma Y, Guo F, Yang Z, Wiggins M, et al. Macrophage CGI-58 deficiency activates ROS-inflammasome pathway to promote insulin resistance in mice. Cell Rep. 2014;7(1):223–35.

Nadal-Casellas A, Proenza AM, Llado I, Gianotti M. Effects of ovariectomy and 17-beta estradiol replacement on rat brown adipose tissue mitochondrial function. Steroids. 2011;76(10-11):1051–6.

Nadal-Casellas A, Bauza-Thorbrugge M, Proenza AM, Gianotti M, Llado I. Sex-dependent differences in rat brown adipose tissue mitochondrial biogenesis and insulin signaling parameters in response to an obesogenic diet. Mol Cell Biochem. 2012;373(1-2):125–35.

Natoli G, Monticelli S. Macrophage activation: glancing into diversity. Immunity. 2014;40(2):175–7.

Nigro M, Santos AT, Barthem CS, Louzada RA, Fortunato RS, Ketzer LA, et al. A change in liver metabolism but not in brown adipose tissue thermogenesis is an early event in ovariectomy-induced obesity in rats. Endocrinology. 2014;155(8):2881–91.

Nozu T, Kikuchi K, Ogawa K, Kuroshima A. Effects of running training on in vitro brown adipose tissue thermogenesis in rats. Int J Biometeorol. 1992;36(2):88–92.

Ogasawara J, Izawa T, Sakurai T, Sakurai T, Shirato K, Ishibashi Y, et al. The molecular mechanism underlying continuous exercise training-induced adaptive changes of lipolysis in white adipose cells. J Obes. 2015;2015:473430.

Oh-ishi S, Kizaki T, Toshinai K, Haga S, Fukuda K, Nagata N, et al. Swimming training improves brown-adipose-tissue activity in young and old mice. Mech Ageing Dev. 1996;89(2):67–78.

Oliveira AG, Araujo TG, Carvalho BM, Guadagnini D, Rocha GZ, Bagarolli RA, et al. Acute exercise induces a phenotypic switch in adipose tissue macrophage polarization in diet-induced obese rats. Obesity. 2013.

O'Rourke RW, White AE, Metcalf MD, Winters BR, Diggs BS, Zhu X, et al. Systemic inflammation and insulin sensitivity in obese IFN-gamma knockout mice. Metabolism. 2012;61(8):1152–61.

Osborn O, Olefsky JM. The cellular and signaling networks linking the immune system and metabolism in disease. Nat Med. 2012;18(3):363–74.

O'Sullivan AJ. Does oestrogen allow women to store fat more efficiently? A biological advantage for fertility and gestation. Obes Rev. 2009;10(2):168–77.

O'Sullivan AJ, Martin A, Brown MA. Efficient fat storage in premenopausal women and in early pregnancy: a role for estrogen. J Clin Endocrinol Metab. 2001;86(10):4951–6.

Park YM, Rector RS, Thyfault JP, Zidon TM, Padilla J, Welly RJ, et al. Effects of ovariectomy and intrinsic aerobic capacity on tissue-specific insulin sensitivity. Am J Physiol Endocrinol Metab. 2016;310(3):190–9.

Patti ME, Butte AJ, Crunkhorn S, Cusi K, Berria R, Kashyap S, et al. Coordinated reduction of genes of oxidative metabolism in humans with insulin resistance and diabetes: potential role of PGC1 and NRF1. Proc Natl Acad Sci U S A. 2003;100(14):8466–71.

Pedersen L, Hojman P. Muscle-to-organ cross talk mediated by myokines. Adipocyte. 2012; 1(3):164–7.

Peirce V, Carobbio S, Vidal-Puig A. The different shades of fat. Nature. 2014;510(7503):76–83.

Petersen AM, Pedersen BK. The anti-inflammatory effect of exercise. J Appl Physiol. 2005;98(4):1154–62.

Ramos RH, Warren MP. The interrelationships of body fat, exercise, and hormonal status and their impact on reproduction and bone health. Semin Perinatol. 1995;19(3):163–70.

Rettberg JR, Yao J, Brinton RD. Estrogen: a master regulator of bioenergetic systems in the brain and body. Front Neuroendocrinol. 2014;35(1):8–30.

Richard D, Labrie A, Rivest S. Tissue specificity of SNS response to exercise in mice exposed to low temperatures. Am J Physiol. 1992;262(5 Pt 2):R921–5.

Ro SH, Semple I, Ho A, Park HW, Lee JH. Sestrin2, a regulator of thermogenesis and mitohormesis in brown adipose tissue. Front Endocrinol (Lausanne). 2015;6:114.

Sanchez-Delgado G, Martinez-Tellez B, Olza J, Aguilera CM, Gil A, Ruiz JR. Role of exercise in the activation of brown adipose tissue. Ann Nutr Metab. 2015;67(1):21–32.

Santosa S, Jensen MD. The sexual dimorphism of lipid kinetics in humans. Front Endocrinol (Lausanne). 2015;6:103.

Saunders TJ, Palombella A, McGuire KA, Janiszewski PM, Despres JP, Ross R. Acute exercise increases adiponectin levels in abdominally obese men. J Nutr Metabol. 2012;2012:148729.

Schmidt S, Monk JM, Robinson LE, Mourtzakis M. The integrative role of leptin, oestrogen and the insulin family in obesity-associated breast cancer: potential effects of exercise. Obes Rev. 2015;16(6):473–87.

Shimizu I, Aprahamian T, Kikuchi R, Shimizu A, Papanicolaou KN, MacLauchlan S, et al. Vascular rarefaction mediates whitening of brown fat in obesity. J Clin Invest. 2014; 124(5):2099–112.

Shinoda M, Latour MG, Lavoie JM. Effects of physical training on body composition and organ weights in ovariectomized and hyperestrogenic rats. Int J Obes Relat Metab Disord. 2002;26(3):335–43.

Singh R, Kaushik S, Wang Y, Xiang Y, Novak I, Komatsu M, et al. Autophagy regulates lipid metabolism. Nature. 2009;458(7242):1131–5.

Sites CK, Brochu M, Tchernof A, Poehlman ET. Relationship between hormone replacement therapy use with body fat distribution and insulin sensitivity in obese postmenopausal women. Metabolism. 2001;50(7):835–40.

Sorisky A, Molgat AS, Gagnon A. Macrophage-induced adipose tissue dysfunction and the preadipocyte: should I stay (and differentiate) or should I go? Adv Nutr. 2013;4(1):67–75.

Speaker KJ, Cox SS, Paton MM, Serebrakian A, Maslanik T, Greenwood BN, et al. Six weeks of voluntary wheel running modulates inflammatory protein (MCP-1, IL-6, and IL-10) and DAMP (Hsp72) responses to acute stress in white adipose tissue of lean rats. Brain Behav Immun. 2014;39:87–98.

Stallknecht B, Vinten J, Ploug T, Galbo H. Increased activities of mitochondrial enzymes in white adipose tissue in trained rats. Am J Physiol. 1991;261(3 Pt 1):E410–4.

Stanford KI, Middelbeek RJ, Townsend KL, An D, Nygaard EB, Hitchcox KM, et al. Brown adipose tissue regulates glucose homeostasis and insulin sensitivity. J Clin Invest. 2013;123(1):215–23.

Stanford KI, Middelbeek RJ, Goodyear LJ. Exercise effects on white adipose tissue: beiging and metabolic adaptations. Diabetes. 2015;64(7):2361–8.

Starkie R, Ostrowski SR, Jauffred S, Febbraio M, Pedersen BK. Exercise and IL-6 infusion inhibit endotoxin-induced TNF-alpha production in humans. FASEB J. 2003;17(8):884–6.

St-Pierre J, Drori S, Uldry M, Silvaggi JM, Rhee J, Jager S, et al. Suppression of reactive oxygen species and neurodegeneration by the PGC-1 transcriptional coactivators. Cell. 2006; 127(2):397–408.

Strawford A, Antelo F, Christiansen M, Hellerstein MK. Adipose tissue triglyceride turnover, de novo lipogenesis, and cell proliferation in humans measured with 2H2O. Am J Physiol Endocrinol Metab. 2004;286(4):E577–88.

Summermatter S, Handschin C. PGC-1alpha and exercise in the control of body weight. Int J Obes (Lond). 2012;36(11):1428–35.

Sun T, Cao L, Ping NN, Wu Y, Liu DZ, Cao YX. Formononetin upregulates nitric oxide synthase in arterial endothelium through estrogen receptors and MAPK pathways. J Pharm Pharmacol. 2016;68(3):342–51.

Sutherland LN, Bomhof MR, Capozzi LC, Basaraba SA, Wright DC. Exercise and adrenaline increase PGC-1{alpha} mRNA expression in rat adipose tissue. J Physiol. 2009;587(Pt 7):1607–17.

Tchernof A, Despres JP. Pathophysiology of human visceral obesity: an update. Physiol Rev. 2013;93(1):359–404.

Tchernof A, Calles-Escandon J, Sites CK, Poehlman ET. Menopause, central body fatness, and insulin resistance: effects of hormone-replacement therapy. Coron Artery Dis. 1998;9(8): 503–11.

Thomas DM, Bouchard C, Church T, Slentz C, Kraus WE, Redman LM, et al. Why do individuals not lose more weight from an exercise intervention at a defined dose? An energy balance analysis. Obes Rev. 2012;13(10):835–47.

Thompson D, Karpe F, Lafontan M, Frayn K. Physical activity and exercise in the regulation of human adipose tissue physiology. Physiol Rev. 2012;92(1):157–91.

Thong FS, McLean C, Graham TE. Plasma leptin in female athletes: relationship with body fat, reproductive, nutritional, and endocrine factors. J Appl Physiol. 2000;88(6):2037–44.

Tiraby C, Tavernier G, Lefort C, Larrouy D, Bouillaud F, Ricquier D, et al. Acquirement of brown fat cell features by human white adipocytes. J Biol Chem. 2003;278(35):33370–6.

Toniolo A, Fadini GP, Tedesco S, Cappellari R, Vegeto E, Maggi A, et al. Alternative activation of human macrophages is rescued by estrogen treatment in vitro and impaired by menopausal status. J Clin Endocrinol Metab. 2015;100(1):E50–8.

Tsatsanis C, Zacharioudaki V, Androulidaki A, Dermitzaki E, Charalampopoulos I, Minas V, et al. Adiponectin induces TNF-alpha and IL-6 in macrophages and promotes tolerance to itself and other pro-inflammatory stimuli. Biochem Biophys Res Commun. 2005;335(4):1254–63.

van Harmelen V, Skurk T, Hauner H. Primary culture and differentiation of human adipocyte precursor cells. Methods Mol Med. 2005;107:125–35.

Varlamov O, Bethea CL, Roberts Jr CT. Sex-specific differences in lipid and glucose metabolism. Front Endocrinol (Lausanne). 2014;5:241.

Velickovic K, Cvoro A, Srdic B, Stokic E, Markelic M, Golic I, et al. Expression and subcellular localization of estrogen receptors alpha and beta in human fetal brown adipose tissue. J Clin Endocrinol Metab. 2014.

Vicente-Salar N, Urdampilleta Otegui A, Roche CE. Endurance training in fasting conditions: biological adaptations and body weight management. Nutr Hosp. 2015;32(n06):2409–20.

Vieira Potter VJ, Strissel KJ, Xie C, Chang E, Bennett G, Defuria J, et al. Adipose tissue inflammation and reduced insulin sensitivity in ovariectomized mice occurs in the absence of increased adiposity. Endocrinology. 2012;153(9):4266–77.

Vieira VJ, Valentine RJ, Wilund KR, Antao N, Baynard T, Woods JA. Effects of exercise and low-fat diet on adipose tissue inflammation and metabolic complications in obese mice. Am J Physiol Endocrinol Metab. 2009;296(5):E1164–71.

Vieira-Potter VJ, Zidon TM, Padilla J. Exercise and estrogen make fat cells "Fit". Exerc Sport Sci Rev. 2015;43(3):172–8.

Villarreal-Molina MT, Antuna-Puente B. Adiponectin: anti-inflammatory and cardioprotective effects. Biochimie. 2012;94(10):2143–9.

Vosselman MJ, Hoeks J, Brans B, Pallubinsky H, Nascimento EB, van der Lans AA, et al. Low brown adipose tissue activity in endurance-trained compared with lean sedentary men. Int J Obes (Lond). 2015;39(12):1696–702.

Wade GN, Gray JM. Cytoplasmic 17 beta-[3H]estradiol binding in rat adipose tissues. Endocrinology. 1978;103(5):1695–701.

Wade GN, Gray JM, Bartness TJ. Gonadal influences on adiposity. Int J Obes. 1985;9 Suppl 1:83–92.

Wallenius V, Wallenius K, Ahren B, Rudling M, Carlsten H, Dickson SL, et al. Interleukin-6-deficient mice develop mature-onset obesity. Nat Med. 2002;8(1):75–9.

Wang H, Eckel RH. Lipoprotein lipase: from gene to obesity. Am J Physiol Endocrinol Metab. 2009;297(2):E271–88.

Wehling M, Schultz A, Losel R. Nongenomic actions of estrogens: exciting opportunities for pharmacology. Maturitas. 2006;54(4):321–6.

Weisberg SP, McCann D, Desai M, Rosenbaum M, Leibel RL, Ferrante Jr AW. Obesity is associated with macrophage accumulation in adipose tissue. J Clin Invest. 2003;112(12):1796–808.

Wiik A, Gustafsson T, Esbjornsson M, Johansson O, Ekman M, Sundberg CJ, et al. Expression of oestrogen receptor alpha and beta is higher in skeletal muscle of highly endurance-trained than of moderately active men. Acta Physiol Scand. 2005;184(2):105–12.

Wohlers LM, Spangenburg EE. 17beta-estradiol supplementation attenuates ovariectomy-induced increases in ATGL signaling and reduced perilipin expression in visceral adipose tissue. J Cell Biochem. 2010;110(2):420–7.

Xu X, Ying Z, Cai M, Xu Z, Li Y, Jiang SY, et al. Exercise ameliorates high-fat diet-induced metabolic and vascular dysfunction, and increases adipocyte progenitor cell population in brown adipose tissue. Am J Physiol Regul Integr Comp Physiol. 2011;300(5):R1115–25.

Xu X, Grijalva A, Skowronski A, van Eijk M, Serlie MJ, Ferrante Jr AW. Obesity activates a program of lysosomal-dependent lipid metabolism in adipose tissue macrophages independently of classic activation. Cell Metab. 2013;18(6):816–30.

Yamashita H, Yamamoto M, Sato Y, Izawa T, Komabayashi T, Saito D, et al. Effect of running training on uncoupling protein mRNA expression in rat brown adipose tissue. Int J Biometeorol. 1993;37(1):61–4.

Yamauchi T, Kamon J, Waki H, Terauchi Y, Kubota N, Hara K, et al. The fat-derived hormone adiponectin reverses insulin resistance associated with both lipoatrophy and obesity. Nat Med. 2001;7(8):941–6.

Yang X, Wang X, Liu D, Yu L, Xue B, Shi H. Epigenetic regulation of macrophage polarization by DNA methyltransferase 3b. Mol Endocrinol. 2014;28(4):565–74.

Chapter 16
Exercise in Menopausal Women

Monica D. Prakash, Lily Stojanovska, Kulmira Nurgali
and Vasso Apostolopoulos

Introduction

Menopause, from the Greek words *men-* (month) and *pausis* (stop), describes the period in a woman's life when menstruation ceases following loss of ovarian follicular function and marks the end of fertility. Also known as climacteric, menopause is not sudden or abrupt and usually occurs over several (5–10) years from the mid 40s to mid 50s of life. During the transition, a number of signs and symptoms may occur as a result of hormonal imbalances. Each woman experiences different symptoms and severity, however hot flushes and irregular periods are the two most common symptoms of menopause. Other symptoms such as night sweats, low libido, headaches, fatigue, itchy skin, back pain and muscle tension, as well as psychological symptoms (mood swings, depression, fatigue, irritability, anxiety, panic attacks, tearfulness, sleep disorder), cognitive symptoms (memory lapses, concentration) and atrophic effects (atrophic vaginitis, bladder irritability, vaginal dryness) are also commonly reported (Philp 2003; Copeland et al. 2004; Freeman and Sherif 2007; Liu et al. 2013; Schiff 2013). The symptoms of menopause can significantly disturb daily activities and in some instances, overall quality of life. Further, many chronic diseases (e.g. osteoporosis, dementia, depression, cardiovascular disease, cancer and diabetes mellitus) commonly strike within 10 years of menopause; hence, making lifestyle changes such as healthier eating, increased exercise and the use of hormone replacement therapy (HRT) necessities to improving quality of life.

M.D. Prakash, Ph.D. • L. Stojanovska, M.Sc., Ph.D. (✉) • V.Apostolopoulos, Ph.D.
Centre for Chronic Disease, College of Health and Biomedicine, Victoria University,
Melbourne, VIC 8001, Australia
e-mail: Lily.Stojanovska@vu.edu.au

K. Nurgali, M.B.B.S., Ph.D.
College of Health & Biomedicine, Victoria University, Melbourne, VIC 14428, Australia

HRT, also known as hormone therapy (HT) or menopause hormone therapy (MHT), uses synthetic hormones; oestrogen and progestin in women with intact uterus, or oestrogen alone for women who have undergone hysterectomy, and is the most effective treatment for the relief of menopause symptoms. However, there are risks associated with HRT use (Utian and Woods 2013). A large randomised trial including 75,343 women with no history of cardiovascular disease or cancer from the Women's Health Initiative reported that significantly higher levels of inflammatory markers, C-reactive protein and interleukin-6 (IL-6) were associated with increased risk of heart disease (Pradhan et al. 2002). Similarly, in a randomised, double-blinded, placebo controlled disease prevention study across 40 US clinics, 10,739 women with prior hysterectomy (aged 50–79 years old) were randomly grouped to receive either oestrogen alone or placebo. Although the study showed no association with increased risk of breast cancer or heart disease, the trial was stopped prematurely due to an increased risk of stroke (Anderson et al. 2004). The Million Women Study from the Cancer Epidemiology Unit, UK and the National Health Services assessed the effects of HRT use in more than one million women, and confirmed that HRT was associated with increased risk of breast cancer, especially when both oestrogen and progestin were used (Banks et al. 2004; Beral et al. 2004; Gray 2003). These findings influenced national policy recommendations on prescribing HRT (Manson et al. 2013). In addition, due to these studies, a large percentage of women have become reluctant to continue or commence HRT due to fear of adverse health risks, even though subsequent studies have shown a significant decrease in the incidence of breast cancer (Clarke et al. 2006; Ravdin et al. 2007). In November 2012, the International Menopause Society conducted a round table discussion involving members of the major regional menopause societies to reach a consensus regarding HRT recommendations. A global consensus statement on HRT was published, which was aimed at women and health care practitioners to aid in making appropriate decisions on the use of HRT (de Villiers et al. 2013). However, as a result of the risks associated with HRT, many women seek other treatment options, particularly complementary and alternative therapies.

Alternative therapies, although a viable approach, claim to provide relief for an array of menopausal symptoms, however in most instances scientific support is lacking. Phytoestrogens (isoflavones), black cohosh, ginseng, evening primrose oil, dong quai, wild yam and *Lepidium meyenii* (maca) have been studied but with inconsistent results (Stojanovska and Kitanovaska 2013). Due to breast cancer risks associated with HRT and conflicting data from alternative treatments, physical activity and exercise has been proposed as another means to improve a women's quality of life during menopausal transition and post-menopause (Daley et al. 2007a, 2009, 2011b).

The Benefits of Exercise

The importance of physical activity for overall health and well-being has been recognised for thousands of years, with records dating back to ancient Greece. Hippocrates (460–370 BC) stated that "Eating alone will not keep a man well; he must also take exercise. For food and exercise, while possessing opposite qualities, yet work together to produce health".

Physical inactivity is ranked second only to cigarette smoking in its detriment to good health, giving rise to enormous economic cost worldwide. The US Department of Health and Human Services Surgeon General published a report on the effects of physical activity on health (USDHHS1996) leading to an international awakening to this important aspect of public health. Exercise has many short- and long-term benefits; it increases endurance, metabolism and energy, the health of muscles, joints and bones, decreases stress, improves cognition and improves sleeping patterns. Participation in regular exercise, either as a lifestyle choice or as part of a disease intervention programme, results in better quality of life and overall health. Indeed, decreased risk and improved health outcomes have been noted in response to cancer, cardiovascular disease, stroke, type 2 diabetes, obesity, osteoporosis and mental health disorders (King et al. 1997; Ainsworth et al. 1998; McMurray et al. 1998; Eriksen and Bruusgaard 2004; Chlebowski 2013).

A 12-week study in obese middle-aged women participating in 1 h of resistance and aerobic exercise 3 days per week showed that metabolic syndrome risk factors (blood pressure, fasting glucose, triglyceride, cholesterol, body fat) were significantly decreased with exercise (Seo et al. 2011). In addition, three classes per week of Bikram yoga improved glucose tolerance (Hunter et al. 2013) and resistance exercise significantly decreased triglyceride levels in the blood (Agil et al. 2010). Furthermore, analysis of 80 independent studies demonstrated a positive correlation between physical inactivity and clinical depression, regardless of gender, age or health status (North et al. 1990). Patients that participated in regular exercise after termination of antidepressants had lower depression scores than those who did not (LaFontaine et al. 1992). Overall, regular physical activity enhances mental health and well-being, including improved mood (Daley et al. 2014) and self-esteem (Daley et al. 2011b), reduced anxiety (Daley et al. 2007c) and reduced stress (Daley et al. 2009).

Menopause is commonly associated with a range of health complaints, most often hot flushes, joint and muscle pain, urinary disorders and psychological distress (Stefanopoulou et al. 2013). In addition, chronic conditions such as osteoporosis and cardiovascular disease are more likely to occur post-menopause than pre-menopause and menopausal women are generally of poorer overall health (Ringa 2000). Physical activity has a positive impact on both bone density and cardiovascular health in menopausal women. In the case of bone density, increased physical activity during both normal, everyday activity and recreationally is associated with higher peak femoral neck strength relative to load in over 1900 menopausal women (Mori et al. 2014). Furthermore, physical activity has a positive effect on the tibial cartilage of the knee during menopause (Fontinele et al. 2013).

It is clear that there are many benefits of exercise: maintenance of healthy bones (Kemmler et al. 2004), cardiovascular health, energy metabolism (Donnelly et al. 2009; Lovejoy et al. 2008), longevity (Lee and Paffenbarger 2000), psychological well-being (Thurston et al. 2006; Elavsky and McAuley 2009), resilience to diabetes (Hu et al. 1999) and cancer, and improved overall better quality of life (Agil et al. 2010). Thus, it is beneficial for women to be physically active throughout menopause and beyond (Stojanovska et al. 2014).

Exercise During Menopause

According to the US Centre for Disease Control and Prevention, regular exercise helps relieve stress, enhances overall quality of life, and reduces weight gain and muscle loss, which are commonly associated with menopause (Warburton et al. 2006). At least 150 min of aerobic activity and 75 min of vigorous activity per week are recommended for the maintenance of cardiovascular health. Strength training is also recommended to build bone and muscle strength, to decrease body fat and increase metabolism, which are also important factors during menopause (Mishra et al. 2011).

In a study of 48 menopausal women aged 55–72 involved in an exercise programme of 3 h per week for 12 months, subjects experienced significantly improved physical and mental health and overall quality of life compared to those who were sedentary (Villaverde-Gutierrez et al. 2006). More importantly, in the group that completed the exercise programme, the proportion of women reporting menopause symptoms dropped from 50 % at the beginning of the study to 37 % at the study's conclusion. Interestingly, in the control group, the proportion of women reporting menopause symptoms rose from 58 % at the beginning of the study to 68 % at the end of the study. Exercise was therefore shown to alleviate menopause symptoms. This study also noted that the woman's ability to choose their preferred physical activity increases the likelihood that they will adhere to exercise as a treatment method. In a more recent study, 108 women were randomised into four groups that participated in either no intervention, nutritional education, aerobic exercise or combined nutritional education and aerobic exercise (Asghari et al. 2016). Outcomes were measured using the Greene and MENQOL (menopause-specific quality of life) symptom scales, and the aerobic exercise intervention group achieved significantly lower symptom scores than control and nutritional education groups (Asghari et al. 2016). Exercise therefore appears to be a cost-effective alternative therapy for menopause, without any adverse side effects. Most importantly, women with greater levels of physical activity report improvements in mental and physical aspects of quality of life (Martin et al. 2009; Moriyama et al. 2008). Such improvements can even be achieved with low intensity aerobic activity, such as walking and dancing (de Souza Santos et al. 2011).

However, not all studies show positive changes to menopause symptoms as a result of exercise (see Tables 16.1 and 16.2). A longitudinal study conducted in Norway of 2002 women over 10 year period demonstrated that there was no correlation between occurrence of symptoms, body mass index (BMI), parity or menarche age and physical exercise (Gjelsvik et al. 2011). Likewise, in a Nigerian cohort there was no association between physical activity and menopausal symptoms and overall health-related problems (Ogwumike et al. 2012). Hence, physical exercise has not consistently been shown to be beneficial in ameliorating symptoms associated with menopause.

Table 16.1 Observational studies on the effect of exercise on menopausal symptoms

	Population	No. subjects	Key observations	Reference
Positive effect	Women aged 45–55 years	151	• Regular physical activity was also associated with significantly lower total Greene score and specifically lower psychological subscore and sexual subscore • Regular exercise was the lifestyle parameter most significantly correlated with a lower total Greene score independent of menopausal status • Regular exercise was significantly correlated with lower psychological and physical subscores • Moreover, the higher the frequency of exercise (both aerobic and non aerobic), the lower the severity of the climacteric symptoms reported, yet the vasomotor and sexual subscores remained unchanged	Haimov-Kochman et al. (2013)
	Women aged 54–63 years, currently experiencing vasomotor symptoms	52	• Greater levels of habitual physical activity, particularly non-leisure time physical activity, are associated with more favourable sleep characteristics • Even relatively modest levels of physical activity characteristic of household physical activity, may be important for women with vasomotor symptoms, a subgroup at high risk for sleep problems	Lambiase and Thurston (2013)
	Premenopausal and early perimenopausal women	1919	• Physical activity in each domain examined (sport, home, active living and work) was associated with higher peak femoral neck strength relative to load in premenopausal and early perimenopausal women	Mori et al. (2014)
	Women aged 45–64 years	1165	• Women whose physical activity increased or remained stable had greater chances for improved quality of life than women whose physical activity decreased • Women whose weight remained stable during follow-up also improved their quality of life compared to women who gained weight	Moilanen et al. (2012)
	Women aged 45–64 years	1427	• Physically active women reported fewer somatic symptoms than did women with a sedentary lifestyle	Moilanen et al. (2010)
	Women aged 45–55 years	336	• The high physical activity group felt better and had less severe climacteric symptoms; 52.08 % of the women had no climacteric symptoms	Skrzypulec et al. (2010)
	Women of mean age 52 years	280	• An increase in physical activity correlated with reporting fewer total menopause symptoms. • When the total menopause symptom score was examined by domain, increased physical activity was related to report of fewer general symptoms attributed to menopause, but had no effect on specific vasomotor and sexual symptoms	McAndrew et al. (2009)
	Middle-aged women	648	• There was a significant positive correlation between the severity of menopausal symptoms and depression • The severity of menopausal symptoms and depression in subjects who exercised more than three times a week were significantly lower than in the subjects who did not exercise	Lee and Kim (2008)
	Menopausal women aged 46–55 years	1206	• Women who were regularly active reported better health-related quality of life scores than women who were not regularly active • No difference in vasomotor symptoms was recorded for exercise status • Women who were obese reported significantly higher vasomotor and somatic symptom scores than women of normal weight	Daley et al. (2007a)
	Women of mean age 51 years	133	• Women who were more physically active reported significantly less severe vaso-somatic and general somatic symptoms	Elavsky and McAuley (2005)
	Women aged 45–55 years	350	• Low exercise levels were significantly associated with reporting bothersome hot flushes • In women reporting hot flushes, the hot flush index score decreased as their age and exercise level increased	Guthrie et al. (2005)

(continued)

Table 16.1 (continued)

	Population	No. subjects	Key observations	Reference
No effect	Women aged 40–60 years	547	• No association between physical activity and menopausal symptoms and overall health-related problems	Ogwumike et al. (2012)
	Women aged 40–44 years	2002	• No correlation between reporting of symptoms, body mass index (BMI), parity or menarche age and physical exercise	Gjelsvik et al. (2011)
	Middle-aged women from the Australian Longitudinal Study on Women's Health	3330	• Physical activity was not associated with total menopausal symptoms, vasomotor or psychological symptoms • There was a weak association between physical activity and somatic symptoms • Weight gain was associated with increased total, vasomotor, and somatic symptoms • Weight loss was associated with a reduction in total and vasomotor symptoms	Van Poppel and Brown (2008)
	Midlife women		• No significant relationship was seen between vasomotor symptoms, sexual function and exercise.	Mirzaiinjmabadi et al. (2006)
	Women aged 48–52	171	• Perimenopausal exercise was not associated with reduced risk of frequent vasomotor symptoms. This lack of relationship was observed in all domains of activity • Physical activity was also not associated with reduced risk of psychologic distress, depressive feelings or somatic symptoms • Vasomotor symptoms were strongly associated with increased risk of psychologic distress, depressive feelings or somatic symptoms	Sternfeld et al. (1999)
	Women aged 45–55	1181	• There was no significant association between levels of physical activity, psychological well-being and women's experience of symptoms during the natural menopause transition	Guthrie et al. (1994)
Negative Effect	Women aged 40–60 years	273	• A negative significant correlation was found between somatic complaints including sexual problems and vaginal dryness as well as joint-muscular discomfort, and the level of physical activity	Javadivala et al. (2013)
	Perimenopausal and postmenopausal women	512	• Highly active women between the ages of 35 and 40 were significantly more likely to report moderate to severe hot flushes and daily hot flushes than minimally active women	Whitcomb et al. (2007)

Table 16.2 Intervention studies on the effect of exercise on menopausal symptoms

	Population	No. subjects	Intervention	Key observations	Reference
Total symptoms	Early menopausal women	108	Nutritional education, aerobic exercise or combined nutritional education and aerobic exercise	• The aerobic exercise intervention group achieved significantly lower symptom scores than control and nutritional education groups	Asghari et al. (2016)
	Menopausal women aged 45–60	36	Aerobic or resistance exercise 3 days/week for 8 weeks	• In the resistance exercise group there were significant improvements in all subscales of Menopausal Rating Scale (MRS), excluding urogenital complaints. There were also significant improvements in all subscales of The Symptom Checklist, excluding the phobic anxiety • Depression levels significantly decreased in both exercise groups • Improvements were observed in all subscales of menopause-specific quality of life (MENQOL) questionnaire in both exercise groups except for sexual symptoms	Agil et al. (2010)
	Menopausal women aged 55–72	48	Two sessions/week of cardiorespiratory, stretching, muscle-strengthening and relaxation exercises totalling 3 h weekly for 12 months	• At the beginning of the study, 50 % of women in the exercise group reported menopausal symptoms, which dropped to 37 % at the study's conclusion • In the control group, the proportion of women reporting menopause symptoms rose from 58 % at the beginning of the study to 68 % at the end of the study	Villaverde-Gutierrez et al. (2006)
Vasomotor symptoms and sleep quality	Perimenopausal and postmenopausal women experiencing hot flushes/night sweats	261	30 min moderate intensity exercise at least 3 days/week increasing to at least 30 min 3–5 days/week by week 24	• This study indicates that exercise is not an effective treatment for hot flushes/night sweats, with neither of the exercise interventions resulting in women reporting significantly fewer hot flushes/night sweats per week compared with controls at the 6- and 12-month follow ups	Daley et al. (2015)

(continued)

Table 16.2 (continued)

Population	No. subjects	Intervention	Key observations	Reference
Women aged 40–62 years in menopausal transition or postmenopause	237	Yoga	• No improvements to vasomotor symptom frequency were noted	Newton et al. (2013)
Midlife women aged 40–60 years	121	30-min moderate-intensity aerobic exercise	• Both total objective and total subjective hot flushes decreased after acute exercise • Daily physical activity was not associated with self-reported hot flushes • Performing more moderate physical activity than usual was associated with more self-reported hot flushes in women with lower fitness levels	Elavsky et al. (2012a)
Symptomatic, sedentary women aged 43–63 years	176	Aerobic training for 50 min 4 times/week for 6 months	• The exercise group had a larger decrease in the frequency of night-time hot flushes and less depressed mood than control women • Changes in depressed mood and menopausal symptoms in the exercise group were dependent on frequency of training sessions	Luoto et al. (2012)
Sedentary women aged 43–63 years with menopausal symptoms	176	Aerobic training for 50 min 4 times/week for 6 months	• Sleep quality improved significantly more in the intervention group than in the control group • The odds for sleep improvement were 2 % per week in the intervention group and a decrease of 0.5 % per week in the control group • The amount of hot flushes relative to sleep diminished by the end of the intervention	Mansikkamaki et al. (2012)
Women aged 45–65 years	173	Walking 4 times/week for 20–30 min for 24 weeks	• After 24 weeks, there were no differences between the walking and control group for change in symptoms • However, frequency of walking along with change in physical symptoms and menopausal status were significant predictors of change in sleep symptoms	Wilbur et al. (2005)

	Postmenopausal, overweight or obese, sedentary aged 50–75 years	173	Year-long moderate-intensity exercise and a low-intensity stretching programme	• Among morning exercisers, those who exercised at least 225 min per week had less trouble falling asleep compared with those who exercised less than 180 min per week • However, among evening exercisers, those who exercised at least 225 min per week had more trouble falling asleep compared to those who exercised less than 180 min per week • Stretchers were less likely to use sleep medication and have trouble falling asleep during the intervention period compared with baseline	Tworoger et al. (2003)
Psychological symptoms	Women aged 57–75 years	121	Moderate intensity walking for 40 min three times/week over 6 months	• Participants in the walking intervention showed a significant decrease in depression as compared with controls	Bernard et al. (2015)
	Late perimenopausal and postmenopausal sedentary women with frequent vasomotor symptoms	106	Moderate intensity aerobic exercise three times/week for 12 weeks	• Exercise did not alleviate vasomotor symptoms, but did result in improved sleep quality, insomnia and depression	Sternfeld et al. (2013)
	Sedentary, sexually active women who had undergone menopause no more than 5 years earlier	32	3-month physical exercise protocol including pelvic floor muscle training	• In the exercise group, there was a significant decrease in the number of women suffering from anxiety, but there was no effect on sexual function	Lara et al. (2012)
	Postmenopausal women aged 60–70 years	60	Mixed physical exercises	• In the exercise group, statistically significant improvements were observed in subjects with moderate and severe depression (18 and 22%, respectively) and in those with symptoms of anxiety. No such changes were observed in the control group	Villaverde Gutierrez et al. (2012)
	Previously low-active middle-aged women of mean age 50 years	164	Walking or yoga	• Walking and yoga were effective in enhancing positive affect and menopause-related quality of life and reducing negative affect • Women who experienced decreases in menopausal symptoms across the trial also experienced improvements in all positive mental health outcomes and reductions in negative mental health outcomes	Elavsky et al. (2012a)

Vasomotor Symptoms

Peri-menopause, women experience vasomotor-related symptoms such as hot flushes, night sweats, sleep disturbances and even chronic insomnia. Symptoms are sometimes so severe that a woman's overall quality of life is disturbed. HRT has been shown to alleviate such symptoms, however prolonged use can have serious side effects (Stuenkel et al. 2012). Lifestyle interventions such as structured exercise and physical activity have the potential to reduce vasomotor symptoms associated with menopause (Daley et al. 2007b, 2009). However, the evidence remains controversial (Sternfeld and Dugan 2011). Intervention studies are largely inconsistent, with about half of the observational studies reporting no effect (Sternfeld et al. 1999; Van Poppel and Brown 2008; Daley et al. 2007c; Gold et al. 2006; Guthrie et al. 1994), and the others suggesting a protective effect (Guthrie et al. 2005; Moilanen et al. 2010; Elavsky and McAuley 2005). Some studies even report increased vasomotor symptoms with increased physical activity (Romani et al. 2009; Whitcomb et al. 2007).

In response to these conflicting reports, the MeFLASH (Menopause Strategies: Finding Lasting Answers for Symptoms and Health) Research Network conducted a 12-week randomised controlled trial of aerobic exercise training in previously sedentary menopausal women (Newton et al. 2014). The study demonstrated that moderate intensity aerobic exercise for 12 weeks did not alleviate vasomotor symptoms, but did result in improved sleep quality, insomnia and depression (Sternfeld et al. 2013). In addition, the type of exercise intervention was analysed amongst 6 eligible studies and compared to HRT (Daley et al. 2011a). There was insufficient evidence demonstrating that exercise was effective in treating vasomotor menopausal symptoms, and it was not clear whether exercise was more beneficial compared to HRT (Daley et al. 2011a). The same research group more recently updated this review with analysis of five additional studies, and again found no evidence for exercise as an effective treatment for menopause associated vasomotor symptoms (Daley et al. 2014). Likewise, the Australian Longitudinal Study on Women's Health reported no improvement in vasomotor or psychological symptoms and only marginal improvements in somatic symptoms upon commencement of physical activity (Van Poppel and Brown 2008). Moreover, in a study of 280 women, increasing their level of physical activity had no effect on vasomotor or sexual symptoms of menopause (McAndrew et al. 2009). In several studies including 16,000 American women from range of backgrounds (Gold et al. 2007), 173 African-American and Caucasian women (Wilbur et al. 2005), and 338 overweight women (Huang et al. 2010), no associations were noted amongst vasomotor symptom severity and physical activity. Similarly, in 164 women participating in moderate physical activity, such as walking and yoga, no improvement was shown in sleep quality (Elavsky and McAuley 2007a). Furthermore, in a randomised controlled study of 237 women participating in yoga classes, no improvements to vasomotor symptom frequency were noted (Newton et al. 2013). Pooled analysis of six pharmacologic and non-pharmacologic interventions showed no effect on vasomotor symptom frequency or severity with either aerobic exercise or yoga (Guthrie et al. 2015). A study comparing at home DVD-based exercise and social exercise to control menopausal women showed no significant decrease in frequency of hot flushes or night sweats in either exercise group (Daley et al. 2015). Another randomised controlled trial at three different sites, where 106 women participated in moderate exercise for 12 weeks and were compared to 142 women with no addition of exercise to their daily routine, showed no improvement to vasomotor symptoms, although slight improvements were sleep quality, insomnia, mood and depressive symptoms were noted in the exercise group (Sternfeld et al. 2013).

However, the longitudinal Melbourne Women's Midlife Health Project, where 438 women were monitored over 8 years, demonstrated that those who exercised daily at baseline were 49% less likely to report hot flushes than those whose exercise levels decreased (Guthrie et al. 1994). Moderate physical activity was associated with decreased objective and subjective hot flushes 24 h post-exercise, although exacerbated symptoms have been noted in women with lower fitness levels (Elavsky et al. 2012a). In a randomised controlled trial, 176 symptomatic sedentary women who were given an aerobic exercise regime of 50 min, four times per week over 6 months, reported a decrease in the frequency of hot flushes (Luoto et al. 2012). These conflicting results may occur due to differences in the type and intensity of the prescribed exercise. A randomised controlled trial is now underway to examine whether resistance training, rather than aerobic exercise, constitutes an effective treatment for menopausal vasomotor symptoms (Berin et al. 2016).

Studies specifically assessing the effects of high intensity exercise on chronic insomnia, while varied in their design, type of exercise prescribed and outcome measures, show overwhelming support for the benefit of exercise (Attarian et al. 2015). A cross-sectional observational study of 339 perimenopausal women demonstrated that high levels of physical activity such as recreational sport was associated with significantly improved sleep quality with fewer disturbances (Kline et al. 2013). Another year-long randomised trial of low intensity stretching versus high intensity exercise also demonstrated improvement in sleep in both groups (Tworoger et al. 2003). In a small trial of 52 perimenopausal women with chronic insomnia and vasomotor symptoms, those that were more physically active reported better subjective sleep and improvement in vasomotor symptoms (Lambiase and Thurston 2013). Another randomised trial of 176 perimenopausal women with chronic insomnia and vasomotor symptoms prescribed subjects either 50 min of aerobic exercise a day, four times per week or sedentary activity for 6 months. The exercise group reported significant improvement in sleep and decreased number of hot flushes (Mansikkamaki et al. 2012). An observational cross-sectional study of 336 menopausal women demonstrated a significant correlation between the absence of vasomotor symptoms and high levels of physical activity, compared to those who had low or moderate levels of physical activity (Skrzypulec et al. 2010). This was not independent of weight as perimenopausal women that were more highly physically active had lower BMI and obesity was associated with increased frequency of chronic insomnia and vasomotor symptoms (Skrzypulec et al. 2010).

In general, it is well accepted that physical activity has positive effects in reducing cholesterol, triglyceride levels, apolipoprotein and blood glucose levels (Hunter et al. 2013; Seo et al. 2011). In 3201 women aged 42–52 years, monitored annually for 8 years, hot flushes were associated with higher cholesterol, triglyceride and apolipoprotein A levels (Thurston et al. 2012a). Furthermore, in 3075 women, a strong correlation between hot flushes and insulin resistance has been shown (Thurston et al. 2012b). Hence, exercise may indirectly be associated with reducing hot flush symptoms (Elavsky et al. 2012b). In addition, sleep disturbances are less prevalent in menopausal women who are physically active (Newton et al. 2013), with fewer awakenings during the night (Lambiase and Thurston 2013) and improved quality of sleep (Mansikkamaki et al. 2012).

Finally, excess body weight is associated with increased menopause symptoms. Indeed, the Australian Longitudinal Study on Women's Health showed in 3330 mid-aged women that although there was no association between physical activity and total menopausal symptoms, but there was an association between reduction in both total and vasomotor symptoms and weight loss (Van Poppel and Brown 2008). In addition, in 1165 Finnish females aged 45–64, followed for 8 years, overall quality of life was improved in those who were physically active and whose weight remained stable during follow-up, compared to those who had gained weight (Moilanen et al. 2012). Vasomotor symptoms such as hot flushes and night sweats are more prevalent in women with higher BMI (Gold et al. 2000), and in an intensive weight loss intervention study which included physical activity, exercise led to an improvement in hot flushes occurrence in obese women (Huang et al. 2010). Conversely, 430 women in a 6-month controlled study demonstrated no correlation between weight change with mental and physical quality of life (Martin et al. 2009). Future studies should involve weight loss by means of physical activity and its effect on menopausal symptoms.

Despite recent efforts to address the issue, inconsistencies remain in the growing body of data examining the effect of exercise on vasomotor symptoms. For this reason, the 2015 position statements of both the North American Menopause Society and the European Menopause and Andropause Society (EMAS) do not recommend exercise or yoga as an alternative therapy for menopause-associated vasomotor symptoms (NAMS 2015; Mintziori et al. 2015).

Psychological Symptoms

Although depression is not caused by menopause, about 75% of women report symptoms of depression (irritability, tearfulness, sadness, fatigue) or anxiety (mood changes, tension, insomnia, heart palpitations, panic attacks, forgetfulness and inability to focus) during this time (Borkoles et al. 2015). Often, such symptoms could be managed through lifestyle changes, including healthy eating, exercise and meditation. In fact, in a study of middle-aged Australian women it was reported that exercise was beneficial for somatic and psychological symptoms including depression and anxiety, but not for vasomotor symptoms or sexual function (Mirzaiinjmabadi et al. 2006). Similarly, a randomised controlled trial of 121 inactive postmenopausal women showed that the group prescribed a walking intervention of 40 min per session, three times a week for 6 months experienced a significant decrease in depression compared to controls (Bernard et al. 2015).

Depression has also been associated with other symptoms of menopause, particularly vasomotor symptoms (Borkoles et al. 2015). In a cross-sectional Korean study of 648 women aged 40–60 years, a positive correlation was shown between severity of menopausal symptoms and depression; those who exercised on a regular basis, were less depressed and less symptomatic than those who were sedentary (Lee and Kim 2008). These findings add to the evidence suggesting that women who are depressed have more severe menopausal symptoms and exercise moderates the psychological symptoms associated with menopause (Elavsky 2009; McAndrew et al. 2009). In addition, habitual physical activities (those that are part of a person's lifestyle) such as gardening, walking, household chores, cycling and work-related physical activities of up to 1 h per day, have positive effects on menopause symptoms and quality of life. Habitual practice improves social outcomes and psychological symptoms and decreases body weight (de Azevedo Guimaraes and Baptista 2011; Elavsky and McAuley 2007b). Likewise, in a cross-sectional study involving 151 physically active women, psychological symptoms improved (Haimov-Kochman et al. 2013), and in 60 postmenopausal women, aged 60–70 years, those who exercised reported improvements in anxiety and depressive symptoms (Villaverde Gutierrez et al. 2012). Exercise is believed to impart psychological benefit on its participants by providing mental distraction and social interaction (Mirzaiinjmabadi et al. 2006; Agil et al. 2010). This is an indirect effect on symptom burden through enhancement of positive disposition and coping efficacy on a day to day basis (Kishida and Elavsky 2015). However, a common barrier for menopausal women considering an exercise regime are the demands of this stage of life, lack of time, safety concerns when exercising outdoors, weather and lack of company (Im et al. 2008). Breaking up exercise regimes into multiple shorter bursts and encouraging social interaction as part of exercise is important in maintaining compliance among midlife women (McArthur et al. 2014).

Somatic Symptoms

Somatic symptoms are those related to the body; distinct from psychological symptoms. They include pressure-like sensation in the head or body, muscle and joint pain, numbness or tingling in the extremities, dizziness, headaches, feeling faint and shortness of breath.

The Health 2000 population-based study of 1427 Finnish women aged 45–64 years, found that those who were physically active reported significantly fewer somatic symptoms and pain than did women with a sedentary lifestyle (Moilanen et al. 2010). Interestingly, smoking showed no correlation with symptoms. Eight years later those that remained physically active exhibited improved quality of life compared to those who were not physically active (Moilanen et al. 2012). Physical activity was also found to improve somatic symptoms, in addition to psychological and urogenital symptoms, in a study of 370 Brazilian women aged 40–65 years old (Gonçalves et al. 2011). In addition, in a large cross-sectional study involving 1206 British women, somatic symptoms were lower amongst active women and those with normal BMI (Daley et al. 2007a). Similarly, in a longitudinal study of 3300 Australian women, increased physical activity was associated with fewer somatic symptoms (Van Poppel and Brown 2008). In the Study of Women's Health Across the Nation (SWAN), a multiethnic observational cohort study of the menopause transition in 3302 women across seven sites in the US, it was noted that physically active women experienced less bodily pain during menopause (Avis et al. 2009). Likewise, a 3-year longitudinal study of over 2400 women from SWAN demonstrated that women who were more physically active at midlife experienced less bodily pain over time regardless of menopausal status (Dugan et al. 2009). This suggests that physical activity significantly improves somatic symptoms in menopausal women and increases their overall quality of life.

Sexual Symptoms

The loss of oestrogen and testosterone following menopause leads to changes in a woman's sexual drive. As a result of depleted oestrogen, there is a significant drop in blood supply to the vagina, leading to vaginal dryness or thinning of the wall, sexual dysfunction or discomfort.

In a study of 42 postmenopausal women, divided into two groups of aerobic or resistance exercise programmes of 3 days per week for 8 weeks, no effects were noted for urogenital complaints and sexual symptoms (Van Poppel and Brown 2008). In another study of 24 women participating in a 3 month exercise regime, no improvements in sexual function were noted, although reduced anxiety and improvement in pelvic floor muscular strength were demonstrated (Lara et al. 2012). Likewise, a cross-sectional study of 1071 postmenopausal Turkish women showed no association between regular exercise and urogenital symptoms (Aydin et al. 2013). However, in another cross-sectional study in 151 women, those who exercised regularly (at least three times a week), reported improved menopausal symptoms including a decrease in sexual symptoms (Haimov-Kochman et al. 2013). Moreover, in 273 Iranian women, a significant negative correlation was noted between sexual problems and vaginal dryness and the level of physical activity (Javadivala et al. 2013). It is clear that the findings with regards to exercise and sexual functioning are ambiguous; it is an area which requires further studies.

Exercise Post-menopause

Habitual physical activity has numerous health benefits, including decreased risk of obesity, cardiovascular disease, type 2 diabetes, stroke, metabolic syndromes, cancer, osteoporosis, psychological symptoms and improved muscle and bone health. The risk of having one of these health issues is greatest post-menopause, independent of traditional risk factors (Sternfeld and Dugan 2011; Kline et al. 2013). Many of these conditions are associated with chronic inflammation; however the link between exercise and inflammation in menopausal women is only now beginning to be explored. In a randomised controlled trial studying the effects of exercise on inflammatory cytokine levels, 28 sedentary postmenopausal women were grouped as controls or prescribed 25–30 min of low-moderate intensity treadmill training 3–4 times a week for 16 weeks (Tartibian et al. 2015). The exercise group showed a significant decrease in proinflammatory cytokines interleukin-1β (IL-1β), IL-6 and tumour necrosis factor-α (TNF-α) and hence, decreased inflammation (Tartibian et al. 2015). Similarly, a study on the effect of resistance training in postmenopausal women showed that high volume resistance training, but not low volume resistance training (where high volume was equal to double low volume) prevented increased inflammation observed in the control group as measured by circulating levels of TNF-α and IL-6 (Nunes et al. 2016).

The incidence of cardiovascular disease is increased in postmenopausal women, but the risk is lower in physically active women (Stevenson et al. 1997). The mechanism is believed to be by improving antioxidant capacity and decreasing body iron burden (Bartfay and Bartfay 2014). For example, blood pressure is lower in physically active postmenopausal women compared to healthy sedentary women (Corrick et al. 2013; Stevenson et al. 1997), and resistance training with an intensity of 60 % once a week for 12 weeks has beneficial effects on blood pressure, heart rate and cholesterol levels (Gelecek et al. 2012). Similarly, a modified relaxation technique used as an intervention in Thai postmenopausal women, lowered blood pressure as early as 4 weeks after treatment commenced (Saensak et al. 2013). Interestingly, whole body vibration exercise training improves systemic and local leg arterial stiffness, leg muscle strength and blood pressure in postmenopausal women with pre-hypertension or hypertension (Figueroa et al. 2014). In addition, cardiorespiratory exercise improves metabolic syndrome factors (waist circumference, blood pressure and blood glucose) in postmenopausal women (Earnest et al. 2013). Furthermore, aerobic exercise and calorie restriction improves insulin sensitivity and reduces the risk of diabetes in postmenopausal women (Ryan et al. 2012).

Decreases in bone mineral density and skeletal muscle regenerative capacity are more commonly observed post-menopause, most likely due to lowered oestrogen levels (Tworoger et al. 2003; Skrzypulec et al. 2010). Regular walking, when continued as an intervention for more than 6 months, improves femoral neck bone mineral density in postmenopausal women (Ma et al. 2013). In addition, combination of low intensity but not high intensity training improves bone mineral density in older frail individuals (Villareal et al. 2004). Long-term periodic resistance training also increases muscle strength and lean body mass and decreases inflammatory markers (leptin and resistin) in postmenopausal women (Botero et al. 2013). Research has started to investigate the effects of exercise with or without HRT to determine the effects of exercise on skeletal muscle regeneration and maintenance of muscle mass in postmenopausal women (Velders and Diel 2013). In fact, an intervention combining HRT and exercise in postmenopausal women showed that exercise in addition to HRT increased positive functional measures to a greater extent than HRT alone (Taaffe et al. 2005).

Concluding Remarks

Physical activity plays a crucial role in maintaining good health and reducing the risk of disease beyond menopause, including cancer, cardiovascular disease and diabetes. Exercise intervention programmes reduce menopause symptoms, particularly psychological and somatic symptoms, and to a lesser extent vasomotor and sexual symptoms. Overall, exercise increases bone and muscle mass, improves mood, cognition and prevents weight gain (Pines 2009). Though exercise has not been shown to treat menopausal symptoms, physically active women are less stressed and have better overall quality of life during and post-menopause. It is therefore imperative for exercise to play a major role in the lives of postmenopausal women, with the aim of decreasing risks of disease and improving overall quality of life. Importantly, exercise is safe with no adverse side-effects. However, due to some inconsistencies between studies on the effects of exercise on menopause symptoms, in particular those relating to vasomotor and sexual symptoms, there is a need for more well-designed and sufficiently powered randomised trials in order to further elucidate the benefits of exercise on menopause symptoms. Possible explanations for the ambiguous findings on vasomotor and sexual symptoms in particular and exercise may be (1) varying sample sizes, (2) non-randomised designs, (3) inadequate specified exercise dose (vigorous vs moderate intensity; frequency, duration), (4) mode (aerobic vs resistance exercise) and (5) inadequate follow-up. Studies have often assessed physical activity and exercise behaviours by means of self-reporting and questionnaires rather than objectively. In addition, some studies included participants who were already physically active, whereas other studies included women who started exercise to alleviate symptoms. Furthermore, different mechanisms might underlie symptom aetiology in those that are active prior to and during menopause compared to those who take up exercise during menopause. Nonetheless, it is clear that exercise has numerous benefits on bone density, muscle mass, cardiovascular health and metabolic and psychological improvements. Regular exercise is also known to boost the immune system (Izzicupo et al. 2013a, b), and decrease chronic inflammation (Phillips et al. 2012) in menopausal women. Moreover, studies relating to physical activity, immunological outcomes and menopausal symptoms, during menopause and beyond are critically needed, as they may hold the key to understanding the underlying mechanisms of menopause symptoms (Apostolopoulos et al. 2014).

References

Agil A, Abike F, Daskapan A, Alaca R, Tuzun H. Short-term exercise approaches on menopausal symptoms, psychological health, and quality of life in postmenopausal women. Obstet Gynecol Int. 2010;2010:Article ID 274261.

Ainsworth BE, Sternfeld B, Slattery ML, Daguise V, Zahm SH. Physical activity and breast cancer: evaluation of physical activity assessment methods. Cancer. 1998;83:611–20.

Anderson GL, Limacher M, Assaf AR, Bassford T, Beresford SA, Black H, et al. Effects of conjugated equine estrogen in postmenopausal women with hysterectomy: the women's health initiative randomized controlled trial. JAMA. 2004;291:1701–12.

Apostolopoulos V, Borkoles E, Polman R, Stojanovska L. Physical and immunological aspects of exercise in chronic diseases. Immunotherapy. 2014;6:1145–57.

Asghari M, Mirghafourvand M, Mohammad-Alizadeh-Charandabi S, Malakouti J, Nedjat S. Effect of aerobic exercise and nutrition education on quality of life and early menopause symptoms: a randomized controlled trial. Women Health. 2016;24:1–16.

Attarian H, Hachul H, Guttuso T, Phillips B. Treatment of chronic insomnia disorder in menopause: evaluation of literature. Menopause. 2015;22:674–84.

Avis NE, Colvin A, Bromberger JT, Hess R, Matthews KA, Ory M, Schocken M. Change in health-related quality of life over the menopausal transition in a multiethnic cohort of middle-aged women: study of women's health across the nation. Menopause. 2009;16:860–9.

Aydin Y, Hassa H, Oge T, Yalcin OT, Mutlu FS. Frequency and determinants of urogenital symptoms in postmenopausal Islamic women. Menopause. 2013;3:3.

Banks, E., Beral, V., Reeves, G. & Million Women Study, C. Published results on breast cancer and hormone replacement therapy in the Million Women Study are correct. Climacteric. 2004;7:415–6. author reply 416-7.

Bartfay W, Bartfay E. A case-control study examining the effects of active versus sedentary lifestyles on measures of body iron burden and oxidative stress in postmenopausal women. Biol Res Nurs. 2014;16:38–45.

Beral, V., Banks, E., Reeves, G. & Million Women Study, C. Effects of estrogen-only treatment in postmenopausal women. JAMA. 2004;292:684. author reply 685-6.

Berin E, Hammar ML, Lindblom H, Lindh-Astrand L, Spetz Holm AC. Resistance training for hot flushes in postmenopausal women: randomized controlled trial protocol. Maturitas. 2016; 85:96–103.

Bernard P, Ninot G, Bernard PL, Picot MC, Jaussent A, Tallon G, Blain H. Effects of a six-month walking intervention on depression in inactive post-menopausal women: a randomized controlled trial. Aging Ment Health. 2015;19:485–92.

Borkoles E, Reynolds N, Thompson DR, Ski CF, Stojanovska L, Polman RC. The role of depressive symptomatology in peri- and post-menopause. Maturitas. 2015;81:306–10.

Botero JP, Shiguemoto GE, Prestes J, Marin CT, Do Prado WL, Pontes CS, Guerra RL, Ferreia FC, Baldissera V, Perez SE. Effects of long-term periodized resistance training on body composition, leptin, resistin and muscle strength in elderly post-menopausal women. J Sports Med Phys Fitness. 2013;53:289–94.

Chlebowski RT. Nutrition and physical activity influence on breast cancer incidence and outcome. Breast. 2013;22 Suppl 2:S30–7.

Clarke CA, Glaser SL, Uratsu CS, Selby JV, Kushi LH, Herrinton LJ. Recent declines in hormone therapy utilization and breast cancer incidence: clinical and population-based evidence. J Clin Oncol. 2006;24:e49–50.

Copeland JL, Chu SY, Tremblay MS. Aging, physical activity, and hormones in women – a review. J Aging Phys Act. 2004;12:101–16.

Corrick KL, Hunter GR, Fisher G, Glasser SP. Changes in vascular hemodynamics in older women following 16 weeks of combined aerobic and resistance training. J Clin Hypertens (Greenwich). 2013;15:241–6.

Daley A, Macarthur C, Stokes-Lampard H, Mcmanus R, Wilson S, Mutrie N. Exercise participation, body mass index, and health-related quality of life in women of menopausal age. Br J Gen Pract. 2007a;57:130–5.

Daley A, Stokes-Lampard H, Mutrie N, Macarthur C. Exercise for vasomotor menopausal symptoms. Cochrane Database Syst Rev. 2007b;4:CD006108.

Daley AJ, Stokes-Lampard H, Macarthur C. 'Feeling hot, hot, hot': is there a role for exercise in the management of vasomotor and other menopausal symptoms? J Fam Plann Reprod Health Care. 2007c;33:143–5.

Daley AJ, Stokes-Lampard HJ, Macarthur C. Exercise to reduce vasomotor and other menopausal symptoms: a review. Maturitas. 2009;63:176–80.

Daley A, Stokes-Lampard H, Macarthur C. Exercise for vasomotor menopausal symptoms (review). Cochrane Database Syst Rev. 2011a;1:39.

Daley A, Stokes-Lampard H, Wilson S, Rees M, Roalfe A, Macarthur C. What women want? Exercise preferences of menopausal women. Maturitas. 2011b;68:174–8.

Daley A, Stokes-Lampard H, Thomas A, Macarthur C. Exercise for vasomotor menopausal symptoms. Cochrane Database Syst Rev. 2014;11, CD006108.

Daley AJ, Thomas A, Roalfe AK, Stokes-Lampard H, Coleman S, Rees M, Hunter MS, Macarthur C. The effectiveness of exercise as treatment for vasomotor menopausal symptoms: randomised controlled trial. BJOG. 2015;122:565–75.

De Azevedo Guimaraes AC, Baptista F. Influence of habitual physical activity on the symptoms of climacterium/menopause and the quality of life of middle-aged women. Int J Womens Health. 2011;3:319–28.

De Souza Santos CA, Dantas EEM, Moreira MHR. Correlation of physical aptitude; functional capacity, corporal balance and quality of life (QoL) among elderly women submitted to a postmenopausal physical activities program. Arch Gerontol Geriatr. 2011;53:344–9.

De Villiers TJ, Gass ML, Haines CJ, Hall JE, Lobo RA, Pierroz DD, Rees M. Global Consensus Statement on menopausal hormone therapy. Maturitas. 2013;74:391–2.

Donnelly JE, Blair SN, Jakicic JM, Manore MM, Rankin JW, Smith BK. American College of Sports Medicine Position Stand. Appropriate physical activity intervention strategies for weight loss and prevention of weight regain for adults. Med Sci Sports Exerc. 2009;41:459–71.

Dugan SA, Everson-Rose SA, Karavolos K, Sternfeld B, Wesley D, Powell LH. The impact of physical activity level on SF-36 role-physical and bodily pain indices in midlife women. J Phys Act Health. 2009;6:33–42.

Earnest CP, Johannsen NM, Swift DL, Lavie CJ, Blair SN, Church TS. Dose effect of cardiorespiratory exercise on metabolic syndrome in postmenopausal women. Am J Cardiol. 2013;111:1805–11.

Elavsky S. Physical activity, menopause, and quality of life: the role of affect and self-worth across time. Menopause. 2009;16:265–71.

Elavsky S, McAuley E. Physical activity, symptoms, esteem, and life satisfaction during menopause. Maturitas. 2005;52:374–85.

Elavsky S, McAuley E. Lack of perceived sleep improvement after 4-month structured exercise programs. Menopause. 2007a;14:535–40.

Elavsky S, McAuley E. Physical activity and mental health outcomes during menopause: a randomized controlled trial. Ann Behav Med. 2007b;33:132–42.

Elavsky S, McAuley E. Personality, menopausal symptoms, and physical activity outcomes in middle-aged women. Personal Individ Differ. 2009;46:123–8.

Elavsky S, Gonzales JU, Proctor DN, Williams N, Henderson VW. Effects of physical activity on vasomotor symptoms: examination using objective and subjective measures. Menopause. 2012a;19:1095–103.

Elavsky S, Molenaar PCM, Gold CH, Williams NI, Aronson KR. Daily physical activity and menopausal hot flashes: applying a novel within-person approach to demonstrate individual differences. Maturitas. 2012b;71:287–93.

Eriksen W, Bruusgaard D. Do physical leisure time activities prevent fatigue? A 15 month prospective study of nurses' aides. Br J Sports Med. 2004;38:331–6.

Figueroa A, Kalfon R, Madzima TA, Wong A. Whole-body vibration exercise training reduces arterial stiffness in postmenopausal women with prehypertension and hypertension. Menopause. 2014;21:131–6.

Fontinele RG, Mariotti VB, Vazzolere AM, Ferrao JS, Kfoury Jr JR, De Souza RR. Menopause, exercise, and knee. What happens? Microsc Res Tech. 2013;76:381–7.

Freeman EW, Sherif K. Prevalence of hot flushes and night sweats around the world: a systematic review. Climacteric. 2007;10:197–214.

Gelecek N, Ilcin N, Subasi SS, Acar S, Demir N, Ormen M. The effects of resistance training on cardiovascular disease risk factors in postmenopausal women: a randomized-controlled trial. Health Care Women Int. 2012;33:1072–85.

Gjelsvik B, Rosvold EO, Straand J, Dalen I, Hunskaar S. Symptom prevalence during menopause and factors associated with symptoms and menopausal age. Results from the Norwegian Hordaland Women's Cohort study. Maturitas. 2011;70:383–90.

Gold EB, Sternfeld B, Kelsey JL, Brown C, Mouton C, Reame N, Salamone L, Stellato R. Relation of demographic and lifestyle factors to symptoms in a multi-racial/ethnic population of women 40, Äì 55 years of age. Am J Epidemiol. 2000;152:463.

Gold EB, Colvin A, Avis N, Bromberger J, Greendale GA, Powell L, Sternfeld B, Matthews K. Longitudinal analysis of the association between vasomotor symptoms and race/ethnicity across the menopausal transition: study of women's health across the nation. Am J Public Health. 2006;96:1226–35.

Gold EB, Lasley B, Crawford SL, Mcconnell D, Joffe H, Greendale GA. Relation of daily urinary hormone patterns to vasomotor symptoms in a racially/ethnically diverse sample of midlife women: study of women's health across the nation. Reprod Sci. 2007;14:786–97.

Gonçalves AKS, Canário ACG, Cabral PU, Da Silva RAH, Spyrides MHC, Giraldo PC, Eleutério JR. Impact of physical activity on quality of life in middle-aged women: a population based study. Rev Bras Ginecol Obstet. 2011;33:408–13.

Gray S. Breast cancer and hormone-replacement therapy: the Million Women Study. Lancet. 2003;362:1332. author reply 1332.

Guthrie JR, Smith AMA, Dennerstein L, Morse C. Physical activity and the menopause experience: a cross-sectional study. Maturitas. 1994;20:71–80.

Guthrie JR, Dennerstein L, Taffe JR, Lehert P, Burger HG. Hot flushes during the menopause transition: a longitudinal study in Australian-born women. Menopause. 2005;12:460–7.

Guthrie KA, Lacroix AZ, Ensrud KE, Joffe H, Newton KM, Reed SD, Caan B, Carpenter JS, Cohen LS, Freeman EW, Larson JC, Manson JE, Rexrode K, Skaar TC, Sternfeld B, Anderson GL. Pooled analysis of six pharmacologic and nonpharmacologic interventions for vasomotor symptoms. Obstet Gynecol. 2015;126:413–22.

Haimov-Kochman R, Constantini N, Brzezinski A, Hochner-Celnikier D. Regular exercise is the most significant lifestyle parameter associated with the severity of climacteric symptoms: a cross sectional study. Eur J Obstet Gynecol Reprod Biol. 2013;170:229–34.

Hu FB, Sigal RJ, Rich-Edwards JW, Colditz GA, Solomon CG, Willett WC, Speizer FE, Manson JE. Walking compared with vigorous physical activity and risk of type 2 diabetes in women: a prospective study. JAMA. 1999;282:1433–9.

Huang AJ, Subak LL, Wing R, West DS, Hernandez AL, Macer J, Grady D, Program to Reduce Incontinence by, D. & Exercise, I. An intensive behavioral weight loss intervention and hot flushes in women. Arch Intern Med. 2010;170:1161–7.

Hunter SD, Dhindsa M, Cunningham E, Tarumi T, Alkatan M, Tanaka H. Improvements in glucose tolerance with Bikram yoga in older obese adults: a pilot study. J Bodyw Mov Ther. 2013; 17:404–7.

Im EO, Chee W, Lim HJ, Liu Y, Kim HK. Midlife women's attitudes toward physical activity. J Obstet Gynecol Neonatal Nurs. 2008;37:203–13.

Izzicupo P, D'amico MA, Bascelli A, Di Fonso A, D'ANGELO E, Di Blasio A, Bucci I, Napolitano G, Gallina S, Di Baldassarre A. Walking training affects dehydroepiandrosterone sulfate and inflammation independent of changes in spontaneous physical activity. Menopause. 2013a;20:455–63.

Izzicupo P, Ghinassi B, D'AMICO MA, Di Blasio A, Gesi M, Napolitano G, Gallina S, Di Baldassarre A. Effects of ACE I/D polymorphism and aerobic training on the immune-endocrine network and cardiovascular parameters of postmenopausal women. J Clin Endocrinol Metab. 2013b;98:4187–94.

Javadivala Z, Kousha A, Allahverdipour H, Asghari Jafarabadi M, Tallebian H. Modeling the relationship between physical activity and quality of life in menopausal-aged women: a cross-sectional study. J Res Health Sci. 2013;13:168–75.

Kemmler W, Weineck J, Kalender WA, Engelke K. The effect of habitual physical activity, non-athletic exercise, muscle strength, and VO2max on bone mineral density is rather low in early postmenopausal osteopenic women. J Musculoskelet Neuronal Interact. 2004;4:325–34.

King AC, Oman RF, Brassington GS, Bliwise DL, Haskell WL. Moderate-intensity exercise and self-rated quality of sleep in older adults. A randomized controlled trial. JAMA. 1997;277:32–7.

Kishida M, Elavsky S. Daily physical activity enhances resilient resources for symptom management in middle-aged women. Health Psychol. 2015;34:756–64.

Kline CE, Irish LA, Krafty RT, Sternfeld B, Kravitz HM, Buysse DJ, Bromberger JT, Dugan SA, Hall MH. Consistently high sports/exercise activity is associated with better sleep quality, continuity and depth in midlife women: the SWAN sleep study. Sleep. 2013;36:1279–88.

Lafontaine TP, Dilorenzo TM, Frensch PA, Stucky-Ropp RC, Bargman EP, Mcdonald DG. Aerobic exercise and mood. A brief review, 1985–1990. Sports Med. 1992;13:160–70.

Lambiase MJ, Thurston RC. Physical activity and sleep among midlife women with vasomotor symptoms. Menopause. 2013;20(9):946–52.

Lara LA, Montenegro ML, Franco MM, Abreu DC, Rosa E, Silva AC, Ferreira CH. Is the sexual satisfaction of postmenopausal women enhanced by physical exercise and pelvic floor muscle training? J Sex Med. 2012;9:218–23.

Lee Y, Kim H. Relationships between menopausal symptoms, depression, and exercise in middle-aged women: a cross-sectional survey. Int J Nurs Stud. 2008;45:1816–22.

Lee IM, Paffenbarger Jr RS. Associations of light, moderate, and vigorous intensity physical activity with longevity. The Harvard Alumni Health Study. Am J Epidemiol. 2000;151:293–9.

Liu HL, Zhao G, Zhang H, Shi LD. Long-term treadmill exercise inhibits the progression of Alzheimer's disease-like neuropathology in the hippocampus of APP/PS1 transgenic mice. Behav Brain Res. 2013;256:261–72.

Lovejoy JC, Champagne CM, de Jonge L, Xie H, Smith SR. Increased visceral fat and decreased energy expenditure during the menopausal transition. Int J Obes (Lond). 2008;32:949–58.

Luoto R, Moilanen J, Heinonen R, Mikkola T, Raitanen J, Tomas E, Ojala K, Mansikkamaki K, Nygard CH. Effect of aerobic training on hot flushes and quality of life—a randomized controlled trial. Ann Med. 2012;44:616–26.

Ma D, Wu L, He Z. Effects of walking on the preservation of bone mineral density in perimenopausal and postmenopausal women: a systematic review and meta-analysis. Menopause. 2013;20:1216–26.

Mansikkamaki K, Raitanen J, Nygard CH, Heinonen R, Mikkola T, Eijatomas-Luoto R. Sleep quality and aerobic training among menopausal women – a randomized controlled trial. Maturitas. 2012;72:339–45.

Manson JE, Chlebowski RT, Stefanick ML, Aragaki AK, Rossouw JE, Prentice RL. Menopausal hormone therapy and health outcomes during the intervention and extended poststopping phases of the Women's Health Initiative randomized trials. JAMA. 2013;310:1353–68.

Martin CK, Church TS, Thompson AM, Earnest CP, Blair SN. Exercise dose and quality of life a randomized controlled trial. Arch Intern Med. 2009;169:269–78.

McAndrew LM, Napolitano MA, Albrecht A, Farrell NC, Marcus BH, Whiteley JA. When, why and for whom there is a relationship between physical activity and menopause symptoms. Maturitas. 2009;64:119–25.

McArthur D, Dumas A, Woodend K, Beach S, Stacey D. Factors influencing adherence to regular exercise in middle-aged women: a qualitative study to inform clinical practice. BMC Womens Health. 2014;14:49.

McMurray RG, Ainsworth BE, Harrell JS, Griggs TR, Williams OD. Is physical activity or aerobic power more influential on reducing cardiovascular disease risk factors? Med Sci Sports Exerc. 1998;30:1521–9.

Mintziori G, Lambrinoudaki I, Goulis DG, Ceausu I, Depypere H, Erel CT. EMAS position statement: non-hormonal management of menopausal vasomotor symptoms. Maturitas. 2015;81:410–3.

Mirzaiinjmabadi K, Anderson D, Barnes M. The relationship between exercise, Body Mass Index and menopausal symptoms in midlife Australian women. Int J Nurs Pract. 2006;12:28–34.

Mishra N, Mishra VN, Devanshi. Devanshi exercise beyond menopause: dos and don'ts. J Midlife Health. 2011;2:51–6.

Moilanen J, Aalto AM, Hemminki E, Aro AR, Raitanen J, Luoto R. Prevalence of menopause symptoms and their association with lifestyle among Finnish middle-aged women. Maturitas. 2010;67:368–74.

Moilanen JM, Aalto AM, Raitanen J, Hemminki E, Aro AR, Luoto R. Physical activity and change in quality of life during menopause—an 8-year follow-up study. Health Qual Life Outcomes. 2012;10:8.

Mori T, Ishii S, Greendale GA, Cauley JA, Sternfeld B, Crandall CJ, Han W, Karlamangla AS. Physical activity as determinant of femoral neck strength relative to load in adult women: findings from the hip strength across the menopause transition study. Osteoporos Int. 2014;25(1):265–72.

Moriyama CK, Oneda B, Bernardo FR, Cardoso Jr CG, Forjaz CL, Abrahao SB, Mion Jr D, Fonseca AM, Tinucci T. A randomized, placebo-controlled trial of the effects of physical exercises and estrogen therapy on health-related quality of life in postmenopausal women. Menopause. 2008;15:613–8.

NAMS. Nonhormonal management of menopause-associated vasomotor symptoms: 2015 position statement of The North American Menopause Society. Menopause. 2015;22:1155–72. quiz 1173–4.

Newton KM, Reed SD, Guthrie KA, Sherman KJ, Booth-Laforce C, Caan B, Sternfeld B, Carpenter JS, Learman LA, Freeman EW, Cohen LS, Joffe H, Anderson GL, Larson JC, Hunt JR, Ensrud KE, Lacroix AZ. Efficacy of yoga for vasomotor symptoms: a randomized controlled trial. Menopause. 2013;21(4):339–46.

Newton KM, Carpenter JS, Guthrie KA, Anderson GL, Caan B, Cohen LS, Ensrud KE, Freeman EW, Joffe H, Sternfeld B, Reed SD, Sherman S, Sammel MD, Kroenke K, Larson JC, Lacroix AZ. Methods for the design of vasomotor symptom trials: the menopausal strategies: finding lasting answers to symptoms and health network. Menopause. 2014;21:45–58.

North TC, Mccullagh P, Tran ZV. Effect of exercise on depression. Exerc Sport Sci Rev. 1990;18:379–415.

Nunes PR, Barcelos LC, Oliveira AA, Furlanetto Junior R, Martins FM, Orsatti CL, Resende EA, Orsatti FL. Effect of resistance training on muscular strength and indicators of abdominal adiposity, metabolic risk, and inflammation in postmenopausal women: controlled and randomized clinical trial of efficacy of training volume. Age (Dordr). 2016;38:40.

Ogwumike OO, Kaka B, Adegbemigun O, Abiona T. Health-related and socio-demographic correlates of physical activity level amongst urban menopausal women in Nigeria. Maturitas. 2012;73:349–53.

Phillips MD, Patrizi RM, Cheek DJ, Wooten JS, Barbee JJ, Mitchell JB. Resistance training reduces subclinical inflammation in obese, postmenopausal women. Med Sci Sports Exerc. 2012;44:2099–110.

Philp HA. Hot flashes – a review of the literature on alternative and complementary treatment approaches. Altern Med Rev. 2003;8:284–302.

Pines A. Lifestyle and diet in postmenopausal women. Climacteric. 2009;12 Suppl 1:62–5.

Pradhan AD, Manson JE, Rossouw JE, Siscovick DS, Mouton CP, Rifai N, Wallace RB, Jackson RD, Pettinger MB, Ridker PM. Inflammatory biomarkers, hormone replacement therapy, and incident coronary heart disease: prospective analysis from the Women's Health Initiative observational study. JAMA. 2002;288:980–7.

Ravdin PM, Cronin KA, Howlader N, Berg CD, Chlebowski RT, Feuer EJ, Edwards BK, Berry DA. The decrease in breast-cancer incidence in 2003 in the United States. N Engl J Med. 2007;356:1670–4.

Ringa V. Menopause and treatments. Qual Life Res. 2000;9:695–707.

Romani WA, Gallicchio L, Flaws JA. The association between physical activity and hot flash severity, frequency, and duration in mid-life women. Am J Hum Biol. 2009;21:127–9.

Ryan AS, Ortmeyer HK, Sorkin JD. Exercise with calorie restriction improves insulin sensitivity and glycogen synthase activity in obese postmenopausal women with impaired glucose tolerance. Am J Physiol Endocrinol Metab. 2012;302:E145–52.

Saensak S, Vutyavanich T, Somboonporn W, Srisurapanont M. Modified relaxation technique for treating hypertension in Thai postmenopausal women. J Multidiscip Healthc. 2013;6:373–8.

Schiff I. Invited reviews: a new addition to menopause. Menopause. 2013;20:243.

Seo DI, So WY, Ha S, Yoo EJ, Kim D, Singh H, Fahs CA, Rossow L, Bemben DA, Bemben MG, Kim E. Effects of 12 weeks of combined exercise training on visfatin and metabolic syndrome factors in obese middle-aged women. J Sports Sci Med. 2011;10:222–6.

Skrzypulec V, Dabrowska J, Drosdzol A. The influence of physical activity level on climacteric symptoms in menopausal women. Climacteric. 2010;13:355–61.

Stefanopoulou E, Shah D, Shah R, Gupta P, Sturdee D, Hunter MS. An International Menopause Society study of climate, altitude, temperature (IMS-CAT) and vasomotor symptoms in urban Indian regions. Climacteric. 2013;17(4):417–24.

Sternfeld B, Dugan S. Physical activity and health during the menopausal transition. Obstet Gynecol Clin North Am. 2011;38:537–66.

Sternfeld B, Quesenberry Jr CP, Husson G. Habitual physical activity and menopausal symptoms: a case-control study. J Womens Health. 1999;8:115–23.

Sternfeld B, Guthrie KA, Ensrud KE, Lacroix AZ, Larson JC, Dunn AL, Anderson GL, Seguin RA, Carpenter JS, Newton KM, Reed SD, Freeman EW, Cohen LS, Joffe H, Roberts M, Caan BJ. Efficacy of exercise for menopausal symptoms: a randomized controlled trial. Menopause. 2013;21(4):330–8.

Stevenson ET, Davy KP, Jones PP, Desouza CA, Seals DR. Blood pressure risk factors in healthy postmenopausal women: physical activity and hormone replacement. J Appl Physiol. 1997;82:652–60.

Stojanovska L, Kitanovaska V. The effect of complementary and alternative therapy at menopause: trick or treat? Curr Top Menopause. 2013;2013:385–413.

Stojanovska L, Apostolopoulos V, Polman R, Borkoles E. To exercise, or, not to exercise, during menopause and beyond. Maturitas. 2014;77:318–23.

Stuenkel CA, Gass ML, Manson JE, Lobo RA, Pal L, Rebar RW, Hall JE. A decade after the Women's Health Initiative—the experts do agree. Menopause. 2012;19:846–7.

Taaffe DR, Sipila S, Cheng S, Puolakka J, Toivanen J, Suominen H. The effect of hormone replacement therapy and/or exercise on skeletal muscle attenuation in postmenopausal women: a yearlong intervention. Clin Physiol Funct Imaging. 2005;25:297–304.

Tartibian B, Fitzgerald LZ, Azadpour N, Maleki BH. A randomized controlled study examining the effect of exercise on inflammatory cytokine levels in post-menopausal women. Post Reprod Health. 2015;21:9–15.

Thurston RC, Joffe H, Soares CN, Harlow BL. Physical activity and risk of vasomotor symptoms in women with and without a history of depression: results from the Harvard Study of Moods and Cycles. Menopause. 2006;13:553–60.

Thurston RC, El Khoudary SR, Sutton-Tyrrell K, Crandall CJ, Gold EB, Sternfeld B, Joffe H, Selzer F, Matthews KA. Vasomotor symptoms and lipid profiles in women transitioning through menopause. Obstet Gynecol. 2012a;119:753–61.

Thurston RC, El Khoudary SR, Sutton-Tyrrell K, Crandall CJ, Sternfeld B, Joffe H, Gold EB, Selzer F, Matthews KA. Vasomotor symptoms and insulin resistance in the study of women's health across the nation. J Clin Endocrinol Metab. 2012b;97:3487–94.

Tworoger SS, Yasui Y, Vitiello MV, Schwartz RS, Ulrich CM, Aiello EJ, Irwin ML, Bowen D, Potter JD, Mctiernan A. Effects of a yearlong moderate-intensity exercise and a stretching intervention on sleep quality in postmenopausal women. Sleep. 2003;26:830–6.

Utian WH, Woods NF. Impact of hormone therapy on quality of life after menopause. Menopause. 2013;20(10):1098–105.

Van Poppel MNM, Brown WJ. "It's my hormones, doctor" – does physical activity help with menopausal symptoms? Menopause. 2008;15:78–85.

Velders M, Diel P. How sex hormones promote skeletal muscle regeneration. Sports Med. 2013;43:1089–100.

Villareal DT, Steger-May K, Schechtman KB, Yarasheski KE, Brown M, Sinacore DR, Binder EF. Effects of exercise training on bone mineral density in frail older women and men: a randomised controlled trial. Age Ageing. 2004;33:309–12.

Villaverde Gutierrez C, Torres Luque G, Abalos Medina GM, Argente del Castillo MJ, Guisado IM, Guisado Barrilao R, Ramirez Rodrigo J. Influence of exercise on mood in postmenopausal women. J Clin Nurs. 2012;21:923–8.

Villaverde-Gutierrez C, Araujo E, Cruz F, Roa JM, Barbosa W, Ruiz-Villaverde G. Quality of life of rural menopausal women in response to a customized exercise programme. J Adv Nurs. 2006;54:11–9.

Warburton DE, Nicol CW, Bredin SS. Health benefits of physical activity: the evidence. CMAJ. 2006;174:801–9.

Whitcomb BW, Whiteman MK, Langenberg P, Flaws JA, Romani WA. Physical activity and risk of hot flashes among women in midlife. J Womens Health (Larchmt). 2007;16:124–33.

Wilbur J, Miller AM, Mcdevitt J, Wang E, Miller J. Menopausal status, moderate-intensity walking, and symptoms in midlife women. Res Theory Nurs Pract. 2005;19:163–80.

Index

A
Acute exercise, 233, 235, 237, 239, 241–244
   effect on genital arousal, 241
   impact women's sexual function, 236
   increases physiological sexual arousal, 243
   on physiological sexual response, 235–236
Acute resistance exercise, 259
Adipocyte lipolysis, 265–267, 279, 280, 283
Adipocytes, 263, 279
Adipokines, 277
Adiponectin, 277
Adipose tissue, 264–268, 270–281, 283
   based hormones, 277
   BAT, 264
   effects of exercise and estrogen, 278–281
   factors affecting distribution, 268–269
   functions overview, 263, 264
   role of estrogen receptors, 270–271
   role of sex in exercise-mediated, 282
   secrets adiponectin proteins, 277
   WAT, 264
Adipose triglyceride lipase (ATGL), 266, 267
Aerobic exercise, 293–295, 297–301, 304–306
Aging
   stress reactivity, 204–205
   thermoregulation, 171
Alberta physical activity and breast cancer prevention trial (ALPHA Trial), 224
ALPHA Trial. *See* Alberta physical activity and breast cancer prevention trial (ALPHA Trial)
AMP-activated protein kinase (AMPK), 280
Anabolic hormones, 252–253, 256, 257, 259
Antepartum depression (APD), 180
Anterior cruciate ligament (ACL), 12, 113
   injury risk and menstrual cycle, 113, 117
Anterior knee laxity, 121
Antidepressant sexual dysfunction, 240–242
Anxiety disorder, 178–183
   mood disorders (*see* Reproductive-related mood disorders)
   PTSD, 177
APD. *See* Antepartum depression (APD)
Arginine vasopressin (AVP), 97, 98
   anterior hypothalamus (AH), 163
   estrogens and progesterone, 164
Atrial natriuretic peptide (ANP), 47

B
BCAA. *See* Branched Chain Amino Acids (BCAA)
BETA Trial. *See* Breast cancer and exercise trial in alberta (BETA Trial)
Biphasic OCs, 9
Blocking estrogen receptors, 74, 76
Blood flow, 233, 235, 236, 243, 268
Body fluid regulation, 164
Body mass index (BMI), 294, 296, 301, 302, 304
Body surface area (BSA), 21
Body water regulation, 162, 163
Branched chain amino acids (BCAA), 104
Breakdown fibrillar collagens, 128
Breast cancer, 292
   postmenopausal, 216, 218
   premenopausal, 216
   RCT, 226
   risk, 216, 218

Breast cancer and exercise trial in alberta (BETA Trial), 225
Brown adipose tissue (BAT), 264, 271–274, 283

C
Calcium, 104, 105
Cancer, 215, 291–293, 304, 306
   androgens, 215
   breast (*see* Breast cancer)
   endometrial (*see* Endometrial cancer)
   estrogens, 215
   GnRH, 217
   2-OHE1, 218
   physical activity, 216, 217
   postmenopausal women, 218
   prepuberty, 218–219
   puberty, 219–221
   SHBG, 216
Carbohydrates (CHO)
   exercise intensity, 36
   and fat, 36
   metabolism, 37–38
   sex-specific steroids, 36
Cardiorespiratory exercise, 297, 305
Cardiovascular disease, 291–293, 304–306
Cardiovascular response, 199
CBG. *See* Cortisol-binding-globulin (CBG)
Central thermoregulatory mechanisms, 96
CGI-58 expression, 279, 280
Childhood sexual abuse (CSA), 239
Chronic diseases, 291
Chronic exercise, 243, 244
Chronic inflammation, 277, 305, 306
Chronic insomnia, 301
CICP, 123, 126 (*see* Collagen synthesis and degradation (CICP))
Clonidine, 238
Collagen synthesis and degradation (CICP), 126
Comorbid anxiety, 178
Condition-dependent system, 140
Contraceptive hormones, 125–127
Corticotropin release hormone (CRH), 201
Cortisol, 256
   HPA, 199
   plasma/salivary, 200
   urinary, 203
Cortisol-binding-globulin (CBG), 203
CRH. *See* Corticotropin release hormone (CRH)
Cutaneous vasodilation, 165, 166
Cycle phase and injury risk, 116–118
Cynomolgus macaque monkeys, 121
Cytokines, 278

D
Dehydroepiandrosterone (DHEA), 215
Dehydroepiandrosterone sulfate (DHEA-S), 215, 252–254, 256–258
Depression, 180–181
   menopause transition, 181–183
   perinatal (*see* Perinatal depression)
DHEA. *See* Dehydroepiandrosterone (DHEA)
DHEAS. *See* Dehydroepiandrosterone sulfate (DHEAS)
Direct Current (DC), 234
DNA methyltransferase (DNAMT), 280
Drug holidays, 241
DSM-V
   MDD, 180
   PMDD, 179
   PPD, 180

E
EAH. *See* Exercise-associated hyponatraemia (EAH)
Endocrine organ, 276–278
Endogenous glucose, 91, 94
Endometrial cancer
   estrogen levels, 216
   risk, 217
Endothelial NO synthase (eNOS), 274
Endotoxin, 281
Endurance exercise, substrate metabolism, 37, 40–44
Energy and macronutrients, 88–95
   habitual diet, 88–89
   nutrient intake and recovery from exercise, 92–93
   nutrient intake before, after and during exercise, 89–91
Epinephrine, 240
Estradiol, 62, 114, 115, 118–121, 123, 124, 126–128, 130, 143, 145, 146, 158, 159, 249, 254–256, 258, 259
Estradiol-β-17, 3
Estrogen, 2, 3, 8, 71, 249, 251, 265–269, 271–273, 275, 277–282
   AVP, 164
   beneficial effects, 80, 81
   estradiol, 158
   fetus, 158
   hormonal contraceptives, 158
   leuprolide/ganirelix, 160
   menstrual cycle phases, 202–203
   muscle damage, 72–73
   muscle inflammation, 73, 74

Index

muscle mass and recovery from atrophy, 78, 79
muscle satellite cells and repair, 76, 78
muscle strength, 79, 80
oral contraception, 203–204
progesterone, 167
progestins, 160
receptors, 270–271, 283
regulate BAT thermogenesis, 273
Estrogen receptor alpha (ERα), 270–272
Estrogen-induced sex differences, 38–40
Estrogen–progesterone ratio, 42
Ethinyl estradiol (EE), 44
Eumenorrheic women, 92, 93, 100, 102, 257–259, 267
Eumenorrhoeic female cyclists, 88
Exercise, 266, 267
  benefits of, 292–293
  estrogen in adiposity reduction, 275
  estrogen on adipocyte lipolysis, 265–267
  estrogen on BAT, 271–273
  intensity, 43
  menopausal symptoms, 295–299
  during menopause, 294–300
  post-menopause, 304–305
  regular, 293–295, 304, 306
  strogen on adipose tissue inflammation, 278–281
Exercise-associated hyponatraemia (EAH), 97, 98
Exogenous glucose, 91

F
Fat metabolism, 38
Female sex hormones, 235, 264
Fibroblast proliferation, 119, 120
Fish oil, 103, 105
Fitness, 235
  ACTH, 207
  HPA axis, 201
  psychosocial stress, 207
Fluid and electrolyte requirements
  aerobic fitness, 169
  electrolyte handling and imbalances, 97
  menopause, ageing and hydration, 98
  sodium concentration, 170
  thermoregulation and body fluids, 95–98
Fluid balance
  cutaneous vasodilation, 165
  temperature regulation, 170–172
Fndc5 gene, 274

Follicle stimulating hormone (FSH), 2
Follicular phase, 249–251, 254–257, 259, 267

G
Gluconeogenesis, 37
Glycogenolysis, 37
GnRH, 160, 161, (see Gonadotropin-releasing hormone (GnRH))
Gonadotropin-releasing hormone (GnRH), 2, 217
Growth hormone (GH), 46–47, 252–255, 258
Growth hormone-inhibiting hormone (GHIH), 258

H
Habitual Diet, 88–89
Heat shock proteins (HSP), 73
Homeostatic mechanisms, 59
Hormonal contraception, 66–67, 158, 159
Hormone profiles in women, 114, 115
Hormone replacement, 71–74, 78–82
Hormone replacement therapy (HRT), 50–51, 74, 282, 291, 292, 300, 305
Hormone sensitive lipase (HSL), 266
Hormone therapy (HT). *See* hormone replacement therapy (HRT)
16α-Hydroxyestrone (16α-OHE1), 218
Hypercapnic ventilatory response (HCVR), 27
  OC use, 30
  sex hormones, 29–30
Hyponatraemia, 87, 97, 98, 159, 163, 167
Hypothalamic–pituitary axis (HPA-axis)
  ACTH, 201
  acute stress, 200
  psychosocial/mental stress, 201
Hypothalamic–pituitary–ovarian (HPO) axis
  estrogen, 2, 3
  female reproductive system, 1, 2
  neuroendocrine basics, 1
  progesterone, 3, 4
  reproductive health, 2
Hypoxic ventilatory response (HVR), 27, 28
Hysterectomy, 239–240

I
Immunometabolism, 264
Inflammation, 274–281, 283, 284
Insulin-like growth factor I (IGF-I), 252, 256
Interleukin-1β (IL-1β), 305

Interleukin-6 (IL-6), 280, 292
Intramyocellular lipids (IMCL), 38, 267
Isoflavones, 101, 102

K
Kiss1 gene, 2
Kisspeptin, 2
Knee laxity
    and ACL Injury, 121–122
    sex hormone effects, 122–125

L
Lactational amenorrhea, 146
Leptin hormone, 269, 276, 277
Life history theory, 140–143
Lipid metabolism, 268
Lipid oxidation, 48
Lipolysis, 279
Lipoprotein lipase (LPL), 266
Lippia citriodora (lemon verbena), 102
Low ovarian steroid levels, 143
Luteal phase, 249–251, 254, 255, 259, 267
Luteinizing hormone (LH), 2

M
Macrophages, 264, 278, 284
Major depressive disorder (MDD), 180
Matt stress reactivity protocol (MSRP), 200
Maximal lipid oxidation rates (MLOR), 48
MDD. *See* Major depressive disorder (MDD)
MeFLASH, 300
Melbourne Women's Midlife Health Project, 301
Menopausal, 49, 71, 81, 292–294, 300–304, 306
    ALPHA Trial, 224
    atrophic effects, 291
    BETA Trial, 225
    BMI and physical activity, 221
    cognitive symptoms, 291
    depression, 303
    exercise during, 294–300
    menstrual dysfunction, 219
    NEW Trial, 224, 225
    psychological symptoms, 291
    RCT, 221–223
    SHAPE Trial, 224
    SHAPE-2 Trial, 225
    symptoms, 292, 293, 303
    transition, 170
    WISER study, 220
    women, 297, 305
Menopause hormone therapy (MHT). *See* Hormone replacement therapy (HRT)
Menopause transition, 182
    MRMD, 187, 188
    reproductive-related mood disorders estradiol, 182
    PROG production, 182
Menstrual cycle, 4, 6, 88–93, 95–102, 104, 105, 114–119, 121, 123, 125, 127, 129, 131, 143, 237, 249, 251, 254, 256–260
    disorders, 256
    effects on strength and weight training, 259
    hormones, 97
    follicular phase, 251
    luteal phase, 251
    motor function, 63–64
    muscle strength during, 251
    nervous system, 61–63
    phase, 250, 254–256, 267
    status, 256–259
    substrate metabolism, 40–44
Menstrual disorders (MD), 254–256, 258, 259
Menstrual dysfunction, 219, 220
Menstrually-related mood disorders (MRMDs)
    gonadal steroid fluctuations, 180
    perinatal depression, 185–187
    physical activity, 184–185
    PMDD, 179
    PMS, 179
    PROG and estradiol levels, 179
Metabolism, 264, 267–272, 275, 276, 279–282
Midfollicular phase, 89, 90
MIST. *See* Montreal imaging stress task (MIST)
Mitochondrial function, 273–274, 279, 280
Mitogen-activated protein kinase (MAPK), 270
Mitohormesis, 272
M1 macrophage, 278, 280
M2 macrophage, 278
Monophasic OCs, 9
Montreal imaging stress task (MIST), 200
Mood disorder, 178–185
    MRMD (*see* Menstrually-related mood disorder (MRMD))
    reproductive-related process (*see* Reproductive-related mood disorders)
Motor performance, 65–66

Index 313

MSRP. *See* Matt stress reactivity protocol (MSRP)
Muscle damage, 71–76
Muscle mass, 71, 78–82
Muscle strength, 64–65, 71, 79, 80, 82
Myogenic differentiation protein D (MyoD), 79
Myokines, 280, 281
Myosin, 80

N

Neuroendocrine system, 205, 258
NEW Trial. *See* Nutrition and exercise for women (NEW Trial)
Non-esterified free fatty acids (NEFAs), 265–267
Non-ovarian hormones, 42
Norepinephrine (NE), 237, 238, 240, 241, 271
Nutrient intake and recovery from exercise, 92–93
Nutrient intake before, after and during exercise, 89–91
Nutrition and exercise for women (NEW Trial), 224, 225
Nutritional status, 43–44, 47–48

O

Oestrogen and antioxidants, 98–101
Oestrogens, 92, 96–101, 103, 105
Oocytes, 5
Oral contraceptive (OC), 123–126
 cardiovascular risk, 10–11
 combinations, 9
 drug interactions, 12–13
 effectiveness, 8
 estrogens, 8
 formulations, 44–45
 gallstone disease symptoms, 12
 metabolic effects, 11
 minor side effects, 12
 neoplastic effects, 11
 non-contraceptive Benefits, 13
 pills usage, 10
 progestins, 9
 at rest and exercise, 23–25
 tryptophan oxygenase activity, 12
 in women, 20
Ovarian hormones, 88–94, 254–256, 258
 menstrual cycle, 40
 and substrate metabolism, 40–48
Ovariectomized female rats, 73

Ovary
 hormone, 5–6
 oocytes, 5
 ovulation, 5–6
Ovulation, 249, 250, 254
Ovulatory cycles, 269
Oxytocin, 2

P

Partial pressure of O_2 (PaO_2), 20
PCOS. *See* Polycystic ovary syndrome (PCOS)
Perimenopausal depression. *See* Menopause transition
Perimenopausal women, 301
Perinatal depression
 APD, 180
 DSM-V, 180
 gonadal steroid hormone, 181
 physical activity (PA), 185–187
 PPD, 180
Peroxisome proliferator-activated receptor gamma coactivator 1 alpha (PGC1-α), 274, 275
Phosphatidylinositide 3-kinase (PI3K) signaling pathway, 76
Physical activity (PA), 292–296, 298, 300–304, 306
 reproductive-related mood disorders, 183
 MRMD, 184, 185
Phytoestrogen, 102, 103
Plasma osmolality (P_{Osm}), 164
Plasma oxytocin, 237
Plasma volume maintenance, 96
PMDD. *See* Premenstrual dysphoric disorder (PMDD)
PMS. *See* Premenstrual syndrome (PMS)
Polycystic ovary syndrome (PCOS), 171, 172
Postmenopausal symptoms, 299
Postmenopausal women, 49–50, 296, 299, 305
Postpartum depression (PPD), 180
Posttraumatic stress disorder (PTSD), 177, 179, 239
PPD. *See* Postpartum depression (PPD)
Predictive adaptive response theory, 145
Premenopausal women, 49–50, 272, 282
Premenstrual dysphoric disorder (PMDD), luteal phase, 179
Premenstrual syndrome (PMS), 103, 179, 184, 251
Prepuberty, 218–219

PROG. *See* Progesterone (PROG)
Progesterone (PROG), 3, 4, 62, 88–90, 92, 93, 95–98, 102, 105, 178, 179, 181, 182, 184, 249–251, 255, 256, 258, 259
  AVP, 164
  endogenous, 158
  hormone therapy, 171
  leuprolide/ganirelix, 160
  progestins, 169
Progestins
  estrogens, 160
  hormonal contraceptives, 158
Progestogens, 97
Protein kinase B (PKB) signaling pathway, 79
Psychological symptoms, 296, 299, 302–304, 306
PTSD. *See* Posttraumatic stress disorder (PTSD)
Puberty. *See* Menopause
Pulmonary gas exchange, effect of sex, 25–26

R
Randomized controlled trial (RCT), 186, 187
RCT. *See* Randomized controlled trial (RCT)
Reactive oxygen species (ROS), 99, 271, 279
Relaxin, 127–131
  and ACL injury epidemiology, 129–131
  and collagen metabolism, 128, 129
Reproductive axis, 2, 14
Reproductive-related mood disorders
  comorbid anxiety, 178
  depression, 178
  menopause transition, 181–183
  MRMD, 179–180
  perinatal depression, 180–181
  physical activity, 183–188
Resistance exercise, 249, 252–260
  dehydroepiandrosterone sulfate, 252, 253
  growth hormone, 252
  hormonal responses, 254–259
  insulin-like growth factor I, 252
  in men, 252
  testosterone, 252
  in women, 252–253
Respiratory system
  alveolar-capillary blood, 20
  neurochemical factors, 20
  oxygen (O_2) transport, 20
  pulmonary capillary blood, 20
  rest and exercise ventilation, 21–23
  terrestrial environments, 20
Rodent model, 269, 270, 272

S
sAA. *See* Salivary alpha-amylase (sAA)
Salivary alpha-amylase (sAA), 200
Selective serotonin reuptake inhibitors (SSRIs), 241, 243
Serum testosterone, 252
Sex hormones, 87, 93, 102, 104, 105, 119–125, 139–147, 250, 251, 259, 260, 269
  effects on, 118–121
    collagen metabolism, 119, 120
    Knee Laxity, 122–125
    ligament laxity, 121
    mechanical properties, 120–121
  estrogens and progesterones, 20, 60
  metabolic intermediaries, 60
  progestogens, 20
  profile variability, 114
  resting and exercise, 21–26
  sulfonated and unsulfonated DHEA, 61
  ventilatory chemoresponsiveness, 27–30
  ventilatory parameters, 20
  ventilatory responses, 22–23
Sex hormones and physical exercise (SHAPE Trial), 224
Sex hormones and physical exercise-2 (SHAPE-2 Trial), 225
Sex steroid hormones
  estrogen, 2, 3
  progesterone, 3, 4
Sexual arousal in women, 233–238, 243, 244
  antidepressant sexual dysfunction, 240–242
  childhood sexual abuse, 239
  with exercise, 236–239
  testosterone, 236
  vaginal photoplethysmograph, 234
  vasocongestion, 233
Sexual symptoms, 295, 304
SHAPE Trial. *See* Sex hormones and physical exercise (SHAPE Trial)
SHAPE-2 Trial. *See* Sex hormones and physical exercise-2 (SHAPE-2 Trial)
SHBG. *See* Sex hormone binding globulin (SHBG)
Skeletal muscles, 251, 259, 266, 267, 273, 275, 281, 282, 305
Somatic symptoms, 295, 296, 300, 302–304, 306
Soy and isoflavones, 101–103
Stress reactivity, 200
  acute exercise, 206
  aging, 204–205

cardiovascular response, 199
cortisol response, 200
estrogen, 202–204
fitness, 207, 208
gender differences, 201, 202
heart rate recovery, 199
homeostasis, 199
HPA axis activity (see HPA axis)
MIST, 200
MSRP, 200
neuroendocrine response, 199
regular exercise, 206–208
TSST, 200
Study of Women's Health Across the Nation (SWAN), 304
Subcutaneous WAT, 268
Substrate metabolism
endurance exercise, 37
estrogen-induced sex differences, 38–40
menstrual cycle, 40–44
sex differences, 49
Supraphysiologic, 119, 120
Sympathetic nervous system (SNS), 236–239, 241–243, 271

T
Tamang women, 145
Temporomandibular joint (TMJ), 130
Testosterone, 236, 237, 250, 252, 256
Thermoregulation, 95–97, 166–167
Thyroid-stimulating hormone (TSH), 2
Training and fitness, 169–170
Trier social stress test (TSST)
ACTH, 207
cardiovascular and epinephrine reactivity, 203
cortisol response, 204
Triphasic OCs, 9

TSST. See Trier social stress test (TSST)
Tumour necrosis factor-α (TNF-α), 305
Type 1 procollagen synthesis, 119
Type 2 diabetes, 274

U
Uterus
anatomy, 6
phases, 7

V
Vaginal blood volume (VBV), 234
Vaginal photoplethysmography, 234–237, 240
Vaginal pulse amplitude (VPA), 234
Vasocongestion, 233, 236
Vasomotor symptoms (VMS), 171, 295–297, 300–302, 306
Ventilatory chemoresponsiveness, chemoreceptors, 27
Ventilatory parameters, 21–26
Ventilatory responses
OC use, 23–25
sex effect, 21–22
Visceral WAT, 268, 269
Vitamin D, 104, 105
VMS. See Vasomotor symptoms (VMS)

W
Water regulation, 161–164
White adipose tissue (WAT), 265, 266, 268, 271–283
Women In Steady Exercise Research (WISER), 220
Women's biological capacity to reproduce, 143
Women's reproductive systems, 144

Printed by Printforce, the Netherlands